3/13

Color Textbook of Pediatric Dermatology

Color Textbook of Pediatric Dermatology

William L. Weston, M.D.
Professor and Chairman
   Department of Dermatology
Professor of Pediatrics
   University of Colorado
   Health Sciences Center
   Denver, Colorado

Alfred T. Lane, M.D.
Associate Professor of Dermatology
   and Pediatrics
   Stanford Medical Center
   Stanford, California
formerly
Professor of Dermatology
   University of Rochester
   Rochester, New York

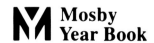

Mosby
Year Book

St. Louis   Baltimore   Boston   Chicago   London   Philadelphia   Sydney   Toronto

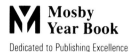
**Mosby
Year Book**

Dedicated to Publishing Excellence

Sponsoring Editor: Nancy E. Chorpenning
Assistant Managing Editor, Text and Reference: Jan
  Gardner
Production Project Coordinator: Carol A. Reynolds
Proofroom Supervisor: Barbara M. Kelly

Mosby-Year Book, Inc.
11830 Westline Industrial Drive
St. Louis, MO 63146

Illustrations by Kemp Weston.
**Color photographs supported in part by an educational grant
from Schering-Plough Corporation.**

1   2   3   4   5   6   7   8   9   0   CLW   94   93   92   91

Library of Congress Cataloging-in-Publication Data
Weston, William L.
    Color textbook of pediatric dermatology / William L. Weston,
Alfred T. Lane.
        p.   cm.
    Includes bibliographical references.
    Includes index.
    ISBN 0-8151-9236-3
    1. Pediatric dermatology.   2. Pediatric dermatology—Atlases.
I. Lane, Alfred T.   II. Title.
    [DNLM: 1. Skin Diseases—in infancy & childhood—atlases.   2. Skin
Diseases—in infancy & childhood—handbooks.   WS   17 W536c]
RJ511.W46   1991
618.92′5—dc20
DNLM/DLC
for Library of Congress
                                                            90-6585
                                                            CIP

Dedication

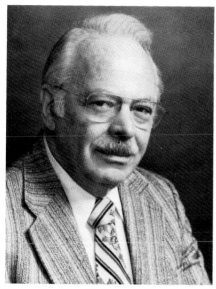

ALVIN H. JACOBS, M.D.

Alvin Jacobs, M.D., is the "very best friend ever" to pediatric dermatology. Like a child in the formative years, pediatric dermatology struggled to find its way as a field of medicine. Al Jacobs was always there to help, to guide, to listen. Any pediatrician worth their salt knows the name of Alvin Hirsch Jacobs, M.D. He has presented hundreds of lectures on pediatric dermatology to national, regional, and local meetings, with never a negative comment. We can think of no others in the field who can match that accomplishment. His seminars on neonatal dermatology are classic, and often the most popular at national pediatric or dermatology meetings. Anyone who hears Al Jacobs talk knows they have heard the master. There are thousands of pediatricians whose first—and often *only*—formal teaching in pediatric dermatology came from Al Jacobs.

We decided to dedicate this book to Al Jacobs for another aspect of his professional career: his work behind the scenes in pediatric dermatology. For a complete appreciation of his contributions we must first examine the man. He was born in Reno, Nevada, and spent his boyhood among the ponderosa pines and broad valleys below the Comstock lode. This was still the Wild West, an invigorating life for an ambitious young man. After

receiving the gold medal at graduation from the University of Nevada in 1933, he ventured east to the famous Johns Hopkins University School of Medicine, where he received his medical degree in 1937. After internship in Pittsburgh, he spent a year in child neurology at the Neurological Institute of New York. He returned West for training in pediatrics and infectious disease at San Francisco County Hospital, then served as chief resident in pediatrics at Stanford University. It was then June 1942, his country was at war, and Dr. Jacobs joined the Navy and was assigned to Navy Medical Research Unit Number 1. By 1946 he was a Lieutenant Commander and ready to return to the practice of pediatrics. In his private practice of pediatrics in San Francisco, Al quickly recognized that 20% of his patients had primary skin complaints and that he was poorly prepared to deal with them. He found his colleagues in pediatrics similarly unprepared, and decided to remedy the situation. After a year's fellowship in dermatology at Stanford he joined the Stanford faculty, and established a career in pediatric dermatology that has spanned three decades. He is now Professor of Dermatology and Pediatrics, Emeritus (active) at Stanford University. He still pursues his love of pediatric dermatology with his usual vigor.

Al Jacobs was a founder of the Society for Pediatric Dermatology and served as its first president. In many ways Al Jacobs was to pediatric dermatology what George Washington was to the establishment of the United States. It is so crucial that the leaders at the founding have the wisdom and vision to create an organization that will grow and be flexible enough to accommodate the changes needed in future generations. The advice and counsel of Al Jacobs was critical for the field of pediatric dermatology.

It is Al Jacobs the man who has endeared himself to so many in pediatrics and pediatric dermatology. He avoided the arrogance that often accompanies positions of importance in academic medicine, and remained the kind, considerate, warm man who always had time to listen to your needs or your problems. It has been his accessibility that has made the field of pediatric dermatology accessible for all who are interested. Who could resist that big smile beneath the cookie-duster moustache or those kind, twinkling eyes? Any personal encounter with Al Jacobs makes one feel they are with their best friend.

It is said that the fulfillment of life is to love, be loved, and have useful work. Al Jacobs loves his charming wife, Opal; his children; his chosen field of pediatric dermatology. In turn, he is loved by his wife and children and the hundreds of physicians whose lives he has touched.

This book is also dedicated to our families: Dr. Janet Atkinson Weston, Betsy and Kemp Weston; Maureen, Amy, Andy, Jeremy, Jordan, and Matthew Lane. We appreciate their support and willingness to provide photographs for this text from their family albums.

WILLIAM L. WESTON, M.D.
ALFRED T. LANE, M.D.

PREFACE

We have written this textbook on pediatric dermatology to meet the specific needs of the clinician responsible for the primary care of children. To understand the requirements of those involved in health care of children, it is best to have firsthand experience. We have practiced pediatrics in private suburban settings, in large urban public hospitals, and in academic centers, and thus meet the requirement of having "served in the trenches." Most important, as Board-certified pediatricians, we learned well the demanding schedule required to care for children. In a busy practice information must be easily accessible and decisive.

In our current positions a major portion of our professional time is devoted to teaching pediatric dermatology to house staff, medical students, and graduate clinicians. We are indebted to our colleagues in pediatrics and family medicine as well as to hundreds of trainees who told us what was needed in a text on skin problems in children. This text evolved from the single-authored text *Practical Pediatric Dermatology*. We incorporated the advice of clinicians, house staff, and students to create a textbook that will serve the clinician in the 1990s. We listened to our friends and included only color photographs. We feared this would price the book too high for the targeted audience, but thanks to the generous support of the publisher and Schering-Plough Corporation for color printing, the cost of the book remains reasonable.

Several unique features are included in this book. A Problem-Oriented Differential Diagnosis Index is provided on the inside of the front cover to allow the busy clinician rapid access when the diagnosis is not clear. The Differential Diagnosis Index provides separate categories for newborns and for older children, recognizing that the conditions encountered are often distinct. A problem-oriented diagnosis algorithm is provided for rapid access to the Differential Diagnosis Index. For use when the diagnosis is known, there is an alphabetical index at the back of the book. A concise and simplified formulary specific for pediatric patients is also available in the back of the book. Useful tables throughout the text deal with, for example, potency of topical steroids, care of premature infants' skin, and workup of sun sensitivity. The patient education information provided at the end of the discussion of each skin condition provides a guide for explanations that can be given to patients. The reader is provided a guide for when to schedule follow-up visits and what to evaluate at the visit. The 20 chapters in this text include novel chapters on drug eruptions in children, hair disorders, nail disorders, and sun sensitivity. All are written in a style that provides the busy clinician with concise, decisive information. Omitted are traditional therapies and ideas that have never been substantiated.

Without the encouragement of our own mentors this book would not be possible. We have dedicated this text to Alvin Jacobs, M.D. who at a time when the world had less than a handful of pediatric dermatologists had the vision of the creation of a new discipline. He provided the impetus to so many young people hesitant to enter the uncertain world of a discipline yet undefined. A special tribute to Dr. Jacobs appears on the dedication page. We thank Drs. Robert Goltz, W. Mitchell Sams, and Lowell Goldsmith for their guidance, protected time, and generous support of our careers. We also thank the officers and members of the Society for Pediatric Dermatology, who provided the collegiality, clinical expertise, scientific interest, and nurture required to make pediatric dermatology a recognized discipline of medicine. We trust with this book we are in some small way repaying the great debt we owe our colleagues.

WILLIAM L. WESTON, M.D.
ALFRED T. LANE, M.D.

CONTENTS

Color Textbook of Pediatric Dermatology

1 _____ Structure and Function of the Skin

A firm understanding of normal skin structure and function is necessary for the recognition and treatment of skin disease. Those providing medical care for children should apply the principles of skin biology to the pediatric patient and master the essentials of the embryology and development of skin.

THE EPIDERMIS

Keratinization

The epidermis functions as a barrier, preventing penetration from outside and retaining substances inside. More than 95% of epidermal cells are keratinocytes. The process of keratinocyte replication and maturation is called *keratinization.* Throughout the life of the keratinocyte, the major proteins that it contains are keratins. The process of keratinization begins with proliferation of new keratinocytes in the region of the basal cell layer, near the dermoepidermal junction (Fig 1–1). As keratinocytes differentiate, they first accumulate granules called *keratohyalin granules* in their cytoplasm. The exact function of the keratohyalin granules is unknown, but they are believed to be important in the organization and formation of a thickened cornified cell membrane. Keratohyalin granules appear within epidermal cells as they emigrate outward from the basal layer and reach the granular layer. Within the granular layer the cells lose their cylindrical and cuboidal shapes and begin to flatten. Cell nuclei are lost and the plasma membranes thicken. The keratinocytes flatten like stacks of plates, and the cell membrane becomes much thicker than the usual cell membrane. This final layer is called the *horny layer,* or *stratum corneum.* The stratum corneum cells accumulate like bricks on a wall, held together by intercellular lipids, which function like mortar. The intercellular lipids are an integral part of the epidermal barrier function. The process of keratinization is ongoing within the skin, and the epidermis is replaced approximately every 28 days.

Epidermal Barrier

It is said that the skin is the interface between humans and their environment. Indeed, the most important function of the epidermis is to provide a skin barrier against microorganisms, irritating chemicals, and electrical charges, as well as to impede the exchange of fluids and electrolytes between the body and the environment. This barrier function resides in the stratum corneum. Although the skin, including the epidermis and dermis, is 1.5 to 4.0 mm thick, the epidermal barrier is only 0.05 to 0.1 mm thick. By the daily shedding of one to two cell layers of stratum corneum, or scale, the epidermal barrier prevents excessive colonization of the skin surface. In addition to continuous shedding, the flattened stratum corneum cells are tightly adherent to each other, so that to obtain entrance into the lower epidermis and dermis, chemicals or microorganisms must pass between tightly compacted epidermal cells.

The water content of the environment greatly influences the epidermal barrier (see Chapter 20, Percutaneous Absorption). Both an excessive and an inadequate water content in the epidermal barrier will cause microscopic and macroscopic breaks in the barrier.

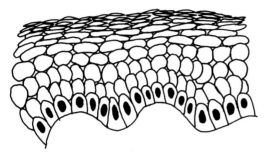

FIG 1–1.
Normal epidermis. The germinative layer with prominent nuclei is at the base of the epidermis and within the same compartment as the fully differentiated cells. As these basal cells differentiate, they migrate up toward the skin surface, shed their nuclei, become flattened, and are shed from the skin surface.

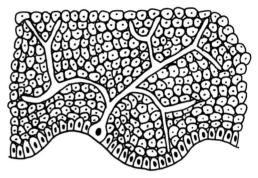

FIG 1–2.
Melanocyte-keratinocyte unit. The dendritic melanocyte, shown here as a clear cell with many branches, provides melanin pigment to many keratinocytes.

In response to friction or other forms of repeated trauma such as ultraviolet light (UVL) or chemical injury, stratum corneum is formed in amounts greater than usual, as can be noted on the palms and soles. The stratum corneum is thinnest over the eyelids and scrotum.

Pigmentation and Ultraviolet Light

Four biochromes in the skin are responsible for clinical pigmentation: melanin, beta carotene, oxyhemoglobin, and reduced hemoglobin. The brown-black pigment melanin is the dominant pigment of the skin. It is the pigment closest to the observer's vision and darkest in color. In dark-skinned individuals, it is difficult to recognize yellow pigment (beta carotene), red pigment (oxyhemoglobin), and blue pigment (reduced hemoglobin). Melanin is produced by the pigment-forming cell, the melanocyte, which is located in the epidermis. Different skin regions contain different numbers of melanocytes. For example, three times as many melanocytes are found in the epidermis of the forehead as in the abdominal skin. Numbers of melanocytes per unit area of skin are the same despite racial differences in pigmentation.

Each epidermal melanocyte has dendritic cytoplasmic extensions that make contact with 35 to 45 epidermal cells. This melanocyte-keratinocyte unit (Fig 1–2) is responsible for clinical pigmentation. The brown-black polymer melanin is produced within the melanocytes in special membrane-bound organelles called melanosomes. The enzyme tyrosinase is contained within the melanosome membrane. Melanosomes develop in stages. Tyrosinase converts the colorless chemical tyrosine to an oxidized quinone compound, which in turn becomes polymerized into the brown-black compound melanin. Clinical pigmentation depends on the stage of the melanosome produced and dispersion of melanosomes from melanocytes to keratinocytes. Keratinocytes actively phagocytize the melanosomes. In black skin, melanosomes are single units of advanced-stage melanosomes, while in lighter skinned persons the melanosomes are aggregated and of earlier developmental stages. Thus the major difference in black and white skin is the stage of the melanosome development and the ability to transfer and disperse melanin pigment, not the number of melanocytes per unit area of skin.

The function of melanin is to protect the deoxyribonucleic acid (DNA) structure of epidermal cell nuclei from damage by UVL irradiation. Melanin dispersed within the cytoplasm of keratinocytes forms a protective cap over the keratinocyte nucleus when the keratinocytes are exposed to UVL (Fig 1–3). Melanin pigment is lost by the daily shedding of stratum corneum cells. Melanin within the dermis, such as that found in dermal melanocytic birthmarks, has no such mechanism available for its elimination.

UVL from the sun increases melanin pigmentation by first oxidizing preformed melanin, increasing cross-linking of the melanin polymer and darkening the color. This effect occurs within minutes after exposure and is called *immediate pigment darkening.* Over the next 4 to 6 days after UVL exposure, both increased melanin pro-

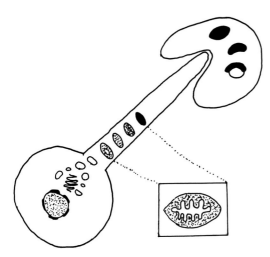

FIG 1–3.
Melanin production and transfer. Melanosomes *(inset)* are organelles formed in the rough endoplasmic reticulum and Golgi area of melanocytes. Their membranes contain the enzyme tyrosinase, responsible for the formation of the brown-black polymer, melanin. At the end of the dendrite, the melanocytes are shown transferring pigment to the keratinocyte, where the melanin moves to form a cap of the keratinocyte nucleus as protection against ultraviolet injury.

duction and melanin transfer to keratinocytes produce tanning. Hormones such as adrenocorticotropic hormone (ACTH) and a polypeptide portion of ACTH called *beta melanocyte–stimulating hormone* are also responsible for increasing pigmentation, presumably by stimulating melanin synthesis within the melanocyte.

Sunlight

The sun produces UVL of numerous wavelengths, which, based on their biologic effects, are arbitrarily divided into three groups: UVA, UVB, and UVC (Table 1–1). Incoming UVL from the sun is scattered by small molecules in the atmosphere and absorbed by the ozone layer; all UVL below 290 nm is absorbed, so that virtually no UVC reaches the earth's surface.

Sunburn is caused by wavelengths of light from 290 to 320 nm. Photons of UVL are absorbed by electrons of chemicals with double bonds and ring structures, such as nucleic acids, DNA, porphyrins, and proteins, producing excited electron states within these molecules or free radical formation. Beta carotene and melanin act by stabilizing the free radicals and are natural photoprotective chemicals found in skin. About 10% of UVB passes through the epidermis and reaches the dermis. The erythema and pain of sunburn are mediated via prostaglandins, and the sunburn wavelengths of UVL are blocked by window glass. The tanning and thickening of the epidermal barrier that result from exposure to sunlight impair the penetration of UVL into the lower epidermis and dermis. Wavelengths of light from 320 to 400 nm (UVA) are responsible for the photosensitivity seen in the porphyrias, many drug photoallergies, and psoralen phototoxicity. Light of these wavelengths passes through window glass and is emitted from fluorescent lamps such as those used as overhead lighting in schools.

THE DERMIS

The dermis is composed predominantly of collagen fibers and some elastic fibers enclosed in a gel continuum of mucopolysaccharides. This fibrous complex gives the dermis its great mechanical strength and elasticity, allowing the skin to withstand severe frictional stress yet still be extensible over joints. Elastin, collagen, and muco-

TABLE 1–1.
Biologic Effects of UVL

Group	Wavelength (nm)	Biologic Effects
UVC	200–290	Cytotoxic (bactericidal, retinal injury)
UVB	290–320	Sunburn, suntan, systemic lupus erythematosus, skin cancers
UVA	320–400	Drug photoallergies, porphyria, phytophotodermatitis, psoralens (PUVA therapy)

polysaccharide gel are all produced and secreted by fibroblasts.

Although the principal mass of the dermis consists of collagen fibers and is acellular, numerous other elements are present, including mast cells, inflammatory cells, blood and lymph vessels, and cutaneous nerves. These elements are responsible for regulation of heat loss, the host defenses of the skin, nutrition, and other regulatory functions. The dermis is thickest on the upper back.

Collagen, Elastin, and Mechanical Properties

Most of the mechanical strength of the skin is derived from the fibrous protein collagen, a macromolecule with a large hydroxyproline content. Mature collagen structure becomes rigid with cross-linking of adjacent protein chains, and young collagen that is without significant cross-linking fails to limit skin distention. Defective collagen cross-linking results in extensive and excessive distensibility of the skin, as seen in Ehlers-Danlos syndrome. Elastin fibers, which are composed of both an amorphous and a fibrillar portion, are responsible for the reversible distensibility that allows the skin to be restored to normal size after stretching. Defective elastin production results in extreme wrinkling and redundant skin as seen in cutis laxa.

Cutaneous Vasculature

Cutaneous arteries course through the subcutaneous fat and give rise to two vascular plexuses that run parallel to the epidermis. These vascular plexuses contain arteriovenous shunts to divert blood from the skin and provide nutrition to it, to regulate heat loss, and to participate in the defense against foreign substances. The epidermis contains no blood vessels and receives its nutrition via the diffusion of plasma into the intercellular epidermal spaces. The stratum corneum has no such nutritive process.

Heat Regulation and Sweating

Skin is important in the control of body temperature. Heat generated in organs and muscles is rapidly transported to the skin vasculature. The cutaneous circulation acts as a "radiator." Varying the rate and volume of blood flow through the skin controls heat loss from this radiator. The blood flow is controlled by the autonomic nervous system. Heat from the skin surface is lost by evaporation of water in the form of eccrine sweat. Heat loss or gain by convection or radiation depends on environmental temperature. At comfortable temperatures, body heat can be regulated by the cutaneous vasculature alone, without sweating. In hot, dry environments, the core body temperature may rise slightly but is stabilized by heat loss via sweating. In hot, humid environments, evaporation of water from the skin surface is restricted, and heat gain occurs in the child's body. If this condition is allowed to continue over a period of time, fever, dehydration, and sodium depletion may occur. In children born with deficient numbers of eccrine sweat glands (hypohidrotic ectodermal dysplasia), heat gain occurs during hot weather or overheating, and recurrent fever is often a presenting feature of the condition.

Cutaneous Nerves

Sensory nerve endings in the skin can elicit all of the principal sensations: touch, pain, itch, warmth, and cold. The skin is supplied by myelinated branches of spinal nerves. Nerve branches enter the dermis from the subcutaneous fat and form both a superficial and a deep nerve plexus. Unmyelinated branches from either plexus terminate in nerve endings that may be simple or specialized. Terminals from a single axon may serve an area as broad as 1 cm^2 and overlap with nerve endings from other axons. Inflow of cutaneous sensory information is strongly controlled and modulated by the cerebral cortex. The skin has a high sensitivity to rapid mechanical stimulation, with positional movements of less than 1 μm detectable. Sensations of cold persist continuously when skin temperature is below 30° C, and sensations of warmth persist continuously when it is above 37° C. Changes in temperature of 0.01° C can be detected, especially if the skin temperature changes faster than 0.007° C/sec. Thermal sensitivity is highest on the face.

At temperatures below 18° C and above 45° C, pain is produced. Pain may also be induced by pressure greater than 50 g/mm^2 and by disruption of skin. A number of chemicals injected into the skin may also elicit pain. Itch is a sensation related to pain and is greatest close to transitions of mucous membranes. Histamine is considered to be the most important mediator of itch, but many other mediators are capable of producing this sensation.

HOST DEFENSES OF THE SKIN

When breaks in the epidermal barrier occur, microorganisms invade the upper epidermis. Plasma proteins, such as complement proteins and immunoglobulins that normally bathe the intercellular epidermal space, initiate an inflammatory response. Cutaneous vasodilation (erythema) occurs early after this initial process, with diffusion of more plasma proteins, followed by the migration of neutrophils, T lymphocytes, B lymphocytes, and monocytes-macrophages into the dermis and later the epidermis. Such cells initially accumulate around dermal blood vessels, but may migrate to the epidermis through the dermoepidermal junction between epidermal cells. For example, in impetigo large numbers of neutrophils accumulate just beneath the stratum corneum. Mast cells containing histamine, heparin, and platelet-activating factors are located around cutaneous blood vessels and play a regulatory role in the immune response of the skin by their influence on cutaneous vascular responses.

The initial response of the skin invasion by microorganisms consists primarily of migration of neutrophilic leukocytes, but by 18 to 24 hours it is characterized by the appearance of lymphocytes and monocytes-macrophages in the dermis. Microorganisms or foreign substances not initially destroyed by neutrophils are presumably further digested by macrophages or destroyed by direct lymphocytotoxicity. A rich lymphatic system is also found in the dermis, and foreign substances are carried to regional lymph nodes, where specific immune responses are generated by T lymphocytes and B lymphocytes. Some antigen recognition probably occurs in the skin, since antigen-processing cells (Langerhans cells) are found in the epidermis, and direct Langerhans–T lymphocyte contact occurs that may be important in the recognition of foreign antigens.

The epidermal barrier remains the primary defense of the skin, but microorganisms that pass through the barrier are destroyed within the midepidermis as the skin defenses attempt to keep them out of deeper tissue.

EPIDERMAL APPENDAGES

Epidermal appendages, which are modifications of epithelium, include hair follicle structures, sebaceous glands, nails, and the apocrine and eccrine sweat glands.

Hair Growth

The hair growth cycle has three phases: the growing phase, anagen; the regressing phase, catagen; and the resting phase, telogen. The cells of anagen hairs have a high mitotic rate and are among the most rapidly replicating cells in humans. The hair growth originates from the hair bulb, which is located in the lower dermis. Human scalp hair grows about 1 cm a month. When growth of the hair ceases, the catagen phase occurs, resulting in cessation of mitosis and upward migration of the hair bulb into the middermis. The hair shaft becomes clubbed at the bottom, causing the catagen hair to become a telogen hair (also called club hair). The telogen hair remains in the follicle for 2 to 3 months and is pushed out when the new hair grows.

There are great differences in the hair growth cycle among the different hair types found in the various body regions. Ambisexual hair follicles are common to both sexes and are androgen dependent. At puberty, androgen converts vellus hairs to terminal hairs in the axilla and the lower pubic triangle. Conversely, conversion of terminal scalp hairs to vellus hairs occurs in the temporal area of the scalp at puberty. Male sexual hair is responsive to high androgen levels, which convert vellus hairs to terminal hairs in the beard area, ears, sternum, and upper pubic triangle. In the occipital and bifrontal areas of the scalp, androgen levels result in a conversion of terminal to vellus hairs, resulting in androgenetic alopecia.

Hair cycles are asynchronous and vary within body sites. In the scalp at any point in time, about 85% of the hairs are growing (anagen), 14% are resting (telogen), and 1% are regressing (catagen). Newborns convert most of their hairs to telogen hairs within the first 6 months of life. Some newborns take several months to develop new anagen hairs, resulting in a "bald baby." Other infants develop new anagen hairs so rapidly that they appear not to lose their hair. After acute febrile diseases in children or adults, many hairs can convert from anagen to telogen hairs, with a subsequent period of months with markedly thinned hair.

Sebaceous Glands

Sebaceous glands are present everywhere on the human skin except the palms, soles, and dorsa of the feet. Generally they are associated with hair follicles, and empty through a short duct into the canal of the hair follicle. The sebaceous sweat glands are holocrine glands that produce sebum, a semiliquid mixture of glanular cell debris containing glycerides, free fatty acids, wax esters, squalene, cholesterol, and cholesterol esters. The largest and most numerous sebaceous glands are found on the face, scalp, chest, and back.

Sebum production is androgen dependent and begins at puberty in skin regions with abundant sebaceous follicles. Sebaceous gland volume, sebaceous cell size, and secretory capacity are all directly androgen dependent. Obstruction of the sebaceous gland is associated with acne.

Eccrine Glands

Humans have 2 to 5 million eccrine glands. These glands function to cool the body through evaporative heat loss of eccrine sweat. In addition, these glands may help to moisten the frictional surfaces of the skin.

Apocrine Glands

Apocrine sweat glands are in the axilla, mons pubis, areola of the breast, circumanal area, and scalp. They are located deep in the subcutaneous tissue and usually open into a hair follicle. Apocrine glands secrete a yellowish, sticky fluid after puberty. The secretion is produced in response to stress or sexual stimulation. In lower animals, these glands function as sex attractors and territorial markers.

Nails

Nails are formed by the fifth fetal month. The nail matrix contains epithelial cells responsible for the production of the nail plate. The nail matrix occupies an area beneath the proximal nail fold, a portion of which may be seen as the lunula. Fingernails grow approximately 1 cm in 3 months; toenails grow more slowly. Newborn nails are spoon-shaped and thin and may remain so until 2 or 3 years of age.

SUBCUTANEOUS FAT

The subcutaneous fat lies just beneath the dermis and is composed principally of lipocytes. It serves as a cushion to trauma, a heat insulator, and a highly important source of energy and hormone metabolism. Premature infants have poorly developed subcutaneous tissues, contributing to thermal instability and metabolic difficulties.

DEVELOPMENT OF SKIN

Periderm

Knowledge of the structure and function of developing fetal skin is invaluable in understanding abnormalities observed in newborn and infant skin. The single layer of ectodermal cells overlaying the developing fetus interacts with the mesoderm below to form the epidermis and dermis, respectively. Through this interaction the appendages develop, and the unique properties of skin at different body sites result.

Between 4 and 5 weeks' gestation, the single layer of ectodermal cells of the fetal epidermis is covered by a layer of flattened cells called the *periderm*. The periderm cells expand across the developing epidermis by active mitosis, becoming rounded, bulging cells uniformly covered by microvilli. The stratum corneum forms beneath the periderm cells during the fifth to sixth month. At this time periderm cells regress and become shrunken remnants that slough into the amniotic fluid and become one component of the vernix caseosa.

The morphologic characteristics of these cells suggest a transport function for periderm cells. It is believed that the periderm may transport fluids, electrolytes, and sugars into the developing embryo.

Epidermis

After 8 weeks' gestation an intermediate cell layer develops between the basal cells and the periderm. In time this layer stratifies and adds additional cell layers. By 24 weeks' gestation granular and cornified cells are present on almost all regions of the body. From this time until birth the stratum corneum matures and thickens, so that at birth the term infant's skin barrier function is comparable to that of an adult. Depending on the gestational age at birth, the premature infant's skin barrier function is more deficient the earlier the premature birth.

The sequence of development of the keratins, the development of the basement membrane zone, and the development of the desmosomes, hemidesmosomes, and antigens of the epidermis has been catalogued. The epidermis follows a sequence of development that is being studied intensively to understand the cellular interactions of normal development and the errors that occur in skin diseases.

Cells That Migrate Into the Epidermis

Although the epidermis is ectodermal in origin, cells from other sources migrate into the epidermis. Langerhans cells are present within the epidermis by 6 weeks' gestation, but they may not be functionally mature until after 12 weeks' gestation. The melanocyte is derived from the neural crest and migrates to the epidermis before the twelfth gestational week. By 16 weeks, melanocytes with melanosomes capable of synthesizing melanin are noted, and by 20 weeks, the epidermis has its full complement of melanocytes. Merkel's cells appear in the epidermis of the fingertips, glabrous skin, and nail beds by 12 weeks and serve as special sensory organs. These cells may develop within the epidermis rather than being an immigrant cell as previously thought.

Epidermal Appendages

Hair follicle or sweat gland development begins earlier in the scalp, palms, and soles than in other body areas. The hair germ begins in the scalp by 12 weeks' estimated gestational age (EGA) as a proliferation of keratinocytes above a collection of fibroblasts. These cells proliferate and invaginate into the dermis, forming the hair peg and the subsequent hair follicle. Granular cells are present within the hair follicle after 14 weeks' EGA, a full 6 to 10 weeks before they are seen in the interfollicular skin. Hair grows at an oblique angle to the skin surface and will erupt caudally, causing the hair to point downward.

Anlagen of eccrine glands may be present on the sole as early as 10 weeks' EGA. The eccrine gland secretory coil forms on the sole at about 16 weeks' EGA, while the secretory and myoepithelial cells differentiate at 22 weeks' EGA. The seba-ceous gland primordia develop off the hair follicle after 16 weeks' EGA. Steroid hormone stimulation of sebaceous glands is so great that these glands are considerably larger in the third trimester fetus than those of a child. Apocrine glands, the last of the appendages to develop, first appear during the sixth month of fetal development.

Nails and Volar Pads.—Development of the fetal nails, the volar pads, skin ridges, and sweat glands is tied together in the developing digit. These structures form simultaneously at 8 weeks, just after the digits separate from one another. By 12 weeks, the proximal and distal nail folds have formed and the volar pads are formed from mounds of mesenchyma and an increased intermediate layer of the epidermis. The distal nail fold is the first epithelial structure to keratinize, beginning at 12 weeks. A nail plate covers the nail bed by 17 weeks' gestation. Primary dermal ridges appear at 12 weeks, and secondary dermal ridges at 16 weeks. Sweat gland buds appear in the fingertips at 12 weeks, but sweating does not occur until after 32 weeks.

Influences of the Dermis on Epidermal Growth and Differentiation

The fetal dermis plays an overwhelmingly predominant role in transformation of the ectoderm into epidermis and maintenance of controlled epidermal appendage development. The continued interaction between the epidermis and the dermis maintains the continued presence of the thickened skin of the palms and soles or the thinner skin of the face. The epidermal appendages are maintained by dermoepidermal interaction, and once full-thickness injury occurs, the reformed scar tissue appears unable to regenerate new appendages. Skin diseases associated with thickening or thinning of the epidermis may be associated with abnormal dermoepidermal communications.

Dermis

The primordial dermis begins as a cellular mesenchyme that is watery and without fibrous structure. By 6 weeks of age, a fine meshwork of collagen fibrils underlies the dermoepidermal junction and adheres to the dermomesenchymal cell surfaces. Extracellular collagen increases with age, and fibrils associate into collagen fiber bundles. Cells of the dermis become spaced farther apart, and their elongated axes become oriented parallel to the skin surface. The fine collagen network persists at the dermoepidermal junction and ensheathes epidermal appendages as they project downward. The dermis increases in thickness from 0.1 mm at 7 weeks to 0.7 mm by 20 weeks' gestation. As the epidermal appendages project deeply into the dermis at 16 weeks of age, the dermis organizes two distinct regions: the papillary dermis with fine fibrillar collagen and the reticular dermis with large collagen bundles. By 20 weeks of age, the fetal dermis is similar to that of the adult in structure, although still smaller in total thickness. Preliminary studies have demonstrated the 8-week-old fetus to contain fibronectin and types 1, 3, and 5 collagen within the dermis. By 14 weeks, recognizable fibroblasts, mast cells, endothelial cells, Schwann cells, and histiocytes are found in the fetal dermis. By 60 days' gestation, anchoring filaments are associated with the basal lamina at the dermoepidermal junction. At 22 weeks of age, the elastic fibers form, but well-developed elastic fiber networks are not observed until after 32 weeks, and the adult form of mature elastic fibers does not occur until after 2 years of age.

Few rigorous studies have been performed on the other components of the dermis, including vasculature, lymphatics, and nerves. Fat initially forms with discrete areas within the dermis at 16 to 18 weeks, followed by demarcation of a distinct fat layer that coincides with the development of hair follicles and their projection into the lower dermis.

Overall, newborn epidermal, hair, sweat, and sebaceous structures are nearly identical to adult structures. The dermis is less mature than adult dermis, being thinner with less organization of collagen and elastic fibers, with a less organized vascular network and cutaneous nerves. The newborn dermis appears as a transition between fetal and adult structures.

BIBLIOGRAPHY

Foster CA, Holbrook KA, Farr AG: Ontogeny of Langerhans cells in human embryonic and fetal skin: Expression of HLA-DR and OKT-6 determinants. *J Invest Dermatol* 1986; 86:240-243.

Goldsmith LA (ed): *Biochemistry and Physiology of the Skin,* ed 2. New York, Oxford University Press, 1990.

Harpin VA, Rutter N: Barrier properties of the newborn infant's skin. *J Pediatr* 1983; 102:419.

Holbrook KA, Odlund GF: Regional development of the human epidermis in the first trimester embryo and the second trimester fetus. *J Invest Dermatol* 1980; 80:161.

Holbrook KA: The biology of human fetal skin at ages related to prenatal diagnosis. *Pediatr Dermatol* 1983; 1:97.

Holbrook KA, Wolff K: The structure and development of skin, in Fitzpatrick TB, et al (eds): *Dermatology in General Medicine,* ed 3. New York, McGraw-Hill, 1987.

Smith LT, Holbrook KA: Embryogenesis of the dermis in human skin. *Pediatr Dermatol* 1986; 3:271-280.

Williams ME: The ichthyoses. Pathogenesis and prenatal diagnosis: A review of recent advances. *Pediatr Dermatol* 1983; 1:1.

2 _____ Evaluation in Children With Skin Diseases

The language of dermatology frequently inhibits students, house officers, and practitioners dealing with children from using the correct terminology for skin disease. It is neither proper nor helpful to simply use the term *rash*. This chapter describes the correct approach to the presenting features, signs, and initial laboratory findings when examining the child with cutaneous disease. The primary lesions should be committed to memory. Particular attention should be paid to the presence of vesicles, pustules, scaling, and color changes. Those four morphologic features will allow identification of the 10 major morphologic groups, which is essential for proper diagnosis and differential diagnosis. A problem-oriented algorithm is included in this chapter and at the front of the book to allow determination of the 10 morphologic groups of skin disease by their cutaneous appearance. Mastering this information will aid in communication with others delivering medical care to children.

MEDICAL HISTORY

The history obtained regarding a child's skin condition should be considered in the same fashion as a general medical history. The onset and duration of each symptom should be recorded. Associated systemic symptoms should be sought, along with a thorough review of systems. A past medical history, complete family history, and information on recent medications should also be obtained.

Health care advice is sought for children for three major concerns regarding the skin: itching (pruritus), scaling, and cosmetic appearance.

Pruritus

Persistent itching of the skin often provides the impetus to seek medical attention. The examiner should note whether the itching is localized or generalized and whether it is associated with skin lesions. Itching without skin lesions suggests biliary obstruction, diabetes mellitus, uremia, lymphoma, or hyperthyroidism. If the pruritus is associated with skin lesions, dermatophytosis, scabies, and the many types of dermatitis should be considered.

Scaling

Normally, one cell layer of stratum corneum, composed of flattened nonviable remnants of keratinocytes packed with protein (keratin), is shed daily. This is not usually visible. Acute injury and resultant separation of 10 to 20 cell layers of stratum corneum result in clinically visible white sheets of scale, such as seen in desquamation after sunburn or thermal burn. Overproduction of stratum corneum by proliferating epidermis, as in psoriasis, results in visible accumulation of excess scale. The scale in psoriasis is thick, in contrast to the thin scale in pityriasis.

Cosmetic Appearance

Parents may be concerned about color change in the child's skin. A history of the time of appearance of skin lesions, sequence of color changes, and course of skin changes should be obtained.

EXAMINATION OF THE SKIN

The evaluation of skin lesions requires careful inspection of the entire cutaneous surface, and many skin diseases are diagnosed only by their morphologic appearance. Examination of the skin should consist of identification of the primary lesion (the earliest lesion to appear) and secondary changes, and a description of the color, arrangement, and distribution of lesions. Often, however, secondary skin changes are seen without primary lesions. For correct diagnosis, a rigorous search should be made for a primary lesion.

Primary Skin Lesions

1. A *macule* (Fig 2–1) is a color change in the skin that is flat to the surface of the skin and not palpable (e.g., a tan macule, café au lait spot, white macule, vitiligo).

2. A *papule* (Fig 2–2) is a solid, raised lesion with distinct borders 1 cm or less in diameter (e.g., lichen planus, molluscum contagiosum).

3. A *plaque* is a solid, raised, flat-topped lesion with distinct borders and an epidermal

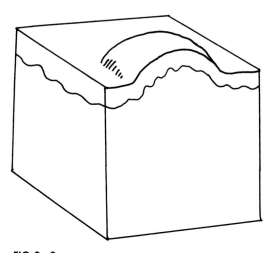

FIG 2–2.
A *papule* is a solid, raised lesion with distinct borders 1 cm or less in diameter (e.g., lichen planus, molluscum contagiosum).

change larger than 1 cm in diameter (e.g., psoriasis).

4. A *nodule* (Fig 2–3) is a raised, solid lesion with indistinct borders and a deep palpable portion. A large nodule is termed a *tumor* (e.g., rheumatoid nodule, neurofibroma). If the skin moves over the nodule, it is subcutaneous; if the skin moves with the nodule, the nodule is intradermal.

5. A *wheal* (Fig 2–4), an area of tense edema

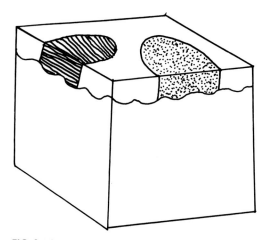

FIG 2–1.
A *macule* is a color change in the skin that is flat to the surface of the skin and not palpable (e.g., a tan macule, café au lait spot, white macule, vitiligo).

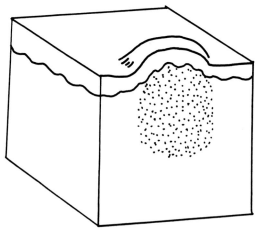

FIG 2–3.
A *nodule* is a raised, solid lesion with indistinct borders and a deep palpable portion. A large nodule is termed a *tumor* (e.g., rheumatoid nodule, neurofibroma).

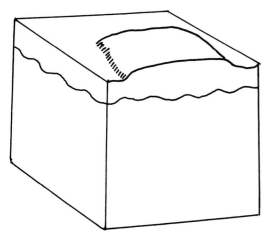

FIG 2–4.
A *wheal,* an area of tense edema in the papillary dermis, produces a flat-topped, slightly raised lesion (e.g., urticaria).

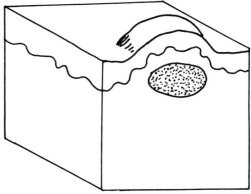

FIG 2–6.
A *cyst* is a raised lesion that contains a palpable sac filled with liquid or semisolid material (e.g., epithelial cyst).

in the upper dermis, produces a flat-topped, slightly raised lesion (e.g., urticaria).

6. A *vesicle* (Fig 2–5) is a raised lesion filled with clear fluid (e.g., varicella, herpes simplex). A *bulla* is a lesion larger than 1 cm in diameter and filled with clear fluid.

7. A *cyst* (Fig 2–6) is a raised lesion that contains a palpable sac filled with liquid or semisolid material (e.g., epithelial cyst).

8. A *pustule* (Fig 2–7) is a raised lesion filled with a fluid exudate, giving it a yellow appearance (e.g., acne, folliculitis).

Secondary Changes

1. *Erosions and oozing.* A moist, circumscribed, slightly depressed area represents a blister base *(erosion)* with the roof of the blister removed (e.g., burns, dermatitis). Because the action of chewing or sucking easily removes the thin blister roof (oral mucosa lacks a stratum corneum), most oral blisters present as erosions (e.g., aphthae, herpes simplex stomatitis).

2. *Crusting* represents dried exudate of plasma combined with the blister roof, which sits on the surface of skin following acute dermatitis (e.g., impetigo, contact dermatitis).

3. In *scaling,* whitish plates are present on the skin surface (e.g., psoriasis, ichthyosis). Des-

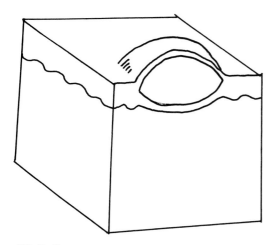

FIG 2–5.
A *vesicle* is a raised lesion filled with clear fluid (e.g., varicella, herpes simplex). A *bulla* is a lesion larger than 1 cm in diameter and filled with clear fluid.

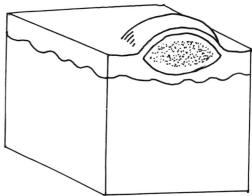

FIG 2–7.
A *pustule* is a raised lesion filled with a fluid exudate, giving it a yellow appearance (e.g., acne, folliculitis).

quamation refers to peeling of sheets of scale following an acute injury to skin (e.g., burn, toxic drug reaction, scarlet fever).

4. In *atrophy* (Fig 2–8), the skin surface is depressed because of thinning or absence of the epidermis, or subcutaneous fat (e.g., atrophic scar, fat necrosis). If the epidermis is thinned, it appears as fine wrinkling.

5. *Excoriations* are oval to linear depressions in the skin with complete removal of the epidermis, exposing a broad section of red dermis. Excoriations are the result of fingernail removal of the epidermis and upper dermis.

6. *Fissures* are characterized by linear, wedge-shaped cracks in the epidermis extending down to the dermis, and narrowing at the base.

Disruption of the Skin Surface

The presence of weeping, crusting, cracking (fissures), or excoriations is characteristic of disruption of the skin surface. Disruption is seen in eczematous lesions but is absent in papulosquamous lesions, and it is an important feature in differentiating the two.

Mobility of Skin

When grasping the skin between thumb and forefinger, the skin should be mobile. Excessive stretching indicates a type of Ehlers-Danlos syn-

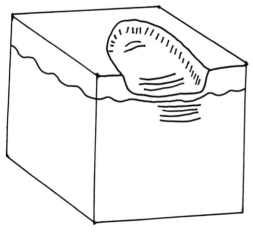

FIG 2–8.
In *atrophy,* the skin surface is depressed because of thinning or absence of the epidermis, or subcutaneous fat (e.g., atrophic scar, fat necrosis).

drome; immobility suggests scleroderma (see Chapter 17).

Color

The color of a skin lesion should be described as skin colored, brown, red, yellow, tan, or blue. Particular attention should be paid to whether the red or red-brown lesion completely blanches; for example, petechiae do not blanch. Red or red-brown color in skin is dependent on the pigment oxyhemoglobin, which is found in red blood cells within superficial cutaneous blood vessels. Compressing the superficial vascular plexus by direct pressure forces red blood cells into deeper vascular channels, and blanching of the skin is observed. If the skin does not blanch with pressure, red blood cells are outside the vascular channels and located in the adjacent dermis.

Melanin is the dominant pigment in the skin. Since it is located in the outer layer of skin closest to the observer's eye, melanin may obscure other pigments located in deeper layers. In dark-skinned black infants and children, a disciplined approach must be used to detect erythema, cyanosis, or jaundice. First, determine the normal skin color and then compare the involved skin area with the normal skin. Erythema will appear dusky red or violet. Cyanosis will appear black. Jaundice will appear diffusely darker, and the sclera must be examined to detect the presence of this disease. Carotenemia will appear golden brown.

Arrangement of Lesions

1. *Linear.* Lesions found in a straight line are called linear (e.g., lichen striatus).

2. *Annular.* Lesions found in a circular arrangement are called annular (e.g., granuloma annulare).

3. *Grouped.* Vesicles, papules, or nodules found closely adjacent to each other in a localized skin area are considered to be grouped (e.g., herpes simplex, herpes zoster).

Distribution of Lesions

It is useful to note whether an eruption is generalized, acral (hands, feet, buttocks, and face), or localized to a specific skin region, such as a dermatome.

RECORDING OF SKIN LESIONS IN THE HEALTH RECORD

Skin lesions should be described in an orderly fashion: distribution, arrangement, color, secondary changes, and primary lesion. For example, guttate psoriasis could be written as generalized, discrete, red, scaly papules. If abnormal, mobility of skin, hair changes, or nail changes should be recorded in addition.

PROBLEM-ORIENTED ALGORITHM

The clinician who has mastered the description of skin lesions can prepare a logical series of steps toward a correct diagnosis, even if the disease is initially unrecognized. Lynch has developed a problem-oriented algorithm for the nondermatologist. It can be applied to infants and children with skin disease, where it has been found to be most useful. This algorithm defines 10 morphologic groups of dermatologic disease that allow differential diagnosis and eventual correct diagnosis of a skin condition. These groups and the chapters in which they are found are listed in Table 2–1. Hair changes and nail changes can be added to make 12 morphologic groups. The 12 morphologic groups can be used for differential diagnosis (see the Problem-Oriented Differential Diagnosis Index, located at the front of this book).

The problem-oriented algorithm requires that three initial objective findings be determined: Are blisters present? Are the lesions red? Are the lesions scaling?

The detection of blisters is the crucial initial step in this diagnostic exercise. If even a single blister is detected, no matter the form of other skin lesions that may be observed, the examiner should consider first the possibility of a blistering disease and proceed to determine whether the blister fluid is clear or pustular.

If no blisters are observed, it should next be determined whether the skin lesions observed are red. If they are not red, it should be determined whether they are skin-colored or another color.

If the skin lesions observed are red, it should be determined whether the individual lesions themselves are scaling or nonscaling. If they are red and nonscaling, it should be determined

TABLE 2–1.

Groups of Dermatologic Disease

Morphologic Group	Chapter
1. Vesiculobullous diseases	4, 5, 7, 8, 9, 11, 18
2. Pustular diseases	3, 5, 6
3. Skin-colored papules and nodules	7
4. White lesions	16
5. Brown lesions	16
6. Yellow lesions	7, 16
7. Inflammatory papules and nodules	3, 5, 6, 7, 9, 18
8. Vascular reactions	13
9. Papulosquamous diseases	9
10. Eczematous diseases	4, 18
11. Hair changes	14
12. Nail changes	15

whether the surfaces of individual lesions are dome shaped or flat. If they are red and scaling, it should be decided whether there is surface disruption.

Starting with these three determinations, then adding up to eight more, the skin disease observed can be placed in one of 10 morphologic groups. Grouping the skin disease observed in this fashion will increase the likelihood of finding a precise diagnosis. The proper diagnosis can be determined with use of the Problem-Oriented Differential Diagnosis Index.

LABORATORY FINDINGS

Exfoliative Cytology

Exfoliative cytology is indicated in any blister-forming disease to detect acantholytic cells (pemphigus) or epidermal giant cells (herpes simplex or herpes zoster). Scrape the blister base with a No. 15 blade and place on a glass microscope slide. Allow to dry, and stain with Wright's or Giemsa stain and examine under the ×40 objective of a microscope.

Skin Biopsy

Biopsy for histopathologic diagnosis should be done of any skin tumor, palpable purpura, persistent dermatitis, or blister that is not diagnosed by morphologic appearance.

Punch Biopsy

Clean the skin for biopsy with alcohol. Inject 0.1 to 0.2 ml of lidocaine 1% intradermally with the use of a tuberculin syringe and a 30-gauge needle. Press a 4 mm Keys' punch firmly downward into the skin, which is stretched perpendicular to wrinkle lines. Rotate the punch until the soft subcutaneous fat is penetrated. Remove the specimen with forceps and scissors and place it in buffered formalin 10% for histologic examination. For immunofluorescence testing, the specimen should be frozen at $-70°$ C in liquid nitrogen or placed in special skin immunofluorescence transport media.

Shave Biopsy

After local anesthesia is achieved, a small elevated lesion may be shaved off with a sterile No. 15 blade or razor blade.

Fungal Scraping

Any red, scaly skin or scaly scalp should be scraped to evaluate the possibility of dermatophyte infection, which can mimic a wide variety of skin disorders (see Chapter 6). Scrape fine scales from the edge of a lesion onto a glass slide. A drop of potassium hydroxide (KOH) 20% added to the scale will dissolve the stratum corneum cells but not the hyphae. Place a coverslip on the slide and examine the scrapings under the $\times 10$ objective of the microscope for long, thin, branching hyphae or spores.

BIBLIOGRAPHY

Arndt KA: *Manual of Dermatologic Therapeutics. II: Procedures and Operations.* Boston, Little, Brown, 1989, pp 171–189.

Burton JL: The logic of dermatological diagnoses. *Clin Exp Dermatol* 1981; 6:1.

Lynch PJ: *Dermatology for the House Officer,* ed 2. Baltimore, Williams & Wilkins, 1987.

Oranje AP, Folkers E: The Tzanck smear: Old, but still of inestimable value. *Pediatr Dermatol* 1988; 5:127.

3 _____ Acne

ACNE

Clinical Features

The common variety of acne, acne vulgaris, is the most prevalent skin condition observed in the pediatric age group. The common forms of acne occur during two major ages, the newborn and the adolescent. Neonatal acne is a response to maternal androgen. It first appears at 2 to 4 weeks of age and lasts until the age of 4 to 6 months. The lesions are primarily on the face and upper parts of the chest and back, in a distribution similar to that of adolescent acne. The individual lesions seen are the same as described for adolescent acne. An oily scalp or face is often seen. It is believed that severe adolescent acne will develop in infants who have severe forms of neonatal acne. Persistence of neonatal acne beyond 12 months of age may be associated with endocrine abnormalities.

Early lesions of acne in the form of microcomedones develop in 40% of children ages 8 to 10 years, primarily on the face. Many authorities believe acne is one of the earliest signs of puberty. Eventually, 85% of adolescents will develop acne. It occurs in sebaceous follicles (Fig 3–1). There are several types of follicular channels present in skin. The sebaceous follicles have large, abundant sebaceous glands and small, vellus hairs. They are located primarily on the face, upper parts of the chest and back, and penis (Fig 3–2).

Obstruction of the sebaceous follicle opening produces the clinical lesions of acne. If the obstruction occurs at the follicular mouth, a wide, patulous opening develops that is filled with a plug of stratum corneum cells. This is the open comedone, or blackhead (Fig 3–3). Open come-dones are the predominant clinical lesion in early adolescent acne. The black color results from oxidized melanin within the stratum corneum cellular plug, not from dirt. Open comedones do not often progress to inflammatory lesions.

Obstruction of the sebaceous follicle just beneath the follicular opening in the neck of the sebaceous follicle produces a cystic swelling of the follicular duct just beneath the epidermis. The stratum corneum produced accumulates continuously within the cystic cavity. This is seen clinically as the microcomedone (closed comedone, or whitehead) (Fig 3–4). It is believed that these microcomedones are the precursors of inflammatory acne. Children 8 to 10 years of age often have microcomedones for months before red papules or pustules are observed. If open and closed comedones are the predominant lesions seen in adolescent acne, it is called comedonal acne.

Inflammatory lesions in acne prompt the adolescent to seek medical attention. These lesions include firm, red papules, pustules, cysts (Fig 3–5), and rarely, interconnecting draining sinus tracts. Most adolescents will have a mixture of microcomedones, red papules, pustules, and blackheads at the time of examination. Excoriation of acne papules and microcomedones is common, and scarring may result. Usually, multiple shallow erosions or crusts are found.

Cystic acne requires prompt medical attention, since ruptured cysts or sinus tracts result in scar formation. New acne scars are highly vascular and have a red or purplish hue. Such scars eventually regain normal skin color after several years. Acne scars may be depressed beneath the skin level, raised, or flat to the skin. In adolescents with a tendency toward keloid formation, keloidal

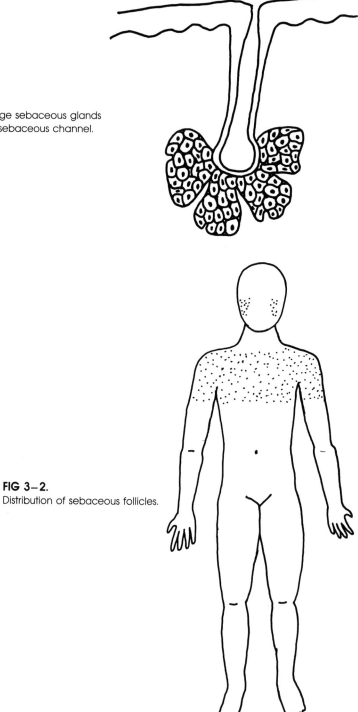

FIG 3–1.
Normal sebaceous follicles. Large sebaceous glands
excrete sebum into cylindrical sebaceous channel.

FIG 3–2.
Distribution of sebaceous follicles.

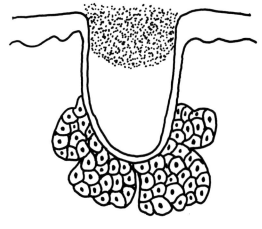

FIG 3—3.
Open comedone; wide, patulous opening of sebaceous channel with plug of stratum corneum cells in follicular mouth.

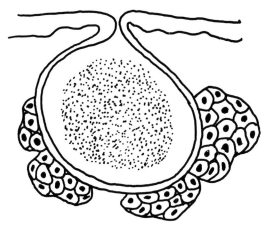

FIG 3—4.
Microcomedone (closed comedone); obstruction of the follicular channel just beneath the opening.

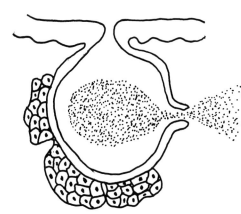

FIG 3—5.
Inflammatory papule; overgrowth of bacteria and rupture of the wall, producing a foreign body reaction surrounding the follicle.

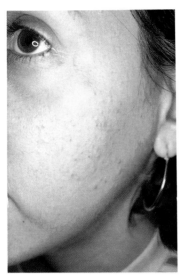

FIG 3–6.
Comedonal acne; multiple microcomedones on the cheek of an adolescent, the most common presentation of acne.

scars can occur following acne lesions, particularly over the sternum. Hypertrophic scars may also occur, even in those adolescents without keloids. In typical adolescent acne, several different types of lesions are present at one time, such as open and closed comedones (Figs 3–6 and 3–7), inflammatory papules and pustules (Fig 3–8), excoriated lesions (Figs 3–9 and 3–10), and nodu-

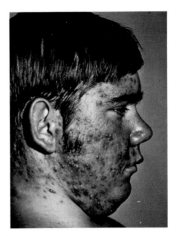

FIG 3–8.
Papulopustular acne; dozens of pustules and red papules on the face.

locystic acne (Fig 3–11). Neonatal acne (Fig 3–12) is characterized by inflammatory papules on the face and chest, with all the lesions in a similar stage.

Drug-induced acne should be suspected if all the lesions are in the same stage at the same time, with involvement of the abdomen, lower part of the back, arms, and legs (Fig 3–13), as well as the usual acne areas (Table 3–1). The presence of hirsutism or symptoms of virilizing syndromes should prompt an endocrine evaluation. Recall that both the adrenal glands and the ovaries contribute to circulating androgens in girls.

Several variants of acne occur in adolescence. Frictional acne from headbands, football helmets, or tight bras or other tight-fitting garments occurs predominantly under the skin area

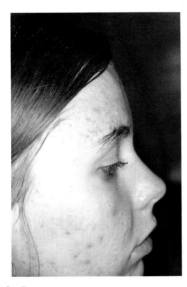

FIG 3–7.
Comedonal acne plus a few inflammatory papules.

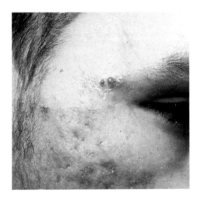

FIG 3–9.
Excoriated acne; oozing from red papule that has been squeezed.

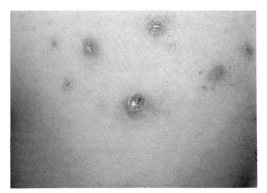

FIG 3–10.
Excoriated acne; atrophic scar from attempted fingernail removal of acne lesion.

where the garment is worn. Oil-based cosmetics may also be responsible for a predominantly comedonal acne, and hair sprays and oil-based mousse produce acne along the hair margin.

Differential Diagnosis

Conditions to be considered in the differential diagnosis of acne are listed in Table 3–2. Rosacea in children can be confused with acne vulgaris. In addition to acne papules and pustules, prominent telangiectasia and a persistent flush to cheeks, nose, or chin are observed. In many instances, rosacea in children results from the use of potent topical glucocorticosteroids on the face (Fig 3–14).

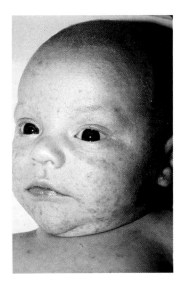

FIG 3–12.
Neonatal acne; red papules and pustules on the face of a 4-week-old infant.

Nevus comedonicus, which may be confused with neonatal acne, is a birthmark consisting of a linear arrangement of open comedones. It is present from birth and is usually unilateral. The anatomic abnormality of nevus comedonicus may also result in obstruction of the sebaceous follicle, with resultant red papules, pustules, or cysts, with

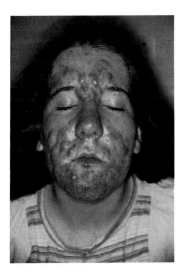

FIG 3–11.
Nodulocystic acne; deep nodules and cysts on the face of an adolescent.

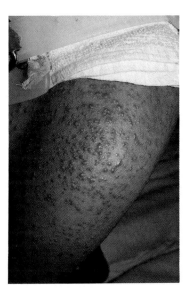

FIG 3–13.
Steroid acne; red papules all in the same stage in an adolescent treated with systemic steroids.

TABLE 3–1.

Drugs Responsible for Acne

Androgens
Adrenocorticotropic hormone (ACTH)
Glucocorticoids
Hydantoins
Isoniazid

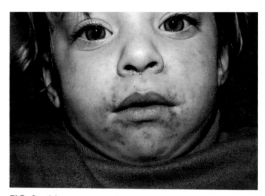

FIG 3–14.
Steroid rosacea; toddler with perioral red papules and pustules from prolonged daily therapy with topical steroid.

inflammatory lesions restricted to the birthmark. Miliaria may also mimic neonatal acne, although the lesions are transient, lasting less than 48 hours, in contrast to neonatal acne lesions, which persist for weeks.

Flat warts occurring on the face are sometimes confused with acne. They are papular, flat topped, and skin colored to slightly darker. The angiofibromas seen in tuberous sclerosis may be confused with acne. They are erythematous soft papules seen in the nasolabial folds and on the cheeks and chin. The onset of these lesions is typically at 7 or 8 years of age. The absence of comedones is an important clue to the diagnosis of angiofibroma, as is the presence of leaf-shaped white macules, seizure disorders, and connective tissue nevi.

Molluscum contagiosum may occasionally be mistaken for acne lesions, but careful inspection will reveal the central umbilication at the top of the papule characteristic of this disease.

Pathogenesis

It is accepted that the primary event in acne is obstruction of the sebaceous follicle. Ordinarily, the lining of such follicles contains one to two layers of stratum corneum cells, but in acne the stratum corneum is overproduced. This phe-

TABLE 3–2.

Differential Diagnosis of Acne

Adolescent
  Rosacea
  Steroid rosacea
  Flat warts
  Angiofibromas of tuberous sclerosis
  Molluscum contagiosum
Newborn
  Miliaria
  Nevus comedonicus

nomenon is androgen dependent in adolescent acne. The sebaceous follicles contain an enzyme, testosterone 5α-reductase, which converts plasma testosterone to dihydrotestosterone (DHT). DHT is a potent stimulus for sebaceous cell nuclear division and, subsequently, of excessive cell production. Thus, obstruction requires the presence of both circulating androgens and the converting enzyme. The interplay of circulating androgens and skin factors is believed to be crucial to the genesis of clinical acne. After the production or the administration of androgens, one would expect a delay of 2 to 4 weeks until cellular proliferation occurs and follicular obstruction appears. This, indeed, is what is seen in androgen-induced acne as well as in acne vulgaris. In a few patients with acne, elevated plasma testosterone is detected, but for the majority, no hormonal abnormality is detected.

The pathogenesis of inflammatory acne is not well understood. Undoubtedly, manipulation of a closed comedone could lead to rupture of the cavity contents into the dermis, with a subsequent inflammatory response (see Fig 3–5). Spontaneous inflammation also occurs in obstructed follicles, but the reasons are unclear. A currently attractive hypothesis is that overgrowth of gram-positive bacteria in the obstructed follicle, either *Propionibacterium acnes* or *Staphylococcus epidermidis,* might produce bacterial chemotactic peptides, enzymes, or other factors that initiate inflammation. Although overproduction of sebum frequently accompanies acne, sebum or metabolites of sebum are an unlikely cause of inflammation in acne as presently understood.

Treatment

Topical Keratolytic Agents.—The mainstay of antiacne therapy is the use of potent topical keratolytic agents applied to the skin to relieve follicular obstruction. Two classes of potent keratolytic agents, retinoic acid and benzoyl peroxide, have been found to be the most efficacious agents for the treatment of acne. Either agent may be used alone once daily, or the combination of retinoic acid applied to acne-bearing areas of skin once daily, in the evening, and benzoyl peroxide applied in the morning may be used. Since the two classes of keratolytics work by different mechanisms, they are synergistic. Topical keratolytic regimens will control 80% to 85% of adolescent acne. Retinoic acid and benzoyl peroxide are most effective in the gel forms; and creams, lotions, and solutions, particularly over-the-counter (OTC) preparations, have little efficacy. Dryness to the skin from using an alcohol- acetone-containing gel may be severe, with the result that the adolescent will often not use the prescribed gel medication. Alternative strategies designed to reduce dryness are use of a noncomedogenic moisturizer such as Moisturel after application of the gel, use of the gel every other day, or use of the cream preparations. The nonprescription lotion forms have minimal or no efficacy. Topical keratolytic therapy is recommended as the primary therapy for comedonal and mild papular forms of acne. Continuous use for several months is often required. Tretinoin should be avoided during pregnancy because of the potential of photoisomerization to isotretinoin. For papular acne, use benzoyl peroxide gel once or twice daily; for comedonal acne, retinoic acid once or twice daily as initial therapy. If no improvement occurs after 4 to 6 weeks, the other form of keratolytic can be added. In inflammatory acne, topical keratolytics plus oral antibiotics are recommended as initial therapy. Topical keratolytics are not used when oral retinoids, such as isotretinoin, are required.

Antibiotics.—Topical antibiotics are used to avoid systemic side effects caused by systemic antibiotics. Antibiotics are less effective when given topically than when given systemically, and at best they are equipotent to 250 mg of oral tetracycline given once a day. Clindamycin phosphate 1% is the most efficacious of all topical antibiotics. Some percutaneous absorption may rarely occur with this drug, resulting in diarrhea and colitis. Topical erythromycin 1%, 1.5%, and 2% solutions, 2% ointment, and 3% gel are quite effective, as is 1% meclocycline cream; topical tetracycline 1% or 2.2% is minimally efficacious (Tables 3–3 and 3–4). Topical antibiotics are most useful for maintenance therapy after improvement from 1 to 2 months of oral antibiotics is observed. The oral antibiotics can be discontinued and improvement maintained with topical antibiotics plus topical keratolytics.

Oral antibiotics that are concentrated in sebum, such as tetracycline and erythromycin, are very effective in inflammatory acne. The usual dose is 500 mg to 1 g of tetracycline or erythromycin taken daily divided into two doses. Tetracy-

TABLE 3–3.

Quick Guide to Initial Acne Therapy

Clinical Appearance	Treatment
Comedones only (Fig 3–6)	Retinoic acid 0.025% cream or benzoyl peroxide 10% gel once daily
Red papules, few pustules (Fig 3–7)	Retinoic acid 0.025% cream in the evening plus benzoyl peroxide 5% or 10% gel in the morning
Red papules, many pustules (Fig 3–8)	Retinoic acid 0.025% cream in the evening, benzoyl peroxide 5% or 10% gel in the morning, plus oral antibiotics: either tetracycline or erythromycin, 500 mg twice daily
Red papules, pustules, cysts and nodules (Fig 3–11)	Retinoic acid 0.05% cream twice daily plus benzoyl peroxide 10% gel twice daily plus oral tetracycline or erythromycin, 1 to 1.5 g daily

TABLE 3–4.

Selected Acne Treatment Products

Product	Size
Topical keratolytics (apply once or twice daily)	
Retinoic acid, tretinoin (Retin-A)	
0.025% cream	20, 45 g
0.05% cream	20, 45 g
0.01% gel	15, 45 g
0.025% gel	15, 45 g
Benzoyl peroxide	
Desquam-X 5% and 10% gel	42.5, 85 g
Desquam-E 5% and 10% emollient gel	42.5, 84 g
Persa-Gel 5% and 10% gel	45, 90 g
Persa-Gel W 5% and 10% gel	45, 90 g
Benzac 5% and 10% gel	60 g
Benzac 5% and 10% gel	60, 90 g
Topical antibiotics (apply twice daily)	
Clindamycin phosphate 1% solution (Cleocin T)	60 mL
Meclocycline sulfosalicylate 1% cream (Meclan)	20, 45 g
Erythromycin 2% solution (T-Stat, Erycette, A/T/S)	60 mL
Systemic antibiotics (1 or 2 capsules twice daily)	
Tetracycline hydrochloride	250 mg capsule; 100/bottle
Erythromycin	250 mg capsule; 100/bottle
Oral retinoids (40 mg capsule twice daily for 16 weeks)	
Isotretinoin (Accutane)	10, 40 mg capsule

cline should be taken on an empty stomach for reliable absorption. Oral antibiotics should be continued for 1 to 3 months until the acne lesions are suppressed. Topical keratolytics should be used in combination with oral antibiotics. Therapy for a period of 4 to 6 weeks is required for clinical improvement.

Oral Retinoids.—The oral retinoid isotretinoin (13-*cis*-retinoic acid) has been very efficacious in nodulocystic acne resistant to standard therapeutic regimens (see Fig 3–11). It is not recommended that isotretinoin be used as the drug of first choice for acne. The precise mechanism of action is unknown, but decreased sebum production, follicular obstruction, and skin bacteria, as well as general antiinflammatory activities, have been described. The initial dosage is 40 mg once or twice daily (0.5 to 1.0 mg/kg/day) for 4 months,

then the drug is stopped. Isotretinoin is neither designed for, nor efficacious in, comedonal acne or other mild forms of acne. Side effects include dryness and scaliness of the skin, dry lips, and, occasionally, dry eyes and nose. Up to 10% of patients experience mild hair loss, but it is reversible. Elevated liver enzymes and blood lipids have rarely been described. Oral retinoids are the most efficacious treatment for severe cystic acne. Teratogenicity restricts the use of isotretinoin in female patients of childbearing potential. The isotretinoin teratogen syndrome is characterized by malformations of the central nervous system, and it has been reported in 25% of women who became pregnant while taking isotretinoin. A negative pregnancy test should be obtained before the drug is considered, with careful adherence to the guidelines provided by the manufacturer, including monthly contraceptive counseling and pregnancy tests. Patients should be encouraged to enroll in the pregnancy prevention program of the manufacturer. Treatment for longer than 4 months is not recommended. At least a 4-month rest period off drug is recommended before a second treatment course is considered.

Other Acne Treatments.—There is no convincing evidence that dietary management, mild drying agents, abrasive scrubs, oral vitamin A, ultraviolet light, cryotherapy, and incision and drainage have any beneficial effects in the management of acne. Although hormonal therapy may have a role in patients with documented endocrine abnormalities or hirsutism, there is but temporary or insignificant benefit in the vast majority of adolescents.

Factors That Aggravate Acne Vulgaris

Acne can be aggravated by a variety of external factors, resulting in further obstruction of partially occluded sebaceous follicles. Avoidance of oil-based cosmetics, hair-styling mousse, face creams, and hair sprays may alleviate the comedonal component of acne 4 to 6 weeks after use of the cosmetics is discontinued. A representative list of nonacnegenic moisturizers and cosmetics is found in Table 3–5. Change of habits such as changing tight-fitting garments may be helpful. Stopping drugs that induce acne should be attempted, if possible.

Patient Education

Acne therapy requires that adequate time and explanation accompany any treatment program. It is important to explain the mechanism of acne and the treatment plan to the adolescent patient. Explain specifically that not much improvement can be expected for 4 to 8 weeks. Time should be set aside at the first visit to answer the patient's questions about acne. One should be certain to

TABLE 3–5.
Nonacnegenic Moisturizers and Cosmetics

Moisturizers
Moisturel
Cetaphil lotion
Cosmetics
Matte Finish (Allercreme)
Matte Makeup for Oily Skin (Almay)
Pore Minimizer Makeup (Clinique)
T-Zone Controller (Charles of the Ritz)

ask what the patient's peers, relatives, and others have advised. Written patient education handouts and lists of useful moisturizers and cosmetics are extremely valuable. The presence of excoriations should prompt an explanation regarding how attempted fingernail removal of acne usually results in scars that are permanent (see Figs 3–9 and 3–10). Suggestions for relief of the nervous habit are useful.

Follow-up Visits

Follow-up visits should initially be every 4 to 6 weeks. The criterion for ideal control is a few new lesions every 2 weeks. Do not expect complete prevention of the appearance of any new acne lesions. Reexplain what the medications you are using are intended to achieve, and question the patient to determine whether the medications are being used properly. At the first visit, a baseline evaluation grading comedones, papules, pustules, and cysts in each affected skin region should be entered on the patients' record to assist with objective measurement (Tables 3–6 and 3–7). At each subsequent visit, the same scoring system should be used for comparison. Objective and subjective evaluations are more likely to differ than correlate in acne patients, and one must rely on objective findings for proper evaluation of response to therapy. Most authorities recommend treatment with oral antibiotics for at least 1 to 3 months. At the follow-up visit, a decision to stop oral antibiotics is made when 90% improvement in red papules and pustules is observed and documented by the scoring system listed in Tables 3–6 and 3–7. When oral antibiotics are stopped, improvement can be maintained by twice-daily application of topical antibiotics. At each follow-up visit, emphasize that therapeutic response is slow in acne and that it is evaluated over weeks to months, not days. Be certain that the red-purple scars that require 6 to 12 months to fade are not the lesions that determine alterations in treatment strategy. Scars are not influenced by antibiotics or keratolytics.

PERIORAL DERMATITIS AND STEROID ROSACEA

Clinical Features

Erythema, slight scaling, telangiectasia, and red papules characterized these closely related conditions. In perioral dermatitis and steroid ro-

TABLE 3–6.

Grading System for Acne

	Baseline (Date)	Follow-up		
		1 (Date)	2 (Date)	3 (Date)
Location and Grade (0–3)				
Face				
Comedones				
Papules				
Pustules				
Cysts				
Chest				
Comedones				
Papules				
Pustules				
Cysts				
Back				
Comedones				
Papules				
Pustules				
Cysts				

0 = no lesions; 1 = 1–19 lesions; 2 = 20–39 lesions; 3 = 40 or more lesions.
Grade each category (comedones, papules, pustules, cysts) for each location (face, chest, back).

TABLE 3–7.

Evaluation of Acne Patients (Example)

	Baseline (10/1/91)	Follow-up		
		1 (11/3/91)	2 (12/8/91)	3 (1/28/92)
Location and Grade (0–3)				
Face				
Comedones	2	1	1	0
Papules	1	1	0	0
Pustules	0	0	0	0
Cysts	0	0	0	0
Chest				
Comedones	0	0	0	0
Papules	0	0	0	0
Pustules	0	0	0	0
Cysts	0	0	0	0
Back				
Comedones	1	1	1	1
Papules	2	2	2	1
Pustules	1	0	0	0
Cysts	0	0	0	0

0 = no lesions; 1 = 1–19 lesions; 2 = 20–39 lesions; 3 = 40 or more lesions.
Grade each category (comedones, papules, pustules, cysts) for each location (face, chest, back).

sacea, lesions are found in the nasolabial folds, just beneath the nose, and on the chin (see Fig 3–14). Often, lesions begin as red macules with a slight scale and are misdiagnosed as dermatitis. A topical steroid is used and the lesions get progressively worse, with redder, telangiectatic skin and red papules or pustules seen. Frequently, the child received the steroid from a relative in the health care field or used an OTC steroid. Superpotent topical steroids are most often associated with steroid rosacea after a few weeks of use, but low-potency steroids, if used daily over many weeks, will also induce the condition. Infants and adolescents are most often involved, although the exact prevalence is not known. Occasionally, in steroid rosacea, pustules and red papules will be found on the lower eyelids in addition to the perioral skin. Rarely, the perioral lesions will have a granulomatous histology and reveal closely spaced skin-colored micronodules in a perioral distribution.

Differential Diagnosis

At the onset of disease, a dermatitis, such as seborrheic or contact dermatitis, is suspected, although careful examination will not detect disruption of the skin surface. This misdiagnosis leads to therapy that worsens the condition. Acne vulgaris may also be restricted to the perioral skin, but the presence of comedones, which are usually absent in rosacea, will help differentiate. Rarely, tinea faciei (see Chapter 6) will involve perioral skin. Scrapings for microscopic identification of fungus and fungal culture will differentiate.

Pathogenesis

Although many authorities believe perioral dermatitis and steroid rosacea are related to acne, the pathogenesis is unclear. Sebaceous gland hyperplasia, obstructed sebaceous follicles, and prominent telangiectasias are pathologic features. In steroid rosacea, the role of topically applied steroids is well established, although the exact mechanism is unknown. Although there is speculation that yeast species have a role, it is yet unproved.

Treatment

The treatment protocols used for common acne are effective in rosacea, perioral dermatitis, and steroid rosacea. Topical steroid preparations must be discontinued, recognizing that the condi-

tion will worsen for about 1 week. In mild cases, topical keratolytics alone will suffice. With many red papules and pustules present, oral erythromycin for 4 to 6 weeks may be required. The use of topical antiyeast agents is controversial.

Patient Education

Many patients are reluctant to stop topical steroids, because their skin is improved for 2 or 3 hours after each application. Insist that topical steroids be stopped, and advise patients that the skin will get worse for 1 week before it begins to improve. Caution them not to use steroids to treat the predicted worsening. It is important to emphasize that this is a form of acne, and treatment is similar to acne treatment. Advice that only certain people are susceptible is useful.

Follow-up Visits

A visit in 4 weeks to evaluate the response to therapy is recommended.

BIBLIOGRAPHY

Benke PJ: The isotretinoin teratogen syndrome. *JAMA* 1984; 251:3267.

Frieden IJ, Prose NS, Fletcher V, et al: Granulomatous perioral dermatitis in children. *Arch Dermatol* 1989; 125:369.

Hirschman JV: Topical antibiotics in dermatology. *Arch Dermatol* 1988; 124:1691.

Lehman PA, Malany AM: Evidence for percutaneous absorption of isotretinoin from the photoisomerization of topical tretinoin. *J Invest Dermatol* 1989; 93:595.

Leyden JJ, Shalita AR: Rational therapy for acne vulgaris: An update on topical treatment. *J Am Acad Dermatol* 1986; 15:907.

Lucky AW: Update on acne vulgaris. *Pediatr Ann* 1987; 16:29.

Lucky AW: Endocrine aspects of acne. *Pediatr Clin North Am* 1983; 30:395.

Peck GL, Olsen TG, Butkus D, et al: Isotretinoin versus placebo in the treatment of cystic acne. *J Am Acad Dermatol* 1982; 6:735.

Rasmussen JE: What causes acne? *Pediatr Clin North Am* 1983; 30:511.

Sheehan-Dare RA, Hughes BR, Cunliffe WJ: Clinical markers of androgenicity in acne vulgaris. *Br J Dermatol* 1988; 119:723.

Swinyer LJ, Baker MD, Swinyer TA, et al: A comparative study of benzoyl peroxide and clindamycin phosphate for treating acne vulgaris. *Br J Dermatol* 1988; 119:615.

4 _____ Dermatitis

Dermatitis, inflammation in the superficial dermis and epidermis characterized by disruption of the skin surface (crusting, weeping, excoriation, and cracking [fissures]), is a common disorder among children and adolescents. The prevalence of dermatitis between 1 and 5 years of age is 34.5 per 1,000; between 6 and 11 years, 26.7 per 1,000; and between 12 and 17 years, 35.5 per 1,000. The terms *dermatitis* and *eczema* are used interchangeably, although eczema was initially used to refer to blistering dermatitis, because the term is derived from a Greek term meaning "to boil over." Dermatitis may vary in intensity from an acute condition, with vesicle formation, oozing, and crusting, to a chronic form, with epidermal thickening, a shiny, flattened epidermal surface, and exaggerated skin creases. In an intermediate form, called *subacute dermatitis*, both vesiculation and epidermal thickening are present. Acute dermatitis implies an intense stimulus; chronic dermatitis suggests a stimulus of low potency repeatedly occurring over time. All forms of dermatitis characteristically involve the epidermis, with inflammation and disruption of epidermal integrity.

The categories of dermatitis are traditional and imprecise. Except for the various forms of contact dermatitis, the pathogenesis is unknown. Therefore, it may be best simply to describe the lesions as dermatitis rather than to apply modifying adjectives such as atopic when the cause is unclear. Some traditional terms are used in this section to avoid confusion with the previous medical literature.

ATOPIC DERMATITIS

Clinical Features

Atopic dermatitis is a hereditary disorder characterized by either a family or a personal history of asthma, allergic rhinitis, or atopic dermatitis. Two thirds of patients with dermatoses morphologically compatible with atopic dermatitis have a family history of asthma or allergic rhinitis. *Atopy* is from the Greek, meaning "without place, unusual," and was first used in 1923 by Coca and Cooke to denote inherited human hypersensitivity as exemplified by asthma and hay fever. The diagnosis of atopic dermatitis is a clinical one, and there is no specific marker for the disorder. The clinical appearance of atopic dermatitis may represent a phenotype resulting from different mechanisms. A variety of terms have been used in the literature to designate the condition. Atopic eczema, allergic eczema, Besnier's prurigo, eczema, and circumscribed neurodermatitis are terms less acceptable and less widely used than atopic dermatitis. Up to 50% of patients with a dermatitis compatible with the diagnosis of atopic dermatitis also have respiratory manifestations of atopy, such as extrinsic asthma or allergic rhinitis. Very rarely does a patient have all three manifestations of the atopic triad.

Atopic dermatitis usually begins at age 1 to 4 months and is less common in premature infants. At the onset, the distribution is primarily on the cheeks, face, trunk, and extensor surfaces of the arms and legs at this age (Fig 4–1). Frequently, the dermatitis seen at this age is a subacute der-

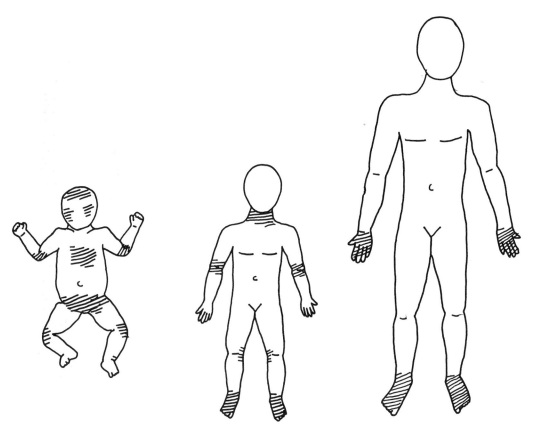

FIG 4–1.
Age-dependent distribution of atopic dermatitis. Involvement of face, scalp, trunk, and extensor surfaces of extremities is seen in infants, flexural skin in toddlers, and hands and feet in preteens and adolescents.

matitis characterized by oozing. Although atopic dermatitis develops in infancy in most patients, it is noted during early childhood in some. By adolescence, more than 90% of patients with atopic dermatitis will already have the disorder. Of all infants in whom atopic dermatitis develops, only a third will continue to have the disease during childhood. Similarly, of those who still have dermatitis during childhood, only a third will have difficulties at adolescence. Thus, one ninth of those who had infantile dermatitis will still have the features and problems of dermatitis in adolescence. Itching has long been recognized as a significant feature of atopic dermatitis. It commonly occurs in paroxysms and can be severe. In most patients, itching is most severe in the evening. The threshold for itching in atopic dermatitis patients is lowered, and their itching is more prolonged than that in normal persons. Scratching frenzies may be reported. The propensity for itch-

ing and the resultant trauma from scratching are central to the genesis of atopic dermatitis (Fig 4–2).

The distribution of dermatitis is largely age dependent (see Fig 4–1). Infantile atopic dermatitis, distributed largely on the cheeks (Fig 4–3), face, trunk, and extensor surfaces of extremities, evolves into the childhood phase, with dermatitis on the feet and in the flexural areas, such as the antecubital fossa, popliteal fossa (Fig 4–4), and neck. By adolescence the distribution is as seen in older adults, with bilateral involvement of the flexural areas and hand eczema. Involvement of the eyelids is common in all phases of atopic dermatitis and may help to make the diagnosis. Foot involvement is common in school-age children and adolescents and may be associated with atopic dermatitis or juvenile plantar dermatosis.

The primary clinical lesion of atopic dermatitis has not been described. In fact, many observ-

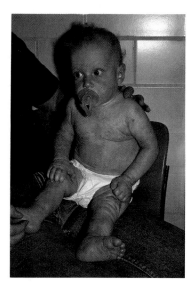

FIG 4–2.
Atopic dermatitis. Itching frenzies may be severe, as seen in this infant.

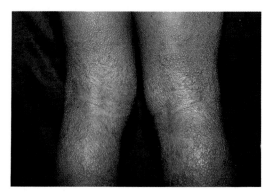

FIG 4–4.
Flexural involvement of popliteal fossae in atopic dermatitis.

ers believe that all visible skin lesions in atopic dermatitis result from scratching. Intense erythema and oozing are absent except in patients with secondary bacterial infection. During exacerbation, dark-skinned patients may demonstrate follicular papules, especially on the trunk. In black skin, hyperpigmented, lichenified nodules are commonly found on the lower arms and legs in addition to flexural involvement (Fig 4–5).

Dry skin is strongly associated with atopic dermatitis, with reduced water content of the stratum corneum. Secretion of sebum and sweat may be suppressed in some patients with atopic dermatitis. Dry skin and horny follicular papules

(keratosis pilaris) are common findings, particularly on extensor surfaces. Microscopic fractures of the stratum corneum during drying result in loss of the epidermal barrier and increased susceptibility to irritants and infection. There is little doubt that dryness of the skin during the winter months in cool climates is a significant factor in exacerbations of atopic dermatitis. Dry, slightly scaly, hypopigmented patches, seen in mild atopic dermatitis, are called *pityriasis alba* (Fig 4–6).

The variety of vasomotor reactions in atopic dermatitis suggests a tendency to vasoconstriction of the skin. The facial skin, particularly around the nose, appears pale, and the peripheral extremities may have a lower skin temperature than that of normal persons. The skin reacts to cold stimuli with marked vasoconstriction. White dermatographism, the production of a white line with surrounding blanching after stroking erythematous

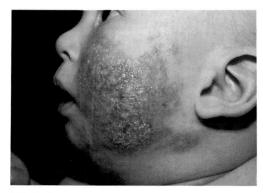

FIG 4–3.
Acute dermatitis of cheeks with oozing and crusting in infant with atopic dermatitis.

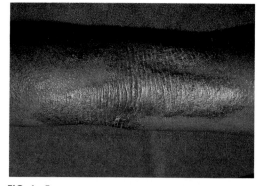

FIG 4–5.
Lichenification from chronic rubbing of the skin in atopic dermatitis.

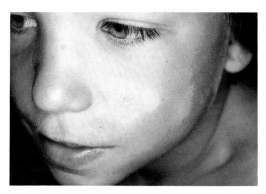

FIG 4–6.
Hypopigmented, slightly scaly patch of mild dermatitis referred to as pityriasis alba.

skin with a blunt instrument, is seen in some children with atopic dermatitis. This blanching is thought to represent edema. There is also a diminished response of atopic skin to intradermal injections of histamine.

Children with atopic dermatitis may be extremely sensitive to certain contactants. They may experience bouts of itching and subsequent exacerbation of dermatitis when wool or an irritant chemical contacts the skin. Detergents and frequent soaping of the skin often result in prolonged itching. Sensitivity to contactants may partially explain localization of dermatitis in certain areas, particularly on the hands and feet.

Emotional stress indisputably leads to increased scratching. This occurs frequently in children, either from heightened awareness of itching or a habit of scratching. The child experiences transient relief after a scratching frenzy. Atopic dermatitis worsens during such episodes. It is important for patients or their parents to recognize that scratching the skin is a means of expressing anxiety. Secondary skin infection with bacteria such as *Staphylococcus aureus* may worsen the dermatitis and worsen itching.

There is no single diagnostic criterion for the phenotype we appreciate as atopic dermatitis; rather, a combination of features must be considered. The major features listed in Table 4–1 are useful in the diagnosis Although many other features may be noted, such as facial pallor, Denny's lines under the eyes, intolerance to wool or occlusive clothing, associated ichthyosis, cataracts, and eosinophilia, they are not considered diagnostic of the disease or necessary for the diagnosis.

TABLE 4–1.

Diagnostic Features of Atopic Dermatitis

Itching
Personal history of asthma or allergic rhinitis
Family history of asthma or allergic rhinitis
Elevated serum IgE level
Dry skin with itching during sweating
Paradoxical vasoconstrictive cutaneous responses

Differential Diagnosis

Differential diagnosis should include any disorder manifested by dermatitis. Thus, contact dermatitis of the primary irritant and allergic type, seborrheic dermatitis, nummular eczema, scabies, juvenile plantar dermatosis, polymorphous light eruption, the dermatitis of human immunodeficiency virus (HIV) infection, or immunodeficiency and tinea constitute the major considerations in the differential diagnosis of atopic dermatitis in childhood. In infants, seborrheic dermatitis may be impossible to distinguish from atopic dermatitis. Serum immunoglobulin E (IgE) levels may be elevated in infantile atopic dermatitis, but clinical findings overlap considerably.

Pathogenesis

Although there are a number of hypotheses as to the mechanism of the generation of atopic dermatitis in children, the exact pathogenesis is unknown. Various forms of both antibody and cellular immunodeficiency, abnormal β-adrenergic receptors and responses, food allergies, and aeroallergens, such as house dust mites, have been evoked, but there is no convincing evidence to substantiate any of these hypotheses. The only method of reproducing a dermatitis is by epicutaneous application of a substance.

Treatment

Atopic dermatitis is a chronic disease and is frustrating for both child and parents. It is tempting for the physician to focus on one or several factors as causes and to regard their elimination as curative. The patient or the family should be told that there is no immediate cure for atopic dermatitis but that spontaneous remissions do occur and that this disorder can be controlled by therapy. Patients and family should pay careful attention to factors that aggravate atopic dermatitis, listed in Table 4–2. The mainstays of therapy are topical steroids, wet dressings, oral antibiotics and avoidance of factors that aggravate the dermatitis.

TABLE 4–2.

Factors That Aggravate Atopic Dermatitis

Dry skin
Tendency for sweat duct obstruction
Contact sensitivity
Stress and anxiety
Secondary bacterial infection

General care instructions are given in Table 4–3.

Abnormal sweating and heat intolerance can be managed by avoiding occlusive clothing, airtight occlusive dressings such as plastic wrap, and overheating. Dry skin can be managed by rehydration of the skin with water and covering the skin generously with a lubricant. Contact sensitivity can be managed by avoiding frequent soaping and washing of the skin, the wearing of wool, and the use of home cleaning agents and any other irritating chemicals that may come in direct contact with the skin. Stress and anxiety can be managed by removing the child to a new environment, such as a hospital. Although hospitalization of a child is generally not desirable, the stress and anxiety of the dermatitis may require such therapeutic intervention. Secondary bacterial infection by *S. aureus* or *Streptococcus pyogenes,* resulting from the frequent breaks in the skin and the excoriations caused by scratching, is treated with systemic antibiotics (Fig 4–7). If lymphadenopathy is present, antibiotics are recommended. Although topical mupirocin has been demonstrated to be efficacious, bacterial resistance is a concern.

Relief of itching is the cornerstone of therapy for atopic dermatitis. Itching may be relieved by removing the factors aggravating atopic dermatitis and by using topical glucocorticosteroids of low or moderate potency or antihistamines. Significant antihistamine sedation often must be achieved before relief of pruritus occurs.

The mainstay of therapy for atopic dermatitis remains topical steroid preparations. They are

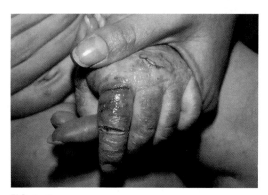

FIG 4–7.
Fissures and many breaks in the skin in atopic dermatitis, with secondary bacterial infection.

central to most treatment strategies for atopic dermatitis. For initial care (Table 4–4) select a moderately potent steroid ointment and use it twice daily for up to 2 weeks; then stop the steroid and switch to long-term management therapy as outlined in Table 4–5. Recommended topical steroid ointments are listed in Table 4–6. For lubrication of skin, select from the preparations listed in Table 4–7.

Short-Term Management.—*Steroids and Wet Dressings.*—Acute weeping dermatitis is best treated by the application of wet dressings,

TABLE 4–4.

Instructions for Initial Care of Atopic Dermatitis

1. Apply moderately potent steroid ointment to wet skin twice daily for 7 to 14 days; then discontinue ointment.
2. Use diphenhydramine or hydroxyzine (2 mg/kg) 1 hour before bedtime.
3. If infected, use antistaphylococcal oral antibiotic (e.g., dicloxacillin, 40 mg/kg/day) three to four times a day for 10 to 14 days.

TABLE 4–3.

General Instructions for Long-Term Management of Atopic Dermatitis

Wear loose-fitting cotton clothing.
Keep fingernails trimmed short.
Avoid overheating of skin.
Avoid frequent soaping of skin (use of soap substitute).
Keep the skin lubricated.

TABLE 4–5.

Instructions for Maintenance Care of Atopic Dermatitis

1. Lubricate wet skin twice daily.
2. Use cetyl alcohol lotion cleanser (Cetaphil) as soap substitute.
3. Continue antihistamines for itching as necessary.
4. If flare up occurs, re-treat with steroid ointment twice daily for 2 or 3 days.

TABLE 4–6.

Moderately Potent Steroids for Use in Childhood Atopic Dermatitis

Mometasone furoate 0.1% ointment (Elocon)
Hydrocortisone valerate 0.2% ointment (Westcort cream)
Fluocinolone acetonide 0.025% ointment (Fluonid, Synalar)

TABLE 4–7.

Lubricants Useful for Atopic Dermatitis*

Apply to wet skin:
Moisturel
Hydrophilic petrolatum
Mineral oil
Cetaphil
Eucerin (do not use on inflamed skin)

the method for which is outlined in Table 4–8. Often, such patients have multiple excoriations, crusting, and secondary bacterial infection; thus, the use of wet dressings in combination with systemic antibiotics is necessary. It may be difficult to treat such patients successfully without the use of antibiotics. Apply a moderately potent steroid ointment or cream to affected areas; cover with a damp cotton dressing followed by a dry cotton dressing (see Table 4–8). In 6 hours, remove all

TABLE 4–8.

Instructions for Wet Dressings

Materials needed
1. Prescription for moderately potent steroid ointment or cream
2. Two pairs of cotton or mostly cotton sleepers or long johns
3. Warm water in a sink or basin
Technique
1. Apply steroid ointment to rash.
2. Wet one pair of cotton sleepers in warm water; wring out until damp.
3. Place damp sleepers on child, the dry sleepers over the damp ones.
4. Be certain room is warm enough and child does not chill.
Duration of treatment
1. Use overnight for 5 to 10 nights.
2. Change every 6 hours for 24 to 72 hours (e.g. reapply steroid; redampen damp sleepers).

dressings and reapply steroids. Follow by applying a redampened dressing, then a dry dressing. Continue this procedure for 24 to 72 hours; then switch to a long-term management strategy. An alternate strategy is to use wet dressings and steroids overnight for 7 to 10 consecutive nights and then use maintenance therapy. Since the evaporation of water results in cooling, be certain to keep the child's room warm when using wet dressings. Use systemic antistaphylococcal antibiotics to treat secondary infection, and oral antihistamines to relieve pruritus.

Long-Term Management.—Wet Method.—Several methods that involve the liberal use of lubricants are equally successful in managing children with acute and chronic atopic dermatitis. A description of two of the more popular methods follows. The child should be bathed in warm water without soap twice a day. While the skin is still wet, the child or parent should liberally apply one of the lubricants listed in Table 4–7. The lubricant can be applied directly to the wet skin as soon as the child leaves the tub, or the lubricant can be applied under water to the skin at the end of the bath. Lubricants should be applied between baths as well. Use of cetyl alcohol lotion cleanser as a soap substitute is recommended. Antihistamines, such as hydroxyzine or diphenhydramine at 2 mg/kg/dose, given 1 hour before bedtime, are useful.

Dry Method.—Again, the frequent and liberal use of lubricants (see Table 4–7) is recommended. Bathe the child only once a week; apply as a lubricant cetyl alcohol lotion (Cetaphil) liberally to the body three or four times a day. Antihistamines are given 1 hour before bedtime.

Lubricants, Antihistamines, Antibiotics, and Intermittent Topical Steroids.—Twice-daily applications of topical steroid ointments and oral antihistamines for 2 to 3 weeks, followed by twice-daily applications of lubricants such as Moisturel and one evening dose of antihistamines may be used. For a flare-up of atopic dermatitis in a child who is controlled on maintenance therapy, re-treat with a topical steroid ointment twice daily for 2 or 3 days and then return to maintenance therapy (see Table 4–5). Oral antistaphylococcal antibiotics used for 2 to 4 weeks may be of great benefit.

Referral for Special Therapy

Children who are not responding to treatment may be referred to a dermatologist for further treatment. Often, therapeutic failures result from not following the treatment plan or in the child who has unrecognized and untreated secondary bacterial infection. Phototherapy with ultraviolet B sunlamps or photochemotherapy with psoralen and ultraviolet A may be efficacious in children with atopic dermatitis who have failed standard therapy. Phototherapy should be supervised by trained, experienced dermatologists.

Alternative Therapies

Although many parents or physicians are convinced that foods induce exacerbations of atopic dermatitis, scientific evidence for reproduction of dermatitis by foods is scanty and unconvincing. This should not become an emotional issue between parents and the treating physician. Restrictive diets have no long-term benefits in atopic dermatitis and may eventuate in nutritional deficiency if too restrictive. Evening primrose oil, desensitization shots, and a number of other remedies have been advocated without obvious benefit. Oral steroids may produce temporary benefits, but high doses are required, and they have no role in the management of a chronic disease because of side effects with long-term use.

Patient Education

It is helpful to instruct the child and the parents in the method of application of the topical medications. One may choose to explain that the child has "sensitive" skin, that heredity plays a role in determining this tendency, but the cause is not known. It should be emphasized that a cure is not possible, but that good control can be achieved so that the child can live a comfortable and normal life. Preventing further skin irritation is also helpful (see Table 4–3), as is emphasis on the five factors aggravating atopic dermatitis, particularly secondary bacterial skin infection. The patient and the parents should be told that the principle underlying good control is the liberal use of lubricants to restore moisture to the skin and protect it from contactants. Using lubricants in this manner avoids the necessity for high-potency topical glucocorticosteroids and long-term steroid medications. Do not make the patient or the parents feel guilty if a flare-up of the eczema occurs. Reinstitute active treatment.

Follow-up Visits

The first follow-up visit should be within the first week, so that therapy can be reviewed. It is often helpful at this time to have the parents or the child demonstrate how medication is applied and to determine how much was used. Have the medication brought back for each visit. Evaluation of the response to antihistamines and the need for antibiotics can be completed at the first follow-up visit. Thereafter, monthly visits will suffice until the patient is using lubricants only, after which he or she should be reevaluated every 3 to 6 months. Be certain that patients know that you will be available when flare-ups occur, and examine the child for secondary infection at the visit related to the flare-up.

CONTACT DERMATITIS

Contact dermatitis, or dermatitis resulting from substances coming in direct contact with the skin, is divided into two subtypes: primary irritant contact dermatitis and allergic contact dermatitis.

Primary Irritant Contact Dermatitis

Strong chemicals that penetrate the epidermal barrier readily, weaker chemicals that penetrate a faulty epidermal barrier, or substances that remove intercellular lipids produce inflammation of the skin (primary irritant contact dermatitis). The form most commonly seen in pediatric patients is diaper dermatitis. Dry skin dermatitis and juvenile plantar dermatosis are other forms commonly seen in children.

DIAPER DERMATITIS

Clinical Features

The exact incidence of diaper dermatitis is unknown, but roughly 7% of all infants younger than age 2 years are believed to develop this condition at any time. Four clinical forms are recognized. The most frequently observed is chafing dermatitis, in which involvement of the convex surface of the thighs, buttocks, and waist area is common. Chafing diaper dermatitis most frequently is observed at 7 to 12 months of age, when the baby's urine volume exceeds the absorbing capacity of the diaper, including the superabsorbent diapers (Fig 4–8). In the second form, the dermatitis is limited to the perianal

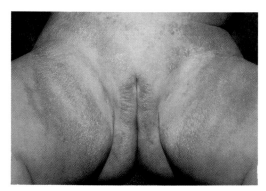

FIG 4−8.
Chafing type of diaper dermatitis.

area. This form is particularly observed in newborns or in children who have experienced diarrhea. The third form is characterized by discrete, shallow ulcerations scattered throughout the diaper area, including the genitalia. In the fourth form, beefy-red, confluent erythema involving the inguinal creases and the genitalia, with satellite oval lesions about the periphery, is seen (Fig 4−9). This fourth form is observed when secondary invasion with *Candida albicans* occurs. Despite major differences in clinical appearance, all four forms share a similar pathogenesis.

Pathogenesis

Diaper dermatitis is a result of prolonged contact of urine and feces with the perineal skin. Airtight occlusion of feces and urine by plastic or rubber diaper covers increases the penetration of these alkaline substances through the epidermal barrier. Diaper dermatitis will not occur without

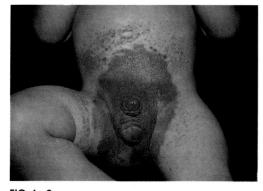

FIG 4−9.
Candidiasis in diaper area. Positive scraping and culture are obtained from satellite pustules.

maceration, and prolonged contact with water is central to the genesis of the dermatitis. Ammonia by itself is not responsible for the dermatitis. If a diaper dermatitis is present for longer than 3 days, there is likely to be secondary *C. albicans* invasion of the inflammatory areas of the skin. *C. albicans* invasion must be suspected in each clinical form of diaper dermatitis.

Differential Diagnosis

Atopic dermatitis or the other forms of dermatitis may begin in the diaper area. Rarely, psoriasis, the Letterer-Siwe form of histiocytosis X, or the eruptions associated with immunodeficiencies or HIV infection may occur in this area. In perianal forms of diaper dermatitis, perianal cellulitis must be distinguished, and a bacterial culture must be obtained.

Treatment

The basis for all treatment programs is to remove the contactants (urine and feces) from the skin surface and eliminate maceration by keeping the diaper area dry. Very frequent diaper changes are useful for this purpose. Diaper changes 1 hour after the baby goes to sleep for the night and reducing fluids just before bedtime may be of benefit. Plastic and rubber pants should be avoided when possible. Let the diaper area skin air dry when practical. When contamination by urine and feces occurs, the skin should be rinsed gently with warm water. A minimum of soap should be used in this area. Alternate use of hydrocortisone 1% cream and nystatin (Mycostatin) cream when changing diapers often results in a dramatic response in 4 to 7 days. Until toilet training is achieved or diaper care changed, recurrences may be frequent. Diaper type does not influence diaper dermatitis, although the incidence decreases with eight or more diaper changes per day.

Patient Education

Reducing the duration of contact of urine and feces with skin is essential. Very frequent diaper changes constitute the best prevention, with careful attention to overnight care. Sleeping on a rubber sheet with the baby not wearing a diaper cover may be helpful. Determining the person actually responsible for diaper changes during the daily routine is very helpful in planning a therapy program. In the 7- to 12-month old, have the parent check the diaper for wetness 1 hour after bedtime and change the baby if wet. Restriction of fluids in the hour just before bedtime may also be helpful.

Follow-up Visits

Routine visits for pediatric care are sufficient for follow-up, but in severe diaper dermatitis, a follow-up visit in 2 days may be useful.

DRY SKIN DERMATITIS

Clinical Features

A dry, rough skin surface with rectangular scales that have erythema on the scale borders is seen in dermatitis due to dry skin (see Fig 4–9). Horny follicular papules on the proximal extremities and buttocks (keratosis pilaris) are also usually seen. Occasionally, the dermatitis will coalesce, and the patient will present with diffuse erythema.

Differential Diagnosis

The differential diagnosis includes all the other forms of dermatitis, the ichthyoses, and scabies. Children with atopic dermatitis have very dry skin.

Pathogenesis

Environmental humidity of less than 30% is the most important factor. Frequent soaping of the skin, removing skin lipids with alcohol or acetone, or the use of drying lotions predisposes to dry skin dermatitis.

Treatment

Therapy is designed to restore moisture to the skin by liberal use of water followed by the application of lubricants. Generally, water-in-oil emulsions (see Chapter 20) two or three times daily are sufficient.

Patient Education

The value of a home humidifier in an area of low environmental humidity and of avoiding frequent soaping of the skin is important to convey to the patient or family. Children with dry skin require daily lubricant therapy.

Follow-up Visits

One visit in 4 weeks to evaluate the therapy program is often sufficient.

JUVENILE PLANTAR DERMATOSIS

Clinical Features

Redness, cracking, and dryness of the weight-bearing surface of the foot is characteristic of juvenile plantar dermatosis (JPD). The great toes are often the first area involved (see Fig 4–5). Involvement of the entire forefoot that can mimic tinea pedis may occur. The involvement is usually quite symmetric. Many, but not all, children with JPD may exhibit features of atopic dermatitis.

Differential Diagnosis

Tinea pedis often mimics JPD. However, JPD is quite common in preadolescence, whereas tinea pedis is uncommon; JPD involves weight-bearing areas while tinea pedis involves the instep. Direct microscopic examination of scale with potassium hydroxide (KOH) and fungal culture will help to distinguish the two conditions. Allergic contact dermatitis involves the dorsum of the foot rather than the weight-bearing surface.

Treatment

Ointment bases such as Aquaphor or petroleum jelly applied two or three times daily are most useful. Attempts to dry the feet often aggravate the condition because the feet are already dry and chapped. Topical glucocorticosteroid ointments of moderate potency may be required if inflammation is severe.

Patient Education

Emphasis that this is neither a fungal infection nor the result of excessive sweating of the foot is important. The patient should recognize that the excessive dryness is similar to chapping of the skin.

Follow-up Visits

A visit 2 weeks after therapy is begun is most useful in evaluating compliance and response.

Allergic Contact Dermatitis

Clinical Features

The exact incidence of allergic contact dermatitis in children is unknown, but some authorities estimate it at 5% to 10% of all dermatitis. In childhood, allergic contact dermatitis usually presents as an acute dermatitis with erythema, vesiculation, and oozing (Fig 4–10). The dermatitis is limited to the area of contact with the external

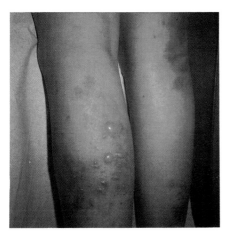

FIG 4–10.
Allergic contact dermatitis due to poison ivy, with blister formation.

substance, such as the stem or leaf of a plant. Less often, children are exposed repeatedly to weaker chemical allergens, resulting in the development of the features of subacute or chronic dermatitis (Fig 4–11). Usually, the contactant is obvious, although considerable detective work is occasionally required to determine the cause. Once the response occurs and a dermatitis is generated, as seen with a strong allergen such as poison ivy, it lasts for 3 weeks, even though the child has not had repeated exposure to the allergen.

Distribution of the dermatitis may provide an important clue to the contact allergen: involvement of the dorsa of the feet in shoe dermatitis; of the earlobes, neck, wrists, and fingers in metal allergy (e.g., due to nickel); of the face and eyelids in cosmetic allergy; of the axilla in deodorant allergy; of the ear canal from medication; of the perioral area from toothpaste or lipstick; or of areas of clothing from exposure to formaldehyde.

Differential Diagnosis

Although all other forms of dermatitis may mimic allergic contact dermatitis, it is usually localized to one area of skin. A sudden onset of dermatitis limited to the hands or feet in children and adolescents is most likely to be contact dermatitis (Fig 4–12). Patch testing (described under Follow-up Visits) may detect the chemical allergen and help distinguish allergic contact dermatitis from other forms of dermatitis.

Pathogenesis

Allergic contact dermatitis is a form of cell-mediated immunity. The process is divided into two distinct but interrelated phases: the sensitization phase and the elicitation phase. The antigens involved in allergic contact dermatitis are incomplete antigens called haptens (Table 4–9). The hapten applied to the skin surface penetrates the epidermis, combines with the antigen-binding site of the epidermal Langerhans cell, and is carried via the lymphatics to the regional lymph node. There, the antigen is processed by macrophages and presented to T lymphocytes. Recognition occurs, as does proliferation of the T lymphocytes specifically programmed to recognize that antigen. These T lymphocytes leave the lymph node and enter the bloodstream, migrating back to the skin. The sensitization phase takes 5 to 7 days to complete in the case of strong chemical allergens;

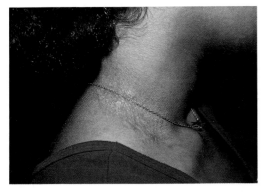

FIG 4–11.
Chronic dermatitis of neck from nickel allergy caused by necklace.

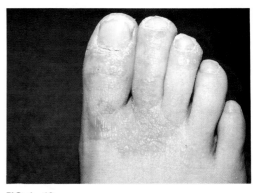

FIG 4–12.
Chronic dermatitis on dorsa of feet and toes due to potassium dichromate allergy from chronic exposure to leather tennis shoes.

TABLE 4-9.

Characteristics of Contact Allergens

1. They are haptens.
2. They can penetrate the epidermis.
3. They can form strong covalent bonds with protein.

with weak allergens, it may take from weeks to months.

In the elicitation phase, antigen-specific T lymphocytes are present in the skin. The next time the allergen comes in contact with the skin surface and penetrates the epidermis, the T lymphocyte combines with the allergen in the skin and releases inflammatory mediators, causing erythema and the accumulation and activation of mononuclear cells, which results in the dermatitis. This phase begins 6 to 18 hours after the antigen is applied.

A great variety of chemicals are responsible for causing allergic contact dermatitis, varying from the simple metal nickel to complex chemicals such as dinitrochlorobenzene. Common sources of contact allergens in children are listed in Table 4-10. However, the allergens have certain features in common, as seen in Table 4-9.

Treatment

Antiinflammatory agents such as glucocorticosteroids are the therapy of choice in allergic contact dermatitis. In localized areas, topical glucocorticosteroids of moderate potency (see Table 4-6 and Chapter 20), applied three times daily for 3 weeks, clear the dermatitis. In generalized skin involvement or in acute vesicular involvement, wet dressings and topical glucocorticosteroids for 2 to 3 days give dramatic relief (see Table 4-8). This is followed by applications of moder-

ate-potency topical glucocorticosteroids three times daily for 14 more days. When greater than 10% of the skin surface is involved, oral glucocorticosteroids, such as prednisone, 1 mg/kg in a single dose every morning for 14 to 21 days, are used. The popular steroid dose packs do not maintain their antiinflammatory effects for a sufficiently long time and often result in a rebound exacerbation of acute contact dermatitis.

Patient Education

Knowledge and avoidance of the offending antigen are central to the care of the child with allergic contact dermatitis. The most common contact allergens are listed in Table 4-11. Emphasize that treatment requires 2 or 3 weeks.

Follow-up Visits

In 3 to 4 weeks, after the allergic dermatitis has subsided, epicutaneous (patch) testing to identify the offending allergen may be desirable in children in whom the cause is obscure. This is not necessary in acute poison ivy or plant dermatitis. Epicutaneous testing has been standardized and is reliable in detecting the suspected allergen. The test is made on the upper part of the back. Finn Chambers mounted on Scanpor tape are used. The suspected antigens are placed on the Finn Chambers, and vertical rows of three to five strips are placed on the upper part of the back and firmly secured with nonirritating occlusive tape (Blenderm). The area is taped securely, so that it is airtight, and the patches are left on for 48 hours without allowing the area to become wet. The patient removes the patches and tape, and the tests are read 72 hours after initial application. Erythema and vesiculation are observed in an allergic reaction, the same clinical and histologic

TABLE 4-10.

Common Sources of Contact Allergens in Children

Jewelry, buckles, clothing snaps (nickel)
Shoes (potassium dichromate)
Topical medications, creams, lotions (neomycin, thimerosal, formaldehyde, Quaternium 15, wool alcohol)
Perfumes, soaps, cosmetics (balsam of Peru, colophony, "fragrances")
Poison ivy, poison oak, poison sumac, mango rind (urushiol)

TABLE 4-11.

Most Prevalent Allergens in Children

Allergen	Percent Sensitized
Neomycin	8
Nickel	8
Potassium dichromate	8
Thimerosal	3
Balsam of Peru	2
Formaldehyde	1
Quaternium 15	1
Colophony	1
p-tert-Butylphenol formaldehyde	1
Wool (lanolin) alcohol	1

features that are seen in allergic contact dermatitis. In allergic reactions, the papules extend beyond the chamber margins, whereas they are limited to the chamber in irritant reactions. The angry back syndrome of hyperreactivity has not been reported in children. Standardized allergens have been developed by the North American Contact Dermatitis Group and may be obtained from the American Academy of Dermatology. Patch testing should be performed by a physician experienced in the interpretation and pitfalls of the procedure.

SEBORRHEIC DERMATITIS

Clinical Features

A chronic dermatitis accompanied by overproduction of sebum may occur on the scalp, face, midchest, or perineum in two age groups: the neonate and the adolescent. With the excessive production of sebum, accumulation of scales entrapped in the sebum, leaving a greasy scale, is an expected finding. In some infants it is limited to the scalp, with a greasy accumulation of scales adherent to the scalp (seborrhea capitis). Many infants also have flexural dermatitis seen in atopic dermatitis. Infants with a tendency to have seborrheic dermatitis may have severe worsening of their dermatitis if they first develop a persistent diaper dermatitis. In the adolescent, erythema and greasy scales in the nasolabial folds and the scalp may be seen. In HIV-infected adolescents, it may be an early sign of acquired immune deficiency syndrome (AIDS).

Differential Diagnosis

Since physiologic overproduction of sebum occurs in many infants during the first 6 months of life, any dermatitis occurring at this age may be mistakenly called seborrheic dermatitis. There is considerable confusion over whether it is necessary to distinguish between atopic dermatitis, contact dermatitis, and seborrheic dermatitis in infants. Most infants with dermatitis eventually demonstrate features consistent with atopic dermatitis, especially if the involvement of the extremities and trunk accompanies the more characteristic lesions of the scalp and face. Scabies may also mimic seborrheic dermatitis in this age group, and scraping unscratched burrows for scabies mites will help distinguish. Seborrheic dermatitis

with petechiae is often seen in the Letterer-Siwe form of histiocytosis X, and this diagnosis may also be excluded by skin biopsy. The immunodeficiency diseases, such as Leiner's disease, severe combined immunodeficiency, and the immunodeficiency that accompanies HIV infection, may be excluded by the history, the presence of signs and symptoms of failure to thrive, severe pulmonary or gastrointestinal infection accompanying the eruption, or the appropriate immunologic or serologic evaluation. Multiple carboxylase deficiency and other biotin-responsive dermatoses also mimic seborrheic dermatitis, and serum biotin levels may be required to distinguish.

Seborrheic dermatitis limited to the scalp (seborrhea capitis) must be distinguished from the diffuse form of tinea capitis due to *Trichophyton tonsurans* and from crusta lactea (cradle cap). A KOH examination of scalp scrapings plus a fungal culture will distinguish tinea capitis, while the absence of redness characterizes cradle cap.

Adolescent seborrheic dermatitis occurs in the nasolabial folds, midface, postauricular area, scalp, and chest. It may be difficult to distinguish from atopic or contact dermatitis, the perioral dermatitis variant of acne, or psoriasis.

Pathogenesis

Although seborrheic dermatitis has been attributed to excessive sebum accumulation on the skin surface, the mechanism is unknown. Similarly, the seborrheic-like dermatitis of immunodeficiency or HIV infection is unknown. Although there are many carboxylase enzymes in skin and biotin may be a cofactor for many skin enzymes, the mechanism of dermatitis is unknown.

Treatment

Topical steroid creams of low potency applied three times daily for 2 weeks often clear the dermatitis. Do not use keratolytic shampoos on the scalp because often these worsen the dermatitis. Bland shampoos left on the scalp for 20 minutes and then rinsed off are useful. Oral biotin therapy should be considered if biotin-responsive dermatoses are suspected. On the face, topical steroids should be of low potency and used two times daily for 2 weeks only; then moisturizers should be substituted. If perioral dermatitis is suspected, antiacne therapy as outlined in Chapter 3 is used.

Patient Education

Patients and parents should be advised that the cause of this disorder is unknown. Although it is tempting to use rigorous methods to remove scale from the scalp, it is unnecessary.

Follow-up Visits

A visit in 1 week to review diagnostic tests that were done and to evaluate response to therapy is recommended. Thereafter, the child should be seen at monthly intervals until the dermatitis resolves.

NUMMULAR ECZEMA

Clinical Features

Symmetrically distributed areas of dermatitis 1 to 10 cm in diameter are seen primarily on the extremities in this condition (Fig 4–13). The Latin word *nummulus,* meaning little coin, is used to describe the shape of the lesions. Two forms occur in children: the wet form, with oozing and crusting (see Fig 4–13), and the dry form, with erythema and scaling. Both forms are persistent, lasting for months if untreated.

Differential Diagnosis

Nummular eczema is important because it frequently mimics two common pediatric conditions: impetigo and tinea corporis. The wet form is frequently confused with impetigo, and multiple courses of antibiotics are given before the diagnosis is suspected. Biopsy of the lesion readily

distinguishes it from impetigo. The dry form can be distinguished from tinea corporis by a KOH examination of skin scrapings or a fungal culture. Some nummular lesions occur in otherwise typical atopic dermatitis or contact dermatitis.

Treatment

The treatment is that outlined for atopic dermatitis, although moderately potent topical steroids are required. Lesions are difficult to resolve, and treatment programs require considerable effort before improvement is seen.

Patient Education

Patients should be informed of the chronicity of nummular eczema and its tendency to recur. They should be told the cause is unknown.

Follow-up Visits

The child should be seen initially in 2 weeks to evaluate the response to therapy.

KERATOSIS PILARIS

Clinical Features

In keratosis pilaris, prominent follicular plugs are noted over the extensor aspects of the extremities, the buttocks, and the cheeks (Figs 4–14 and 4–15). Individual lesions represent plugs of stratum corneum in separate follicular openings. A dermatitis may surround the plugs. The affected skin surface feels rough and dry. Keratosis pilaris is worsened by drying of skin and is frequently associated with dry skin, ichthyosis vulgaris, and atopic dermatitis. Some children

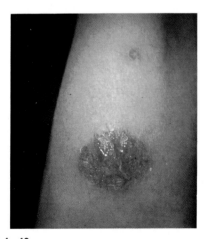

FIG 4–13.
Oozing coin-shaped area of dermatitis in nummular eczema.

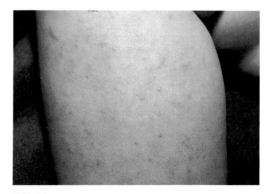

FIG 4–14.
Dry, pinpoint, white, discrete papules on extensor surfaces of upper arms in keratosis pilaris.

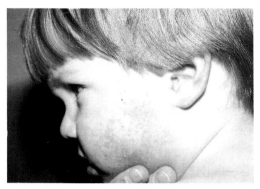

FIG 4–15.
Papules with associated erythema on cheeks of patient with keratosis pilaris. Same patient as in Fig 4–14.

may present with extensive keratosis pilaris with no evidence of the other conditions, however. In these children, the keratosis pilaris is extensive and often involves the forearms, the lower legs, and much of the face.

Differential Diagnosis

Keratosis pilaris may be confused with microcomedones of acne, molluscum contagiosum, warts, milia, psoriasis, or, occasionally, folliculitis. Since it is not seen at birth, it should be easily distinguished from neonatal acne and erythema toxicum.

Pathogenesis

The pathogenesis is unknown. Some authorities regard keratosis pilaris as a disorder of keratinization. They believe that the keratinous plug is produced through abnormal keratinization of the follicular channel. Other authorities believe it is a response to drying of the skin surface, which results in a dry plug of scale lodged in follicular openings. It is more severe in cold, dry climates.

Treatment

In the very mild forms of this disease, the use of lubricants applied to wet skin may be sufficient to control the condition. In more extensive keratosis pilaris, topical keratolytics may be required, frequently in combination with lubricants. Lactic acid 12% cream (Lac-Hydrin) and a urea cream 10%, each applied once daily, are frequently beneficial. All treatment strategies require many weeks of therapy to see improvement. Therapy must be continued after improvement is seen.

Topical tretinoin (Retin-A) is also effective, but it may cause significant irritation to the skin, particularly if the child has ichthyosis or an associated atopic dermatitis. Often when the child moves to a more humid climate, the condition spontaneously improves.

Patient Education

The patient should be informed of the nature of this disease and its likelihood of becoming chronic if untreated. The patient should also be advised of the slow response to therapy and the necessity for long-term treatment.

Follow-up Visits

A follow-up visit in 2 weeks, to determine response to therapy, is usually indicated. Thereafter, follow-up every 3 or 4 months is sufficient.

BIBLIOGRAPHY

Atherton, DJ, Carabutt F, Glover MT, et al: The role of psoralen photochemotherapy (PUVA) in the treatment of severe atopic eczema in adolescents. *Br J Dermatol* 1988; 118:291.

Beck HI, Korsgaard J: Atopic dermatitis and house dust mites. *Br J Dermatol* 1989; 120:245.

Bergstresser P: Contact allergic dermatitis. Old problems and new techniques. *Arch Dermatol* 1989; 125:276.

Burks AW, Mallory SB, Williams LW, et al: Atopic dermatitis: Clinical relevance of food hypersensitivity reactions. *J Pediatr* 1988; 113:447.

Campbell RL, Bartlett AV, Sarbaugh FC, et al: Effects of diaper type on diaper dermatitis associated with diarrhea and antibiotic use in children in day-care centers. *Pediatr Dermatol* 1988; 5:83.

Ewing CI, David TJ: Atopic eczema and preterm birth. *Arch Dis Child* 1988; 63:435.

Graham-Brown RAC: Atopic dermatitis. *Semin Dermatol* 1988; 7:37.

Hellgren L, Mobacken H: Nummular eczema: Clinical and statistical data. *Acta Derm Venereol (Stockh)* 1969; 48:189.

Hyams JS, Carey DE: Corticosteroids and growth. *J Pediatr* 1988; 113:249.

Lever R, Hadley K, Downey D, et al: Staphylococcal colonization in atopic dermatitis and the effect of topical mupirocin therapy. *Br J Dermatol* 1988; 119:189.

MacKie RM, Husain SL: Juvenile plantar dermatosis. A new clinical entity? *Clin Exp Dermatol* 1976; 1:253.

Menni S, Piccinno R, Baietta S, et al: Sutton's

summer prurigo: A morphologic variant of atopic dermatitis. *Pediatr Dermatol* 1987; 4:205.

Podmore P, Burrows D, Eedy DT, et al: Seborrheic eczema: A disease entity or a clinical variant of atopic eczema? *Br J Dermatol* 1986; 115:341.

Prose NS, Mendez H, Menikoff H, et al: Pediatric human immunodeficiency virus infection and its cutaneous manifestations. *Pediatr Dermatol* 1987; 4:67.

Raimer SS: The use of topical steroids in children. *Pediatr Dermatol,* in press.

Rasmussen JE: Advances in nondietary management of children with atopic dermatitis. *Pediatr Dermatol* 1989; 6:210.

Rehder PA, Eliezer ET, Lane AT: Perianal cellulitis. Cutaneous group A streptococcal disease. *Arch Dermatol* 1988; 124:702.

Turpeinen M, Lehtokoski-Lehtiniemi E, Leisti S, et al: Percutaneous absorption during and after the acute phase of dermatitis in children. *Pediatr Dermatol* 1988; 5:276.

Vickers CFH: The natural history of atopic eczema. *Acta Derm Venereol [Suppl] (Stockh)* 1980; 92:113.

Werner Y: The water content of the stratum corneum in patients with atopic dermatitis. *Acta Derm Venereol (Stockh)* 1986; 66:281.

Weston WL: The use and abuse of topical steroids. *Contemp Pediatr* 1988; 5:57.

Weston JA, Hawkins K, Weston WL: Foot dermatitis in children. *Pediatrics* 1983; 72:824.

Weston WL, Lane AT, Weston JA: Diaper dermatitis. *Pediatrics* 1980; 66:532.

Weston WL, Weston JA, Kinoshita J, et al: Prevalence of positive epicutaneous tests among infants, children and adolescents. *Pediatrics* 1986; 78:1070.

Yates VM, Kerr REI, MacKie RM: Early diagnosis of infantile seborrheic dermatitis and atopic dermatitis: Clinical features. *Br J Dermatol* 1983; 108:633.

Yates VM, Kerr REI, Frier K, et al: Early diagnosis of infantile seborrheic and atopic dermatitis: Total and specific 1gE levels. *Br J Dermatol* 1983; 108:639.

Yohn J, Weston WL: Topical glucocorticosteroids. *Curr Probl Dermatol* 1990; 2:29.

5 _____ Bacterial Infections of Skin (Pyodermas) and Spirochetal Infections

Bacteria constantly colonize the skin surface and occasionally invade the epidermal barrier to replicate within the skin. The majority of skin microorganisms are nonpathogenic. The two major pathogens found on children's skin are *Staphylococcus aureus* and *Streptococcus pyogenes*. The former is found in 5% of children and the latter in 1%. However, during epidemics and in endemic areas, either of these organisms may be recovered from the skin of 50% to 80% of children. In humid climates, pyodermas are common in childhood.

IMPETIGO AND ECTHYMA

Clinical Features

Erosions covered by moist, honey-colored crusts are suggestive of impetigo (Fig 5–1). Impetigo begins as small (1 to 2 mm) vesicles with a fragile roof that is quickly lost. Multiple lesions are often present, and exposed areas such as the face and extremities are the most common sites of involvement. The term *bullous impetigo* has been used to describe lesions with a central moist crust and an outer zone of blister formation (Fig 5–2). Whether small blisters or large, *impetigo* is the preferred term. Impetigo has a high attack rate, and its spread is enhanced by crowding and poor socioeconomic conditions. In contrast, ecthyma is characterized by a firm, dry, dark crust with surrounding erythema and induration. Direct pressure on the crust results in the extrusion of purulent material from beneath the crust.

Both ecthyma and impetigo may occur simultaneously in the same patient. The clinical features are so characteristic that bacterial culture is not routinely performed.

Differential Diagnosis

Subacute dermatitis, such as nummular dermatitis, herpes simplex infections, and a kerion resulting from dermatophyte infections, may have moist crusts and mimic impetigo. Nummular dermatitis has dozens of symmetrically distributed lesions as opposed to impetigo, which has a few nonsymmetric lesions. Herpes simplex is usually a distinct group of lesions that, even when crusted, demonstrate a group of individual papules or vesicles beneath. Viral culture or Tzanck smear may be required to differentiate. A potassium hydroxide (KOH) examination or fungal culture may be required to distinguish a kerion from impetigo. A second-degree burn, cutaneous diphtheria, or cutaneous anthrax may be confused with a solitary lesion of ecthyma. Bacterial culture of the purulent material beneath the crust may be required.

Pathogenesis

Invasion of the epidermis by pathogenic *S. aureus* or group A streptococci occurs in impetigo and ecthyma. The depth of invasion in impetigo is superficial (into the papillary epidermis), while the entire epidermis is involved in ecthyma (Figs 5–3 and 5–4). Microscopic breaks in the epidermal barrier, such as the trauma of scratching dermatitic skin, predispose to im-

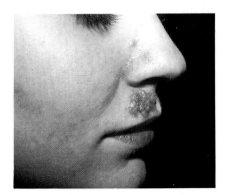

FIG 5–1.
Impetigo. Honey-colored, moist crust just above the upper lip.

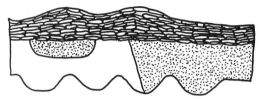

FIG 5–3.
Difference between impetigo and ecthyma. Superficial neutrophilic collection in middermis *(shaded area on left)* in impetigo in contrast to full-thickness involvement *(shaded area on right)* in ecthyma.

petigo, while staphylococci or streptococci penetrate the lower epidermis in ecthyma after injury to the midepidermis and upper epidermis. Often, colonization of the skin surface with the two major pathogens occurs several days to a month before the appearance of clinical lesions. It is now recognized that in many areas of North America penicillinase-producing staphylococci are more likely to be responsible for impetigo than streptococci. For impetigo secondary to an underlying skin disease such as dermatitis, scabies, psoriasis, or varicella, staphylococci are virtually always responsible. Poststreptococcal glomerulonephritis may follow such infections of the skin if nephritogenic strains of streptococci are involved.

Treatment

Systemic antibiotics to eradicate staphylococci and streptococci are the treatment of choice. In order to treat both pathogens, dicloxacillin, 15 to 50 mg/kg/day, or cloxacillin, 50 to 100 mg/kg/day orally for a total of 10 days may be used. Erythromycin, 40 mg/kg/day orally for 10 days is an alternative, but in many areas of North America strains of staphylococci resistant to erythromycin have been encountered. If streptococci are cultured, penicillin V, 125 mg to 250 mg four times daily for 10 days, may be used. Topical antibiotics may result in clinical improvement but may prolong the carriage state of the pathogen on the skin. Topical pseudomonic acid cream, while efficacious, should be reserved for serious staphylococcal infections, since resistant strains are reported. Removal of crusts and scrubbing the impetigo skin lesions with antibacterial soaps have not been shown to be effective. Hand washing with a surgical soap may reduce the likelihood of spread.

The risk of nephritogenic strains of streptococci varies considerably throughout North America, but an active program in which both patients

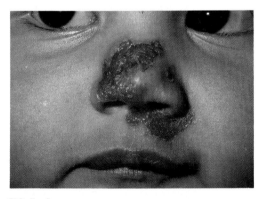

FIG 5–2.
Impetigo. Spread of infection to top of nose from beneath the nose in an infant with impetigo.

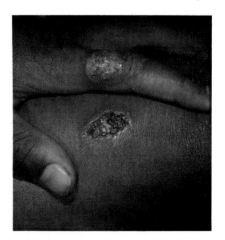

FIG 5–4.
Dry crust with indurated border in child with ecthyma.

and contacts are treated will significantly reduce the incidence of acute glomerulonephritis in endemic areas.

Patient Education

Good hand washing techniques and good general personal hygiene are useful in preventing further infection of contacts and reducing the chances for future infections. The highly contagious nature of these infections should be strongly emphasized, and contacts should be examined if feasible.

Follow-up Visits

A visit 10 days to 2 weeks after therapy has begun is useful to determine the therapeutic response and possible spread of the organism to contacts.

CELLULITIS

Clinical Features

Tender, warm, erythematous plaques with ill-defined borders are seen in cellulitis. Occasionally, linear red macules proximal to the large plaque are seen. Regional lymphadenopathy and fever are common findings. A preceding puncture wound or other penetrating trauma to the skin is often noted (Fig 5–5). Cellulitis of the fingertips in infants is called blistering dactylitis, and several fingers may be involved. Perianal cellulitis in infants is increasingly recognized in North America and is characterized by tender perirectal

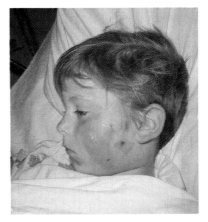

FIG 5–5.
Puncture wound with surrounding cellulitis of cheek.

erythema. Cellulitis over large joints such as the hip, shoulder, or knee may be observed in infants and toddlers. Septicemia follows cellulitis in untreated patients. Extension into the joint cavity and bone is seen, with cellulitis overlying a joint, particularly in infants. A bluish hue within the lesion in infants is seen particularly with *Haemophilus influenzae* cellulitis, but is also observed in cellulitis due to other bacteria. Cellulitis of the cheeks or over joints in children 3 months to 3 years of age is predominantly due to *H. influenzae* infection, whereas in older children it may result from streptococci or staphylococci. Streptococcal cellulitis spreads rapidly, within hours, in contrast to staphylococcal cellulitis. Perianal cellulitis in infants is virtually always due to streptococci. Periorbital cellulitis is of great concern because of spread to the brain.

Pathogenesis

Invasion of bacteria into the reticular dermis and subcutaneous fat, with subsequent spread via the lymphatics, is responsible for the clinical features of cellulitis. Pathogenic streptococci account for most cases of cellulitis; *H. influenzae* and *S. aureus* may also be responsible. Blood cultures are most likely to reveal the responsible bacteria. Aspiration of the center or advancing edge of the cellulitis is rarely positive.

Differential Diagnosis

Erythematous swellings overlying an unrecognized bony fracture may mimic cellulitis, although they may not feel warm. Similarly, pressure erythema, giant urticaria, and contact dermatitis in the early stages may be difficult to distinguish from cellulitis, but they are not tender. The redness and swelling over a septic joint may also mimic cellulitis. Acute cold injury to the fat of the cheeks of infants (popsicle panniculitis) may mimic facial cellulitis. Herpetic whitlow may mimic blistering distal dactylitis, and diaper dermatitis may mimic perianal cellulitis.

Treatment

In an acutely ill child or a child with periorbital cellulitis, hospitalization is recommended. Prompt administration of antibiotics is essential. If a streptococcal infection is suspected, systemic penicillin is given, either as benzathine penicillin, 600,000 to 1,200,000 units intramuscularly, or oral penicillin V, 30 to 60 mg/kg/day for 10 days. In an acutely ill febrile infant or child, hospitalization and intravenous penicillin, up to 2 million units per day, is recommended. If staphylococcal cellulitis is suspected, oral dicloxacillin, 50 to 100 mg/kg/day, is recommended. With blue cellulitis, suggestive of *H. influenzae,* a blood culture should be obtained before starting antibiotics. Ampicillin, 100 to 200 mg/kg/day, is given intravenously in combination with chloramphenicol, 50 to 85 mg/kg/day. If ampicillin- or chloramphenicol-resistant strains of *H. influenza* are found in your locale, use of third-generation cephalosporins, such as ceftriaxone, 50 mg/kg intramuscularly every 12 hours, or cefotaxime or cefuroxime is recommended.

NECROTIZING FASCIITIS (STREPTOCOCCAL GANGRENE)

Clinical Features

Diabetic children with ketoacidosis are susceptible to streptococcal gangrene. This condition is rare, but prompt recognition is lifesaving. The lesion begins as cellulitis, with tender erythematous plaques, usually on the leg. Within 2 hours, bullae appear on the erythematous surface, accompanied by severe pain. A purulent center develops, followed by the appearance of a black eschar and the subsidence of the acute pain (Fig 5–6). The decrease in pain correlates well with destruction of the cutaneous nerves as they

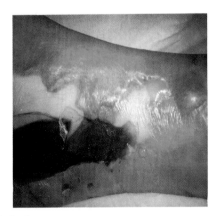

FIG 5–6.
Central black painless necrosis; painful yellow purulent lake and surrounding erythema in necrotizing fasciitis on leg of diabetic adolescent.

course through the fascia and subcutaneous tissue. Over the next 2 days, frank gangrene may be observed. Culture of the deep tissues yields group A streptococci.

Pathogenesis

Invasion by group A streptococci through the dermis and subcutaneous fat into the deep fascial compartments occurs because of the faulty host defenses of the diabetic patient. Often, trauma to the skin precedes the appearance of these lesions. Rapid spread and destruction of tissue occur.

Differential Diagnosis

Cellulitis may mimic necrotizing fasciitis early in the disease, but the rapid evolution of necrotizing fasciitis to form necrotic areas within hours after the onset helps distinguish the two. With the development of gangrene, arterial embolism or thrombosis should be considered. Metastatic calcification with occlusion of major skin vessels may also mimic necrotizing fasciitis, but its slow onset and lack of acute pain are important differentiating features.

Treatment

Prompt surgical debridement down to the fascia is essential and the most important aspect of therapy. Penicillin is the treatment of choice; from 4 to 10 million units per day is given intravenously. Correction of the metabolic abnormalities of diabetic ketoacidosis is important. Even with prompt surgical intervention, mortality is high.

Patient Education

It should be emphasized that good diabetic control and good personal hygiene are essential to prevent such episodes. Prompt cleansing of cuts or skin abrasions and topical antibiotics are suggested, and the patient should be strongly advised to seek prompt medical attention when the early signs of infection appear.

Follow-up Visits

After hospitalization, a follow-up a week later is most helpful to evaluate the patient's progress. Weekly visits may be required to assess healing of the devitalized skin and deeper tissues.

SCARLET FEVER

Clinical Features

Scarlet fever occurs most often in children between 2 and 10 years of age. The portal of entry of the streptococci may be either the pharynx or a skin wound. The exanthem appears 24 to 48 hours after infection and consists of erythematous macules and papules, beginning on the neck and spreading downward over the trunk to the extremities (Fig 5–7). In severe cases the exanthem may be petechial, and a positive tourniquet test is common. Petechiae in a linear pattern are seen along the major skin folds in the axillae and antecubital fossa (Pastia's sign). The palms and soles are characteristically uninvolved, and a facial flush with circumoral pallor is common. Tongue involvement (a thick white coat with hypertrophied red papillae) is helpful in the differential diagnosis, since "strawberry tongue" is seen with streptococcal but not with staphylococcal scarlet fever. Generalized lymphadenopathy is common, with the inguinal lymph nodes particularly enlarged. Desquamation occurs as the eruption fades, progressing in the same manner as it began. In black skin, tiny, slightly erythematous papules called gooseflesh are found. Although it is difficult to observe the erythema and the papular nature of the eruption in black children, scarlet fever in these children is identical to that seen in the white child.

Pathogenesis

Three immunologically distinct scarlet fever–producing toxins have been identified from cultures of *Streptococcus.* Toxin release from streptococci is mediated by viral infection of the streptococcus. The mechanism of action by the toxin on the skin is thought to be dependent on receptor-mediated activation of skin cells.

Differential Diagnosis

The scarlatiniform eruption is seen in other infectious diseases, such as that appearing in the early stages of viral hepatitis, infectious mononucleosis, the mucocutaneous lymph node syndrome, toxic shock syndrome, and rubella. Drug-associated eruptions may also mimic scarlet fever. Drugs that result in scarlatiniform eruptions include the sulfonamides, penicillin, streptomycin, quinine, and atropine. Drug eruptions are more likely to produce mucosal erosions and crusts, which may be a helpful distinguishing sign.

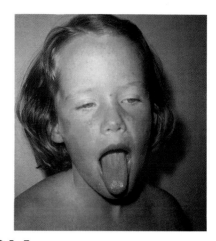

FIG 5–7.
Bright red erythema and strawberry tongue in scarlet fever.

Treatment

Penicillin, in the same doses as used for impetigo and streptococcal pharyngitis, is the treatment of choice for scarlet fever. Erythromycin is used in penicillin-allergic patients. If staphylococcal scarlet fever is suspected, dicloxacillin, 15 to 50 mg/kg/day orally for 10 days, is recommended. Prompt treatment virtually eliminates the complications of scarlet fever (bacteremia, rheumatic fever, pneumonia, and meningitis).

During the later stages of desquamation, bland lubricants applied to wet skin will restore the skin surface integrity.

Patient Education

The association of scarlet fever with rheumatic fever is of great patient concern. It is important to reassure the patient that prompt treatment has virtually eliminated this association. Identification and cultures of patient contacts are essential.

Follow-up Visits

Seven to 10 days after the first visit, another visit is helpful to observe the response to therapy and to assess further any other sources of streptococcal infection in the household.

FOLLICULITIS, FURUNCULOSIS, AND CUTANEOUS ABSCESSES

Clinical Features

The manifestations of infection of the hair follicle vary clinically with the depth of bacterial

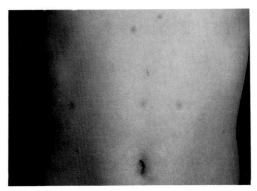

FIG 5—8.
Superficial bacterial folliculitis of trunk of adolescent.

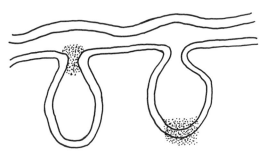

FIG 5—10.
Superficial folliculitis *(left)* with inflammation of follicular mouth, compared with deep folliculitis *(right)* with involvement of base of follicle and adjacent reticular dermis.

invasion. Infection at the follicular orifice (superficial folliculitis) appears as tiny pustules, 1 to 2 mm in diameter (Fig 5—8). Furunculosis (deep folliculitis) appears as a tender, erythematous nodule (Fig 5—9). Confluence of several adjacent areas of furunculosis produces a tender erythematous tumor that becomes soft and fluctuant after several days. Abscesses are commonly found on the buttocks and trunk, but may appear in any location.

S. aureus is regularly cultured from furuncles and abscesses, although gram-negative organisms may occasionally be found. Superficial folliculitis is often found to contain the normal skin flora.

Pathogenesis

Invasion of the follicular wall by bacteria is the usual cause of the disease (Fig 5—10). Obstruction of the follicular orifice is an important factor in the development of the bacterial infection.

Differential Diagnosis

Acne pustules and chemical folliculitis from tars and other compounds contacting the skin may mimic superficial folliculitis. Occasionally, dermatophyte infections due to animal ringworm or *Candida albicans* infections will produce follicular pustules.

Treatment

Superficial folliculitis may be treated with topical keratolytics, such as the benzoyl peroxide gels, applied twice daily for 4 to 5 days. Furunculosis and abscesses are best treated by incision and drainage. Systemic antistaphylococcal antibiotics such as dicloxacillin, 15 to 50 mg/kg/day orally for 7 to 10 days, may be required in more severe cases.

Patient Education

Good personal hygiene is important in preventing follicular skin infections. Thorough hand washing and daily skin cleansing with an antibacterial soap are most useful. Avoiding chemicals that have resulted in follicular obstruction is beneficial.

Follow-up Visits

Poor personal hygiene is the most likely cause in children with recurrent episodes of furunculosis. Reemphasizing good hygiene at the follow-up visit is most important. Evaluation for diabetes mellitus and immunodeficiency is not warranted without recurrent or systemic infection of other organ systems such as the lungs (e.g., pneumonia), central nervous system (e.g., encephalitis), or bone.

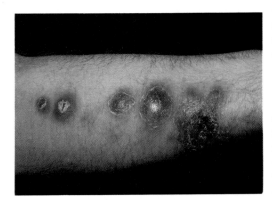

FIG 5—9.
Deep bacterial folliculitis (furunculosis) on arm.

STAPHYLOCOCCAL SCALDED SKIN SYNDROME

Clinical Features

A spectrum of clinical presentations of staphylococcal scalded skin syndrome (SSSS) is now recognized, ranging from purely localized forms to generalized involvement.

Localized Form.—Large (1 to 3 cm) bullae filled with clear or slightly purulent fluid are seen primarily over the extremities or lower area of the abdomen in infants and children. Frequently, the blister base with a rim of desquamating epidermis is observed (Fig 5–11). Neonates are particularly susceptible. Culture of *S. aureus* of phage group II is possible from the blister fluid. Multiple bullae will appear if the disease is not treated. In varicella, secondary infection by such staphylococci results in bullous impetigo in some, but not all, of the varicella lesions.

Generalized Form.—Following an upper respiratory infection, a faint erythematous eruption begins on the central part of the face, neck, axillae, and groin. The skin rapidly becomes acutely tender, with crusting around the mouth, eyes, and neck. Mild rubbing of the skin results in epidermal separation, leaving a shiny, moist, red surface. In infants and preschool children, the lesions are usually limited to the upper part of the body, but in the newborn the entire cutaneous surface may be involved (Ritter's disease) (Fig 5–12). SSSS is uncommon after the age of 5 years.

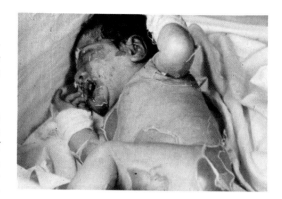

FIG 5–12.
Diffuse erythema and extensive peeling in newborn with Ritter's disease.

Differential Diagnosis

Localized Form.—Bullous impetigo must be differentiated from second-degree burns and from the uncommon bullous diseases seen in childhood, such as linear IgA dermatosis, bullous pemphigoid, and bullous forms of erythema multiforme.

Generalized Form.—Toxic epidermal necrolysis, which is often drug induced, may be differentiated from SSSS by skin biopsy and by a preceding history of urticarial or target lesions occurring 2 to 3 days before the appearance of bullae. Pathologic examination of tissue from a patient with toxic epidermal necrolysis shows full epidermal necrosis with a prominent perivascular dermal infiltrate of inflammatory cells. SSSS shows no epidermal necrosis nor inflammatory cells on microscopic examination. Occasionally, SSSS may resemble exfoliative erythroderma, sunburn, toxic shock syndrome, or streptococcal scarlet fever.

Pathogenesis

S. aureus of phage group II elaborates a toxin that is carried via the circulation to the skin, where it acts on the cell surface of the epidermal granular cells. Injury to these cells results in intraepidermal separation of the cells within the granular layer and subsequent shedding of the entire granular layer and stratum corneum when minor trauma occurs.

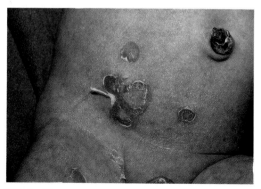

FIG 5–11.
Erosions with peeled scale at rim on abdomen of an infant with localized staphylococcal scalded skin syndrome.

Treatment

Oral dicloxacillin, 15 to 50 mg/kg/day, is the treatment of choice. Newborns require intravenous antistaphylococcal antibiotics. The skin should be handled minimally, especially during the first 24 hours. Newborns may require burn therapy, with careful attention to fluid and electrolyte losses and prevention of secondary infection of affected skin. During the desquamation stage, bland lubricants used twice daily may be helpful in restoring the skin surface.

Patient Education

It is important to emphasize to the patients that such lesions are not like a burn and that they heal without scarring. In children with normal host defenses, neutralizing antitoxins to the staphylococcal exfoliation are rapidly formed, and the child recovers promptly. It should also be stressed that only certain staphylococci are capable of producing this condition and that household carriers should be investigated. Nursery outbreaks require prompt investigation and culturing of all those entering the nursery.

Follow-up Visits

Routine follow-up care in regular pediatric visits is recommended.

TOXIC SHOCK SYNDROME

Clinical Features

A typical presentation of the toxic shock syndrome (TSS) would involve a menstruating adolescent female who presents with a high fever, a scarlatiniform rash, and hypotension, with a systolic blood pressure less than 90 mm Hg or orthostatic syncope. Prominent desquamation of the palms and soles follows the acute onset of the eruption by 1 to 2 weeks. These four features are the major diagnostic criteria for diagnosis of TSS (Table 5–1). Vomiting and diarrhea frequently precede the hypotensive state, and laboratory signs of liver, kidney, or muscle injury may be present. Diffuse redness of the conjunctival, oral, and vaginal mucosa may be observed. Swelling of the hands and feet may be prominent. Although the majority of cases have been described in adolescent females, TSS was first noted in infants and children of either sex. The circulatory collapse may be mild or severe, and a fatality rate of 3% has been reported.

TABLE 5–1.

Case Definition of Toxic Shock Syndrome

1. Fever (temperature greater than 39.9° C)
2. Rash (diffuse macular erythroderma)
3. Desquamation 1 to 2 weeks after the onset of illness, particularly of the palms and soles
4. Hypotension (systolic blood pressure less than 90 mm Hg for adults or below the fifth percentile for children, or orthostatic syncope)
5. Involvement of three or more of the following organ systems:
   a. Gastrointestinal (vomiting or diarrhea at onset of illness)
   b. Muscular (severe myalgia or creatine phosphokinase level greater than two times normal)
   c. Mucous membrane (hyperemia)
   d. Hepatic (total bilirubin, aspartate aminotransferase (AST), alanine aminotransferase (ALT), two times normal)
   e. Hematologic (platelets less than 100,000/mm^3)
   f. Renal (blood urea nitrogen [BUN] or creatinine greater than two times normal)
   g. Central nervous system (disorientation or alterations in consciousness without focal neurologic signs when fever and hypotension are absent)
6. Negative results
   a. Blood, throat, and cerebrospinal fluid cultures
   b. Serologic tests for Rocky Mountain spotted fever, leptospirosis, or measles

Differential Diagnosis

Rocky Mountain spotted fever, meningococcemia, and leptospirosis may each present with high fever, dizziness, and a rash. In each, the eruption is acral and purpuric and not scarlet fever–like. Blood cultures and specific serologic tests will help to distinguish these conditions. The staphylococcal scalded skin syndrome has considerable overlapping cutaneous features with TSS. The presence of skin tenderness and a positive Nikolsky's sign favor the scalded skin syndrome. Kawasaki disease is more likely to occur in patients under age 5, lacks hypotension, and has prominent mucous membrane involvement. The fever in Kawasaki disease lasts for a week or more rather than the 2 or 3 days in TSS. The scarlatiniform skin eruption and desquamation may be the same in both TSS and Kawasaki disease.

Pathogenesis

S. aureus infection of the vagina or other tissues initiates the disease. Prolonged tampon use with positive cultures obtained from tampons in adolescent females is very frequent. Positive blood cultures for *S. aureus* may be obtained. Most authorities consider the staphylococcal toxin designated TSS-1 or enterotoxin C as responsible for the skin eruption and the systemic symptoms. Both of these two distinct exotoxins have been implicated, but the precise mechanism is unknown.

Treatment

Prompt replacement of fluids to correct the hypotension is recommended, as are other general supportive measures for shock. Treatment with an antistaphylococcal antibody, usually given intravenously, is recommended. Bland lubricants may be used on the desquamating skin.

Patient Education

It is important to emphasize the conditions that might favor the growth of the pathogenic organism. In adolescent females, discontinuing the use of tampons is advisable. It is unknown whether other antibacterial measures to reduce skin or mucous membrane colonization of staphylococci are useful.

Follow-up Visits

The hypotension and acute illness at the onset usually result in hospitalization. Daily examination with documentation of the sequence of events is often necessary to confirm the diagnosis. After discharge, a 1-week follow-up is advisable, as is a visit during the next anticipated menses for follow-up bacterial cultures.

CAT-SCRATCH DISEASE

Clinical Features

A primary inoculation papule on skin or mucous membrane after the scratch of a cat is found in 58% of patients (Fig 5–13). Persistent tender regional lymphadenitis of the lymph nodes draining the site of the cat scratch is observed in virtually all patients. The lymph nodes become swollen about 2 weeks after the scratch and remain enlarged for about 3 months, but may be enlarged for up to a year later. If the scratch involves the conjunctiva, granulomas may appear in the site. About one third of patients will experience a few days of fever, but occasionally fever persists

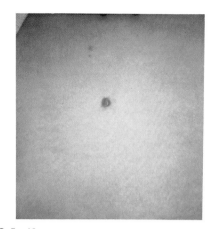

FIG 5–13.
Solitary papule at site of cat scratch in cat-scratch disease.

for several weeks. Fatigue, headache, anorexia, vomiting, splenomegaly, sore throat, a morbilliform exanthem, purulent conjunctivitis, and parotid swelling are uncommon findings in children with cat-scratch disease. Quite rare are Parinaud's syndrome, encephalitis, and erythema nodosum.

Differential Diagnosis

Bacterial lymphadenitis caused by *S. aureus, s. pyogenes,* atypical mycobacteria, *Francisella tularensis,* or *Brucella* infection may mimic cat-scratch disease. Biopsy of a papule or lymph node and staining for microscopic examination with a Warthin-Starry silver impregnation stain will reveal the cat-scratch bacillus within areas of necrosis or granulomas. Other causes of persistent lymphadenopathy in children include lymphomas, cytomegalovirus, Epstein-Barr virus, human immunodeficiency virus, *Toxoplasma,* and deep fungus infection; the lymphadenopathy is more often bilateral. Kerion due to dermatophyte infection will produce local lymphadenopathy, but the kerion is much larger than an inoculation papule of cat-scratch disease.

Pathogenesis

The bacillus believed responsible for cat-scratch disease is detected in the dermis of inoculation papules or the microabscesses of enlarged lymph nodes if obtained within 1 month of the onset of symptoms. The host response may obscure the bacillus in long-standing disease.

Treatment

In most patients, spontaneous resolution of the disease in 2 to 4 months occurs. There is no known effective antibacterial therapy. Needle aspiration of a tender lymph node abscess is recommended by some authorities. Surgical excision of the lymph node is often done, especially when the diagnosis is in doubt.

Follow-up Visits

Follow-up 1 week after the first visit is useful to ascertain the growth rate of enlarged nodes or to discuss biopsy results. Further visits are dictated by the child's recovery.

Patient Education

Disposal of the healthy cat suspected of being the vector is not recommended. About 5% of household contacts may develop cat-scratch disease, usually within 3 weeks of the first case.

SPIROCHETAL DISEASES

Lyme Disease

Clinical Features

The earliest feature of Lyme disease is the unique skin eruption, called erythema chronicum migrans (ECM). ECM begins 4 to 20 days after the bite of a tick, although only one third of patients distinctly recall a tick bite. A red papule begins at the site of the tick bite and then slowly enlarges over several weeks to form an annular ring with a flat, red border that clears in the center. Sometimes the center remains a red, edematous plaque that feels hot. Fifty percent of patients will develop multiple secondary annular rings, which begin 1 to 6 days after the primary lesion appears (Fig 5–14). Untreated ECM lasts about 3 weeks and then spontaneously resolves. It may recur for up to a year or more, accompanied by arthritis or other symptoms. Skin lesions are associated with headaches, fatigue, myalgias, and low-grade fever. Sometimes nausea, vomiting, sore throat, and lymphadenopathy will accompany ECM.

Joint, central nervous system (CNS), and cardiac abnormalities begin about 4 weeks after the tick bite, after the ECM has resolved. Fifty percent of untreated Lyme disease patients will develop arthritis. The onset is abrupt, usually monarthric (knee, shoulder, elbow, temporomandibular joint, ankle, wrist, or hip), and the affected joint is warm, swollen, and tender, but not red. The first

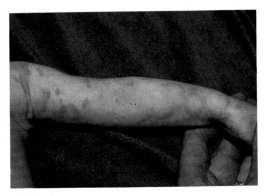

FIG 5–14.
Lyme disease. Multiple annular red rings in erythema chronicum migrans.

episode lasts 1 week, but up to three recurrences is common. CNS disease occurs in 10% to 15% of untreated patients with the classic triad of meningitis, cranial nerve palsies, and peripheral radiculoneuropathy. The meningitis is characterized by an excruciating headache and stiff neck, and may include changes in behavior. The seventh nerve is most frequently involved, with recurrent episodes of facial palsy. Neuritic pain or focal weakness is seen with the peripheral radiculoneuropathy of Lyme disease. Less than 10% of patients experience cardiac involvement, with atrioventricular block or myopericarditis reported. A great variety of additional neurologic and other organ symptoms are occasionally reported. The erythrocyte sedimentation rate is usually elevated, but other routine laboratory studies are variable.

Differential Diagnosis

ECM may mimic ringworm or be diagnosed as erythema multiforme or erythema marginatum. ECM evolves slowly, over days; erythema marginatum is transient, often changing hourly. A negative KOH examination and a skin biopsy will help distinguish. In ECM, a dense mononuclear cell accumulation around blood vessels and adnexal structures without epidermal changes is seen. Serologic tests for Lyme disease with the use of enzyme immunoassays for IgM are helpful when noncutaneous symptoms develop. The organism can be cultured on modified Kelly's medium, but yields are too low for practical use.

Pathogenesis

The spirochete *Borrelia burgdorferi* is carried by a variety of ticks, predominantly the deer tick, *Ixodes dammini*. The ticks may be carried by rodents or house pets or attach themselves to grasses or bushes. Humans are incidental hosts. The spirochete has irregular coils, is 10 to 30 μm long, and is found worldwide, although most cases come from northern Europe or the eastern United States. Within a few days after a tick bite, the spirochete migrates within the skin or enters the bloodstream. It appears that all symptoms and signs are directly related to the presence of the spirochete in affected tissues or the immune response to the organism.

Treatment

For children over age 8, oral tetracycline, 25 to 50 mg/kg/day for 10 days, is the treatment of choice. Younger children are treated with oral phenoxymethyl penicillin, 50 mg/kg/day for 10 days. The ECM will disappear within 3 days with successful treatment, and secondary complications are often prevented. Parenteral penicillin is recommended for secondary complications.

Patient Education

Avoidance of the tick vector is the basis of prevention. Avoidance of high-risk areas, such as wooded, grassy areas during tick season, wearing protective clothing, using insect repellent, and periodic examination for ticks are required. Parents of children with ECM should be advised about the possibility of secondary complications of arthritis or neurologic disease.

Follow-up Visits

After successful treatment, monthly visits for 3 months are useful to check for late complications. A second antibiotic course may be required if secondary symptoms occur.

Syphilis

Clinical Features

Acquired and congenital syphilis are uncommon in industrialized countries but are common in Third World countries. Acquired syphilis has three distinct stages. Primary acquired syphilis is characterized by the chancre, a painless, shallow ulcer surrounded by a red, indurated border that appears about 3 weeks after exposure (Fig 5–15). If untreated, the chancre heals spontaneously in 1 to 2 months. Secondary syphilis is usually seen as a morbilliform, generalized eruption accompanied by lymphadenopathy, fatigue, headache, and,

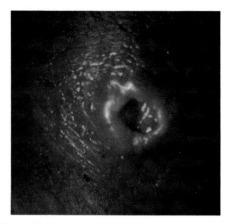

FIG 5–15.
Syphilitic chancre. Painless scrotal ulcer with indurated borders in 11-year-old boy.

sometimes, low-grade fever. Involvement of the palms and soles is frequently observed (Fig 5–16). Nodular, pustular, annular, and papulosquamous lesions are occasionally seen. Mucous patches are seen as weeping, erosive areas on oral or genital mucosa. Tertiary stages are rare in childhood.

Congenital syphilis is usually observed as a persistent rhinorrhea that develops during the newborn period or, in severe cases, as hydrops fetalis. The newborn is usually small for gestational age and has mild hepatosplenomegaly. Usually the newborn symptoms are so mild as to be overlooked, and signs of late congenital syphilis are the first clue to maternal-fetal transmission of syphilis. Late signs begin around 6 years of age

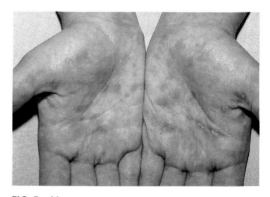

FIG 5–16.
Secondary syphilis. Ham-colored palmar macules on palms of hands of adolescent with secondary syphilis.

and include cloudy corneas (interstitial keratitis) accompanied by photophobia and pain, bilateral eighth nerve deafness, notching of small central and lateral incisors (Hutchinson's teeth), painless swelling of the knees (Clutton's joint), perforation of the nasal septum leading to a saddle nose deformity and perforated palate, saber tibia, and radial scarring about the mouth (rhagades).

Differential Diagnosis

Syphilis is known as the great mimic, and a high index of suspicion for syphilis should be maintained. The primary chancre of acquired syphilis must be distinguished from bacterial ulcers, herpes simplex infections, chancroid, or lymphogranuloma venereum. The absence of pain is a useful distinguishing feature, and identification of *Treponema pallidum* by dark-field microscopic examination of smears of the ulcer base is definitive. Secondary acquired syphilis must be distinguished from pityriasis rosea, infectious mononucleosis, many other viral exanthems, and a number of papulosquamous diseases. A serologic test for syphilis is required. Biopsy of a secondary syphilis lesion will reveal numerous plasma cells within a perivascular dermal infiltrate and swelling of the vascular endothelium.

Hydrops fetalis due to congenital syphilis must be differentiated from blood group incompatibility, the rhinorrhea from upper respiratory bacterial or viral infections. Hepatosplenomegaly and intrauterine growth failure in the newborn must be distinguished from other congenital infections such as herpes simplex, cytomegalovirus, rubella, and toxoplasmosis. Serologic test results for maternal syphilis and the fluorescent treponemal antibody (FTA)–IgM test results should be positive in the affected infant.

Pathogenesis

T. pallidum is the spirochete responsible for syphilis. It is spread primarily through sexual contact and invades the bloodstream in the early phase of infection. The chancre of primary syphilis develops at the time the blood-borne infection is maximal, and the morbilliform rash of secondary syphilis represents spirochetes that have left the bloodstream and entered the skin. Congenital syphilis represents a more massive infection than acquired syphilis, being blood borne in the fetus from the fourth month of pregnancy onward. The rhinorrhea represents tissue infection of the nasopharynx, and late signs of congenital syphilis represent effects on developing tissues or osteomyelitis due to *T. pallidum*.

Treatment

Penicillin is the treatment of choice. Parenteral penicillin given intramuscularly in the form of benzathine penicillin in doses of 2.4 million units is recommended for children and adolescents with primary or secondary syphilis. Penicillin, 50,000 units/kg/day intramuscularly or intravenously for 10 days is recommended for congenital syphilis.

Patient Education

Children and adolescents with primary or secondary syphilis should be thoroughly educated on the transmission of disease. Routine serologic testing for syphilis during pregnancy and the importance of prenatal care for prevention should be emphasized for congenital syphilis. The long-term prognosis with prompt treatment is good in congenital syphilis, but delayed treatment may result in developmental delays and the complications of late congenital syphilis.

Follow-up Visits

Following treatment, children should be seen monthly for 6 months to observe for recurrences and to monitor serology. In congenital syphilis, serologic tests should be obtained at 6 months, 12 months, and 2 years of age. Otherwise, follow-up during routine well-child care will suffice.

BIBLIOGRAPHY

Barton LL, Friedman AD: Impetigo: A reassessment of etiology and therapy. *Pediatr Dermatol* 1987; 4:185.

Barton LL, Friedman AD, Portilla MG: Impetigo contagiosa: A comparison of erythromycin and dicloxacillin therapy. *Pediatr Dermatol* 1988; 5:88.

Berkowitz FE: Bacterial exotoxins: How they work. *Pediatr Infect Dis J* 1989; 8:42.

Chawla V, Pandit PB, Nkrumah FK: Congenital syphilis in the newborn. *Arch Dis Child* 1988; 63:1393.

Dagan R, Bar-David Y: Comparison of amoxicillin and clavulanic acid (Augmentin) for the treatment of nonbullous impetigo. *Am J Dis Child* 1989; 143:916.

English CK Wear DJ, Margileth AM et al: Cat-scratch disease. Isolation and culture of the bacterial agent. *JAMA* 1988; 259:1347.

Hansen RC: Staphylococcal scalded skin syndrome, toxic shock syndrome, and Kawasaki disease. *Pediatr Clin North Am* 1983; 30:533.

Harnden A, Lennon D: Serious suppurative group A streptococcal infections in previously well children. *Pediatr Infect Dis J* 1988; 7:714.

Howe PM, Fajardo JE, Orcutt MA: Etiologic diagnosis of cellulitis: Comparison of the aspirates obtained from the leading edge and the point of maximal inflammation. *Pediatr Infect Dis J* 1987; 6:685.

Leyden JJ: Pyoderma. Pathophysiology and management. *Arch Dermatol* 1988; 124:753.

McCray MK, Esterly NB: Blistering distal dactylitis. *J Am Acad Dermatol* 1981; 5:592.

Margileth AM: Dermatologic manifestations and update of cat scratch disease. *Pediatr Dermatol* 1988; 5:1.

Murono K, Fujita K, Yoshioka H: Microbiologic characteristics of exfoliative toxin-producing *Staphylococcus aureus*. *Pediatr Infect Dis J* 1988; 7:313.

Powell KR, Kaplan SB, Hall CB, et al: Periorbital cellulitis. *Am J Dis Child* 1988; 142:853.

Rehder PA, Eliezer ET, Lane AT: Perianal cellulitis: Cutaneous group A streptococcal disease. *Arch Dermatol* 1988; 124:702, Committee on Infectious Disease, American Academy of Pediatrics: *1988 Red Book*. Elk Grove Village, IL, The Academy, 1988.

Rizkallah MF, Tolaymat A, Martinez JS, et al: Toxic shock syndrome caused by a strain of *Staphylococcus aureus* that produces enterotoxin C but not toxic shock syndrome toxin-1. *Am J Dis Child* 1989; 143:848.

Schachner L, Gonzalez A: Impetigo: A reassessment of etiology and therapy. *Pediatr Dermatol* 1988; 5:139.

Stechenberg BW: Lyme disease: The latest great imitator. *Pediatr Infect Dis J* 1988; 7:402.

Tunnesen WW Jr: Cutaneous infections. *Pediatr Clin North Am* 1983; 30:515.

6 _____ Fungal and Yeast Infections of Skin

DERMATOPHYTES

Dermatophytes are fungi that invade and proliferate in the outer layer of the epidermis (stratum corneum). In addition to invading the stratum corneum, some species may also invade the hair and nails. Dermatophyte infections are common and increase in frequency with increasing age; in hot, humid climates; and in crowded living conditions. In one United States urban area, 4% of children had a positive fungal culture for scalp dermatophytes.

HAIR INFECTIONS (TINEA CAPITIS)

Clinical Features

Scalp hair involvement is usually limited to prepubertal children and is largely due to infections with either *Microsporum canis* or *Trichophyton tonsurans*. Each infection has a noninflammatory stage lasting 2 to 8 weeks, followed by an inflammatory stage. Hair loss is a regular feature of tinea capitis. *M. canis* infections are characterized by one or several patches of broken hairs that appear thickened and white (Fig 6–1). The hairs fluoresce yellow-green with Wood's light. In contrast, *T. tonsurans* produces one of three distinct clinical presentations: hairs that break off at the follicular orifice in a circumscribed area of the scalp, which leaves small, dark hairs in the follicles, or so-called black-dot ringworm (Fig 6–2); diffuse, fine scaling of the scalp without obvious broken hairs (Fig 6–3); and multiple triangular, scaly bald areas with indistinct margins (Fig. 6–4). *T. tonsurans* does not fluoresce with Wood's lamp.

The diagnosis in the noninflammatory stage should be confirmed by the following steps: (1)

Wood's light examination, (2) potassium hydroxide (KOH) examination, and (3) fungal culture.

Wood's Light Examination.—Wood's light examination is best performed with a hand-held ultraviolet black lamp with two fluorescent bulbs. The lamp should be held within 6 inches of the scalp to observe for yellow-green fluorescence of the thickened scalp hairs. Lint from clothing fluoresces white from the addition of optical brighteners, and scale entrapped in sebum appears a dull yellow. These may be confused with fungal fluorescence. *M. Canis* fluoresces, but the epidemic form of tinea capitis due to *T. tonsurans* does not. The Wood's lamp examination cannot be used to exclude the diagnosis of tinea capitis nor for screening children during epidemics.

Potassium Hydroxide Examination.— KOH examination should be performed in every case of hair loss associated with broken hairs and in children with diffuse scaling of the scalp. If the hair fluoresces, hold the Wood's lamp in one hand and a curet in the other. Gently remove the fluorescent hairs by scraping the scalp with the curet for KOH examination and culture. The involved hairs are loosened in the follicles and will be included in the scrapings, without pain to the child. If the hair does not fluoresce, use the curet to scrape the follicular openings in the involved area of the scalp hair loss. If a kerion is present, scrape the border of the lesion. Place the scrapings that include infected hair on a glass microscope slide, partially dissolve in KOH 20%, and place under a coverslip. Wait 20 to 40 minutes to examine the specimen, under the ×10 and the ×40 lenses. In fluorescent hairs, the outer surface of the hair is coated with mats containing billions of tiny spores (Fig 6–5), and hyphae may be seen

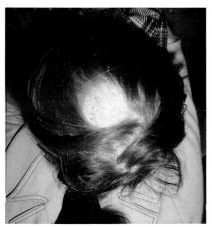

FIG 6–1.
Circumscribed patch of scalp hair loss with thick scales due to *M. canis* infection.

within the hair shaft. In nonfluorescent hairs, hyphae and spores are seen within the hair shaft (Fig 6–6).

Culture.—Fungal culture should be routinely performed in children with suspected tinea capitis. A modified Sabouraud's dextrose agar (dermatophyte test medium) makes this procedure simple. Broken hairs or scrapings are inoculated so as to break the agar surface; the bottle cap is loosely applied, and the culture bottles are left at room temperature. If a dermatophyte is present, the agar medium turns from yellow to red in 4 to 5 days. A positive culture can be subcultured on Sabouraud's dextrose agar for precise identification.

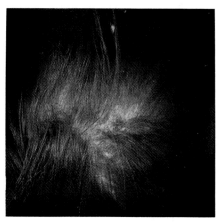

FIG 6–3.
Diffuse scaling in a dandruff-like pattern in *T. tonsurans* infection.

Inflammatory lesions produce a kerion, which is an erythematous boggy nodule with superficial pustules (Fig 6–7). These lesions are almost completely devoid of hair and will lead to scarring and permanent hair loss if untreated (Fig 6–8). A kerion will appear 2 to 8 weeks after infection begins, and represents an exaggerated host response to the invading fungus. Approximately 40% of untreated tinea capitis caused by *M. canis* or *T. tonsurans* may eventuate in a kerion.

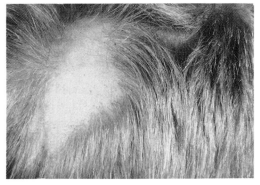

FIG 6–2.
Circumscribed area of hair loss without scalp change and with hairs broken off at follicular orifice. This is the black-dot pattern of *T. tonsurans* infection.

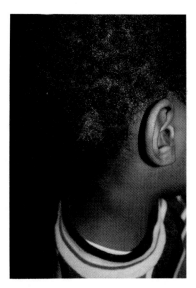

FIG 6–4.
Numerous triangular patches of hair loss accompanied by pustular kerion formation and enlarged lymph node in *T. tonsurans* infection.

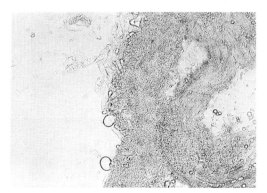

FIG 6–5.
Photomicrograph of hair dissolved in KOH. Mats containing billions of small spores coat the outside of hair, with hyphae seen within hair shaft in *M. canis* infection.

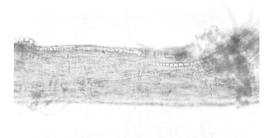

FIG 6–6.
Photomicrograph of hair dissolved in KOH. Hyphae and spores of *T. tonsurans* appear as chains within the hair shaft. There are no spores coating the hair.

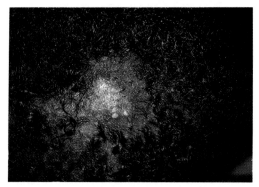

FIG 6–7.
Boggy, red scalp nodule with superficial pustules in kerion.

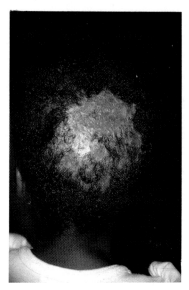

FIG 6–8.
Scarring hair loss in child with previously undiagnosed tinea capitis and kerion.

Differential Diagnosis

Alopecia areata and trichotillomania are the major considerations in the differential diagnosis of tinea capitis in children. Alopecia areata may be distinguished by the total absence of hair in a circumscribed patch, without any associated scalp change. In trichotillomania, scalp excoriations, perifollicular petechiae, and hairs broken off at differing lengths are the distinguishing features. Seborrheic dermatitis may mimic the diffuse forms of *T. tonsurans* scalp infection.

In inflammatory tinea capitis (kerion), bacterial pyodermas are often mistaken for kerion. The pustules in kerion are sterile, however, and incision produces only serosanguineous fluid. Bacterial culture of the skin surface may yield *Staphylococcus aureus* and lead to the incorrect diagnosis of pyoderma, but one should recall that *S. aureus* frequently colonizes the skin surface, and such cultures would not detect bacterial invasion. Less commonly, traction alopecia, scleroderma, lichen planus, psoriasis, lupus erythematosus dandruff, or porokeratosis of Mibelli may be confused with tinea capitis.

Pathogenesis

M. canis is harbored by cats, dogs, and certain rodents, and children handling such animals are susceptible to infection. Humans appear to be a terminal host for *M. canis,* and human-to-human transmission does not occur. When there is delayed hypersensitivity to the organism, a kerion may develop. Histologic study of this lesion shows a mononuclear cell infiltrate consistent with that seen in delayed hypersensitivity reactions. *M. canis* accounts for 70% of the tinea capitis in suburban and rural areas (Table 6–1).

T. tonsurans is transmitted from human to human, and presumably entered the United States from Central and South America. It is most prevalent in areas of crowding, and accounts for 90% of tinea capitis in inner-city children. It has recently been shown that 4% of asymptomatic inner-city children are carriers of *T. tonsurans*.

Treatment

Griseofulvin in a micronized form, 10 to 20 mg/kg/day for a minimum of 6 weeks, is the treatment of choice. Often treatment for 2 to 3 months is required. Topical antifungal agents cannot reach the hyphae within the hair shaft and are ineffective. In *M. canis*, with successful treatment the lesions become nonfluorescent 13 days after the administration of griseofulvin is begun. Although griseofulvin has many side effects, including agranulocytosis and aplastic anemia, it is a relatively safe drug in children. Absorption is enhanced by a fatty meal; taking griseofulvin twice a day with ice cream or whole milk is a popular prescription. Oral ketoconazole is a second alternative to griseofulvin. Side effects with this agent are more frequent than with griseofulvin, and oral ketoconazole should be used only for resistant cases. In addition to oral griseofulvin, some authorities advocate 2.5% selenium sulfide shampoo, applied twice weekly to the scalp, to reduce infectivity and to hasten the child's return to school or child care setting.

Kerion may well respond to griseofulvin alone. Severely inflamed or long-standing kerions may require a short course of oral steroid therapy to reduce inflammation and prevent scarring alopecia. Prednisone, 1 to 2 mg/kg/day for 5 to 10 days, is most efficacious.

Patient Education

If *M. canis* is found, animal sources should be identified and the animal treated by a veterinarian to prevent infection of other children. In *T. tonsurans*, identification of the likely contacts is necessary. Patients should be instructed that hair regrowth is slow, often taking 3 to 6 months. If a kerion is present, some scarring and permanent hair loss may result.

Follow-up Visits

A visit in 2 weeks is helpful to ascertain the effectiveness of the griseofulvin therapy. Reexamination for fluorescence and a repeat culture will serve as guidelines for increasing the therapeutic dosage. If at 2 weeks the lesions are not fluorescent or culture is negative, or both, a total of 6 weeks' therapy may be all that is required. Treatment 4 to 6 weeks after the lesions are culture negative is a useful rule of thumb. With the use of selenium sulfide shampoo plus griseofulvin, the child can usually return to school in 1 week. A follow-up visit every 2 to 4 weeks until hair growth begins is advised.

FUNGAL INFECTION INVOLVING SKIN ONLY

Tinea Corporis

Clinical Features

Dermatophyte infections on the body often consist of one or several circular erythematous

TABLE 6–1.

Organisms Responsible for Tinea Capitis

Feature	M. canis	T. tonsurans
Source	Cats and dogs	Other children
Fluorescence	Yellow-green	None
Contagious	No	Yes
Hair loss	Yes	Yes
Kerion	Yes	Yes
Children infected	Rural and suburban	Urban
Clinical patterns	Thickened hairs	Black-dot, dandruff-like, or multiple areas of alopecia

patches (Fig 6–9). The patches may have a papular, scaly, annular border and a clear center (Fig 6–10) or may be inflammatory throughout, with superficial pustules (Fig 6–11). *M. canis* and *Trichophyton mentagrophytes* are the dermatophytes most commonly responsible for tinea corporis. Diagnosis is confirmed by KOH examination of scrapings of thin scales obtained from the border of the lesion. Cultures are not usually done routinely.

Differential Diagnosis

The herald patch of pityriasis rosea may mimic tinea corporis, as may any of the forms of dermatitis. It is not unusual to confuse the annular nodules of granuloma annulare with tinea corporis. Psoriasis, parapsoriasis, secondary syphilis, and lupus erythematosus can also mimic tinea corporis.

Tinea Pedis (Athlete's Foot)

Clinical Features

The three clinical forms of tinea pedis are found almost exclusively in the postpubertal adolescent and rarely in children. The most common form consists of vesicles and erosions on the instep of one or both feet (Fig 6–12). The dermatophyte may be identified by removing the vesicle roof, scraping the underside of the roof, and examining the scrapings under a microscope for hyphae. Occasionally, fissuring between the toes, with scaling and erythema in the surrounding skin, is seen. Rarely, diffuse scaling of one or both feet, with exaggerated scaling in the skin creases ("moccasin foot" tinea pedis), is seen. The organ-

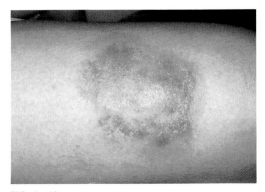

FIG 6–10.
Red, scaly plaque with partial clearing in center in tinea corporis due to *M. canis*.

isms most commonly responsible for tinea pedis are *T. mentagrophytes* and *Trichophyton rubrum*.

Differential Diagnosis

Atopic dermatitis mimics tinea pedis in prepubertal children. The diagnosis of athlete's foot before adolescence should be viewed with suspicion. Contact dermatitis and other forms of dermatitis may also mimic tinea pedis. Contact dermatitis usually involves the top of the feet, whereas tinea pedis involves the weight-bearing surface. Juvenile plantar dermatosis (JPD) is characterized by redness, dryness, and fissures of the weight-bearing surface of the foot, and may be easily confused with tinea pedis. Fungal scrapings and culture are needed to distinguish tinea pedis from JPD. Scabies, granuloma annulare, and psoriasis may also mimic tinea pedis.

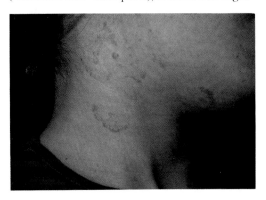

FIG 6–9.
Annular, red, scaly borders with clear center in tinea corporis.

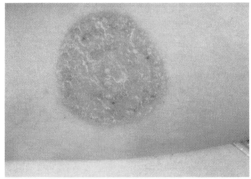

FIG 6–11.
Plaque, red throughout with prominent pustules, in tinea corporis due to the cattle ringworm, *T. verrucosum*.

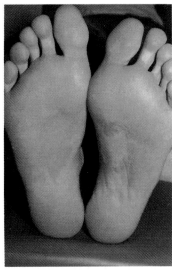

FIG 6–12.
Annular erythema with vesicles on instep of feet of an adolescent youth is tinea pedis due to *T. rubrum.*

Tinea Faciei

Clinical Features

Dermatophyte infections on the face are common in children. They are erythematous and scaly and may have a "butterfly" distribution (Fig 6–13). KOH examination of the scaly border will confirm the diagnosis. *M. canis* and the cattle ringworm, *T. verrucosum,* are the most commonly involved fungi of tinea faciei in children.

Differential Diagnosis

Tinea faciei may mimic lupus erythematosus and other collagen vascular diseases. A KOH examination for hyphae should always be performed in children in whom the butterfly rash of lupus erythematosus is considered. Atopic dermatitis, contact dermatitis, and seborrheic dermatitis should also be considered.

Tinea Cruris

Clinical Features

An erythematous, scaly eruption on the inner thighs and inguinal creases characterizes tinea cruris. Sometimes an elevated papular, scaly border is present and suggests the diagnosis. KOH examination of the border for hyphae will confirm the diagnosis. Tinea cruris is unusual before adolescence. *T. mentagrophytes* and *Epidermo-*

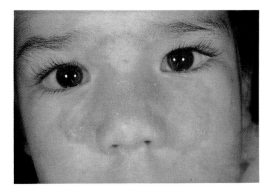

FIG 6–13.
Tinea faciei due to *M. canis.* Annular, red, scaly lesions of the nose and malar skin in this girl were misdiagnosed as lupus erythematosus.

phyton flocossum are the organisms most often responsible.

Differential Diagnosis

Diaper dermatitis and candidiasis may mimic tinea cruris, but these usually are seen in infants. Yeast infection in the perineal area may be distinguished by involvement of the scrotum. Several forms of dermatitis also occur in this area. Rarely, erythrasma, a superficial bacterial infection due to *Corynebacterium minutissimum,* may be confused with tinea cruris. Wood's light examination in erythrasma produces a coral-red fluorescence.

Pathogenesis of Tinea Corporis, Pedis, Faciei, Cruris

Dermatophytic invasion of the stratum corneum but not the remainder of the epidermis or dermis is responsible for superficial dermatophyte infections. The exact mechanism of the inflammation is not known, but toxins released by the dermatophyte are thought to be important in initiating the inflammatory response.

Treatment of Tinea Corporis, Pedis, Faciei, Cruris

Topical therapy is the treatment of choice. Clotrimazole, econazole, miconazole, ciclopiroxin, and tolnaftate creams are all efficacious against 90% of dermatophyte species. They are applied twice daily, either as cream or solution, to the entire area until the lesions have cleared. This often takes 2 to 4 weeks of therapy. Rarely is griseofulvin required.

Patient Education for Tinea Corporis, Pedis, Faciei, Cruris

Knowledge that these fungi are found in soil or animals may help identify the source and prevent other family members from being infected. Be certain to instruct the patient to treat the entire lesion plus an area of about 1 cm around it. Efforts to keep the affected skin area dry after successful treatment and changing habits regarding family pets (e.g., keeping the pets out of the child's room and not allowing the child to carry the pet) may be useful in preventing reinfection, until the pet is cured.

Follow-up Visits for Tinea Corporis, Pedis, Faciei, Cruris

A visit 2 weeks after therapy is started is helpful to ascertain its efficacy. If no response has occurred, either the diagnosis is incorrect or a resistant dermatophyte has been encountered. At this point it is useful to culture the lesion and perhaps prescribe a different class of topical antifungal agent.

INFECTION OF THE NAILS (ONYCHOMYCOSIS)

Clinical Features

Distal thickening and yellowing of the nail plate are regular features of onychomycosis (tinea unguium). The yellowing represents separation of the distal nail plate from the nail bed and entrapment of air between these two structures. Usually only one or two nails, most often the toenails, are involved. It is uncommon to find onychomycosis in children; it is almost exclusively limited to adolescents. With toenail involvement, concurrent tinea pedis is usually present.

Differential Diagnosis

Psoriasis also causes distal yellowing and thickening of the nail, but eventually all 20 nails are involved and superficial nail pitting is also present. Lichen planus and 20-nail dystrophy also usually involve all 20 nails. Hereditary nail disorders associated with ectodermal defects are sometimes confused with onychomycosis. Bacterial and candidal nail involvement characteristically results in proximal rather than distal nail plate disease.

Pathogenesis

Dermatophytes may invade nails as well as the stratum corneum. They proliferate within the nail plate, destroying its integrity.

Treatment

Successful therapy of onychomycosis is uncommon. Only 10% to 30% of patients treated respond, and then only after 6 to 12 months of griseofulvin therapy. The consequences of prolonged therapy should be weighed against the poor success rate. Topical agents generally are not successful unless used in combination with griseofulvin.

Patient Education

The difficulty in curing onychomycosis should be thoroughly explained to the patient and the parents. They may not desire griseofulvin therapy simply to achieve improvement.

Follow-up Visits

Visits at 6-month intervals are useful to follow the course of the illness and to observe for the possible involvement of other nails.

YEAST INFECTIONS

Tinea Versicolor

Clinical Features

In tinea versicolor, multiple oval macules with a fine scale are found on the neck, chest, upper back, shoulders, and upper arms of children and adolescents (Fig 6–14). Occasionally the le-

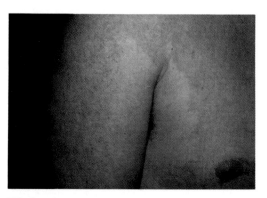

FIG 6–14.
Pink macules with a fine scale over the chest and arm of an adolescent with tinea versicolor.

sions are confluent and appear as a continuous sheet. Their color depends on the state of pigmentation. In well-tanned or darkly pigmented adolescents, the lesions appear as hypopigmented macules. In the winter months, as normal pigment fades, the lesions may appear as tan or dark brown macules, hence the term *versicolor.* The infection tends to be persistent. KOH examination of scrapings reveals numerous short, curved hyphae and circular spores ("spaghetti and meatballs"). Occasionally Wood's light examination reveals orange fluorescence of the lesions. Biopsy of these lesions will show periodic acid–Schiff (PAS)–positive hyphae and spores within the stratum corneum.

Differential Diagnosis

Seborrheic dermatitis, contact dermatitis, and tinea corporis can mimic tinea versicolor. Vitiligo, pityriasis alba, and other hypopigmented states are also sometimes confused with it.

Pathogenesis

The yeastlike organism *Malassezia furfur,* which in its culture phase is called *Pityrosporum orbiculare,* invades the stratum corneum to produce the lesions of tinea versicolor. The organism thrives in hot, humid climates.

Treatment

Miconazole, clotrimazole, or haloprogin creams applied twice daily for 2 to 3 weeks may be efficacious, but all are costly, considering the amount required to cover the trunk of an adolescent. Overnight applications of selenium sulfide or sodium hypochlorite once weekly for 2 months will result in temporary clearing, but the recurrence rate is high. After initial clearing, prevention of recurrence by once-monthly treatment may be considered. Irritation is a problem with overnight applications. As an alternative, 10- to 15-minute daily applications for 7 to 14 days may be tried.

In tropical and subtropical climates, oral ketoconazole given in a single dose once daily for 2 weeks may be considered in difficult cases.

Patient Education

Patients should be instructed that repigmentation of the hypopigmented areas will not occur until they are exposed to the sun, and that a recurrence is likely.

Follow-up Visits

A follow-up visit in 1 month to evaluate therapy should be considered.

Candidiasis

Clinical Features

In regions of the body where warmth and moisture lead to maceration of the skin or mucous membranes, the tissue is predisposed to invasion by the pathogenic yeast *Candida albicans.* Candidiasis in different body sites has distinct clinical features. In neonates and infants, white plaques on an erythematous base (thrush) are commonly seen on the buccal mucosa and other sites in the oral cavity. In this same age group, intertriginous involvement of the body folds, such as in the diaper area, is also common.

Fully established diaper candidiasis demonstrates beefy red erythema with elevated margins and satellite red plaques (Fig 6–15). However, erosions, pustules, erythematous papules, and vesicles may also be features of candidiasis of the diaper area. *C. albicans* colonizes the diaper area within 3 days of the development of diaper dermatitis, and should always be considered as a secondary infection in long-standing diaper dermatitis.

Intertriginous candidiasis involving the inframammary, axillary, neck, and inguinal body folds may also be seen in obese children and adolescents.

A rare form of candidiasis (congenital can-

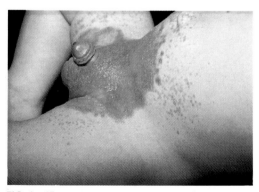

FIG 6–15.
Beefy red central erythema with satellite pustules in candidiasis of diaper area. Positive cultures can be obtained only from satellite lesions, not central erythema.

didiasis) acquired in utero results in generalized erythema of the newborn, with scaling and pustule formation (Fig 6–16).

Paronychia due to candidiasis is a common result of thumb sucking. The erythema and swelling around the base of the nail are usually not tender (Fig 6–17).

Vaginal candidiasis appears as a cheesy vaginal discharge, with whitish plaques on erythematous mucous membranes.

The rare candidal granulomas are oval red plaques with a thick yellow crust. They are found on the head and neck and other areas of skin in children with defective host defenses. In chronic mucocutaneous candidiasis (Fig 6–18), seen in patients with defective host defenses, persistent thrush with extensive involvement of the tongue and lips and chronic paronychia are present. Patients receiving long-term glucocorticosteroid, antibiotic, or oral contraceptive therapy (in adolescent girls) appear unusually susceptible to candidiasis. Similarly, children with diabetes mellitus and reticuloendothelial neoplasms are also predisposed to candidiasis.

The diagnosis can be established by scraping the skin or mucosal lesions and observing the single budding yeast in a KOH preparation under the microscope. *C. albicans* is readily cultured on Sabouraud's dextrose or corn meal agar.

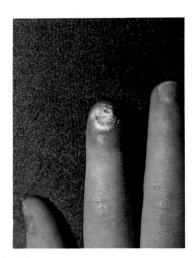

FIG 6–17.
Cuticular, nontender swelling and erythema with thickened, disrupted nail surface in paronychia caused by *C. albicans.*

Differential Diagnosis

Herpes simplex, aphthous stomatitis, epidermolysis bullosa, geographic tongue, burns, and erythema multiforme of the oral cavity may mimic thrush.

Diaper dermatitis, bacterial infection of intertriginous areas, Letterer-Siwe disease, linear IgA

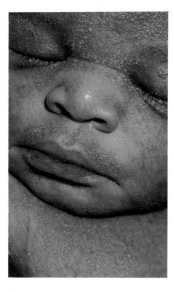

FIG 6–16.
Hundreds of pinpoint pustules with an erythematous base on the face of a newborn infant with congenital candidiasis.

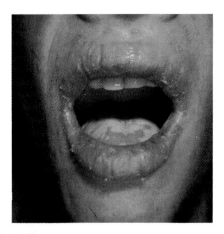

FIG 6–18.
Thick white coating of tongue with scaling and fissuring of lips in chronic mucocutaneous candidiasis.

dermatosis, and maceration may mimic the intertriginous forms of candidiasis.

Congenital candidiasis may be confused with severe erythema toxicum, miliaria, transient neonatal pustular melanosis, infantile acropustulosis, the ichthyosiform erythrodermas, and congenital syphilis or other intrauterine infections.

Paronychia due to *S. aureus* may mimic candidal paronychia, but usually has an acute onset, and the affected nail is tender and fluctuant. Psoriasis, lichen planus, and pachyonychia congenita should also be considered. Gonorrhea, *Trichomonas* infections, and chemical vaginitis may mimic vaginal candidiasis. Psoriasis, impetigo, and deep fungal infections such as sporotrichosis may be similar to candidal granulomas.

Acrodermatitis enteropathica and vitamin deficiency states may be confused with chronic mucocutaneous candidiasis.

Pathogenesis

C. albicans may be considered a part of the normal flora of the skin and mucous surfaces in certain body areas. Moisture, warmth, and breaks in the epidermal barrier allow overgrowth and invasion of the epidermis by the organism. It has been demonstrated that *C. albicans* generates inflammation by activation of the complement system within the skin and attraction of neutrophils to skin sites of *Candida* invasion. Keratolytic proteases and other enzymes in *C. albicans* species allow them to penetrate the epidermal barrier more easily than other organisms.

Treatment

Topical therapy with one of several anticandidal agents is usually efficacious. Nystatin, haloprogin, miconazole, and clotrimazole in a cream vehicle applied four times daily will result in prompt clearing of the lesions in 3 to 5 days. In the diaper area, application with each diaper change for 2 to 3 days is useful. The antifungal creams may sting or burn if there are breaks in the skin surface. Antiyeast ointments may be substituted.

Correction of the predisposing factors, such as good care of the diaper area, drying of intertriginous areas, and withdrawal of broad-spectrum antibiotics or glucocorticosteroids, is also important in the management of candidiasis. Treatment of candidal vaginitis or candidal infections of the nipples in nursing mothers is valuable in the therapy of thrush.

The following specific treatment protocols may be utilized:

Thrush.—Apply nystatin solution topically to the area four times daily for 5 days. With recurrence, another course of this therapy or with haloprogin, miconazole, or clotrimazole may be helpful. Simultaneous therapy of *Candida* vaginitis or nipple infection in the mother is most helpful in reducing surface colonization with *C. albicans*.

Diaper Candidiasis.—Application of nystatin (or one of the three other agents listed) in a cream form with each diaper change for 2 to 3 days is most useful if combined with the usual measures to keep the diaper area dry and cool.

Paronychia.—Nystatin cream applied nightly under occlusion (a plastic glove covered by a cotton stocking) for 3 to 4 weeks will often clear candidal paronychia.

Patient Education

The patient or parents should understand that *C. albicans* is part of the normal skin flora in certain persons and will reinvade susceptible tissue sites if the predisposing factors favoring overgrowth are not eliminated. Thus, careful attention to the treatment of intertrigo and good diaper area care are essential to the long-term satisfactory results.

Follow-up Visits

An examination 5 to 7 days after initiating therapy is useful to evaluate the therapeutic response and reinforce the measures to diminish warmth and moisture in intertriginous areas. Most therapy failures are due to poor compliance, not to host defense defects.

BIBLIOGRAPHY

Allen H, Honig P, Leyden J, et al: Selenium sulfide: Adjunctive therapy for tinea capitis. *Pediatrics* 1982; 69:81.

Borelli D: Treatment of pityriasis versicolor with ketoconazole. *Rev Infect Dis* 1980; 2:592.

Butler KM, Baker CJ: Candida: An increasingly important pathogen in the nursery. *Pediatr Clin North Am* 1988; 35:543.

Faergemann J, Fredriksson T: Tinea versicolor:

Some new aspects on etiology, pathogenesis and treatment. *Int J Dermatol* 1982; 21:8.

Gan VN, Petruska M, Ginsburg CM: Epidemiology and treatment of tinea capitis: Ketoconazole vs. griseofulvin. *Pediatr Infect Dis J* 1987; 6:46.

Gelgor I: LE-like tinea of the face. *JAMA* 1971; 215:2091.

Ginsburg CM, Gan VN, Petruska M: Randomized controlled trial of intralesional corticosteroid and griseofulvin vs. griseofulvin alone for treatment of kerion. *Pediatr Infect Dis J* 1987; 6:1084.

Herbert AA: Tinea capitis. Current concepts. *Arch Dermatol* 1988; 124:1554.

Jacobs AH, O'Connell BM: Tinea in tiny tots. *Am J Dis Child* 1986; 140:1034.

Leyden JI, Kligman AM: The role of microorganisms in diaper dermatitis. *Arch Dermatol* 1978; 114:56.

Nanda A, Kaur S, Bhakoo OK, et al: Pityriasis (tinea) versicolor in infancy. *Pediatr Dermatol* 1988; 5:260.

Prevalence of dermatologic disease among persons 1–74 years of age: United States. USD-HEW Advance Data. Washington, D.C.: U.S. Department of Health, Education, and Welfare, 1977.

Provost T: The rise and fall of fluorescent tinea capitis. *Pediatr Dermatol* 1983; 1:127.

Rockoff AS: Fungal cultures in a pediatric clinic. *Pediatrics* 1979; 63:276.

Rudolph N, Tariq AA, Reale MR, et al: Congenital cutaneous candidiasis. *Arch Dermatol* 1977; 113:1101.

Sharma V, Hall JC, Knapp JF, et al: Scalp colonization by *Trichophyton tonsurans* in an urban pediatric clinic. *Arch Dermatol* 1988; 124:1511.

Stein DH: Superficial fungal infections. *Pediatr Clin North Am* 1983; 30:545.

7 _____ Infestations

Arthropods are constantly present in the human environment, and hundreds of species are known to cause skin disease. Biting and stinging insects may produce wheals, erythema, and even bullae from contact with the skin. The erythematous papule with a central punctum is a common feature of insect bites. In this chapter, scabies, pediculoses, and papular urticaria are discussed in detail, since they are the most common forms of infestations and often require therapeutic intervention. Cutaneous eruptions related to ticks, spiders, mites, and helminths are also considered briefly. Arthropods may be divided into arachnids, which have eight legs (mites, ticks, spiders), and hexapods, with six legs (lice, mosquitoes, fleas, bedbugs, ants, bees, and other insects).

SCABIES

Clinical Features

Pruritic papules on the abdomen, dorsa of the hands and feet, elbows, periaxillary skin, genitalia, and interdigital webs of the hands and feet, are seen in scabies (Fig 7–1). In infants, eczematous eruptions of the face and trunk are seen in addition (Fig 7–2). In contrast, the head and neck regions are almost never involved in older children, adolescents, or adults. Most infants have acute dermatitis that is characterized by excoriations, erythematous papules, honey-colored crusts, and pustules. Secondary impetigo is common. When present, S-shaped burrows are diagnostic (Fig 7–3). They are usually found on the wrist, palm, interdigital webs, or genitalia. Nocturnal pruritus is severe. Within one household the disease may vary in severity from asymptomatic infested children to a child with a few nonpruritic papules to hundreds of lesions. Infants are likely to have numerous lesions (Fig 7–4). A high index of suspicion should be maintained in any patient with pruritic skin disease. Children who are severely retarded and unable to scratch effectively may be infested with thousands of scabies mites, which produce a diffuse hyperkeratosis of the skin and lichenification that may be confused with ichthyosis. This form of scabies is designated *Norwegian scabies.*

Differential Diagnosis

The diagnosis is confirmed by scraping an unscratched burrow that is covered with a drop of microscope immersion oil and placing the scrapings on a glass slide. Under the X10 objective of a microscope, the female mite, *Sarcoptes scabiei* (Fig 7–5), or her eggs or feces should be visible (Fig 7–6). Examination of skin scrapings from the fingerwebs, wrists, or ankles is most likely to show positive findings. Findings in excoriated and crusted lesions are often negative. In children with Norwegian scabies, scraping of the thick scales will often yield several viable mites. Atopic dermatitis, lichen planus, dermatitis herpetiformis, and other severely pruritic skin conditions mimic scabies. Scabies should be suspected in any infant in whom the onset of dermatitis was acute and who has no history of atopic dermatitis. A careful inspection for burrows and identification of household members who may have a history of itchy bumps are necessary.

Pathogenesis

Scabies is caused by the eight-legged human mite, *S. scabiei,* which may be up to 4 μm in length. The female mite remains in the stratum corneum, which she traverses at a rate of 0.5 to 5 mm/day. She deposits her eggs during her journey and dies after 30 or 40 days. Her eggs reach

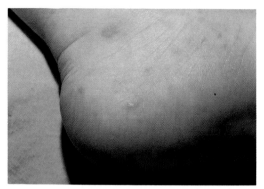

FIG 7–1.
Scabies. Papules and burrows on foot of an infant.

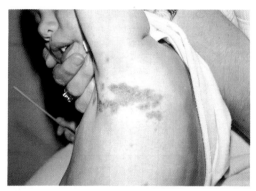

FIG 7–2.
Scabies. Nonspecific eczematous lesions in a child's axilla.

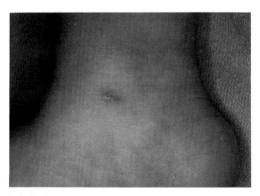

FIG 7–4.
Scabies in infant. Hundreds of lesions present.

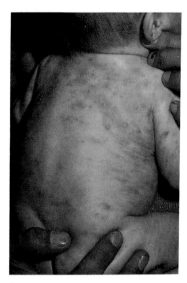

FIG 7–5.
Photomicrograph of female scabies mite recovered from scrapings of burrow. (Original magnification ×10.)

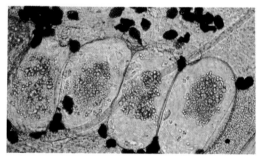

FIG 7–3.
S-shaped burrow diagnostic of scabies. This is the preferred lesion for obtaining a scraping.

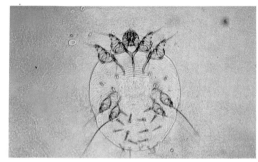

FIG 7–6.
Photomicrograph of oval eggs and dark brown scybala in skin scraping from infant with scabies. (Original magnification ×10.)

maturity in 10 to 14 days, and a new cycle begins. Transmission of scabies requires close personal contact, although female mites can survive 2 to 3 days off the human body. A pandemic of scabies has followed each major war of the twentieth century. Human scabies is quite contagious because newly infested individuals may not experience itching for the first 3 weeks of infestation, and only casual contact is required for spread of mites to others. Humans are the reservoir for scabies, and infestation of children with animal mites (e.g., dog, cat, chicken) is rare.

Treatment

Application of a scabicide, such as 1% gamma benzene hexachloride lotion, is curative. The lotion is available in 60 and 480 mL bottles. It should be dispensed as the calculated dose needed for therapy. In children and adolescents, one 2-hour application followed by a bath is curative in approximately 82% of cases; one 6-hour application results in a cure rate of 96%. Prolonged contact with the skin may result in significant percutaneous absorption. Gamma benzene hexachloride is concentrated in the central nervous system if absorbed; percutaneous absorption with central nervous system symptoms has been reported in a few infants. In infants under 6 months of age, an alternative scabicide such as sulfur, 6% to 10% ointment twice daily for 3 days, or crotamiton, applied to the entire body for a single 24-hour period and then reapplied for a second 24-hour period, may be substituted. Gamma benzene hexachloride remains the most effective scabicide, however, and cautious use in infants under 6 months of age may be required. In any infant or toddler, covering the hands with clothing to prevent licking the scabicide from the skin is recommended. One retreatment in 2 weeks may be necessary. In infants with extensive involvement, several retreatments may occasionally be required.

Even with the elimination of all viable scabies mites and eggs, itching may persist for 7 to 10 days after successful therapy. Simultaneous treatment of household contacts is required. Treatment failures are often the result of poor compliance or failure to treat an infested household member.

Patient Education

One should emphasize the mode of transmission of scabies and identify all household contacts. Instructions on the treatment schedule should be specific, and the persistence of itching even after scabicidal therapy and the importance of treating all household contacts should be emphasized.

Follow-up Visits

A follow-up visit in 2 weeks is important to ascertain success or failure of therapy. Any new lesions that may have appeared should be rescraped to determine whether infestation has persisted or that the child is reinfested. If the mite or her products are found, retreatment is suggested. Infants, who tend to have hundreds of lesions, may require several retreatments.

TICKS

Clinical Features

Tick bites are usually painless and inapparent to the child. Usually, the tick is noted several days after contact with the skin when pruritus begins. Localized urticarial reactions can be found. A diagnosis is usually made by identifying the presence of the tick in particular cutaneous locations. The most common sites for tick attachment are the occipital area of the scalp, ear canal, axilla, groin, and vulva. Rarely, a systemic reaction to a tick bite, characterized by fever, nausea, abdominal cramping, and headache, may occur, as may a paralysis similar to the Guillain-Barré syndrome, with ascending symmetric paralysis. A persistent, pruritic nodule, sometimes surrounded by hair loss, may be the result of an incompletely removed tick, leaving mouth parts remaining in the skin. Since ticks in certain areas of North America and Europe may carry *Borrelia burgdorferi,* the spirochete responsible for Lyme disease, observation for expanding rings of erythema about the site of the bite is advised for 3 weeks after the bite (see Chapter 5).

Differential Diagnosis

Most tick bite reactions are obvious, since the tick is found attached to the skin. If the mouth parts are left in and a pruritic nodule remains, the diagnosis may be quite difficult to distinguish from scabies, lichen simplex chronicus, or other infestations. The expanding annular red rings of erythema chronicum migrans may be confused with ringworm, urticaria, or other annular conditions.

Pathogenesis

Tick bites may occur when children play in the woods and when ticks are transferred from dogs to children. The tick attaches itself to the skin by its head in an effort to suck blood. The tick cuts the skin surface, introduces its proboscis, and secretes saliva into the wound. The saliva may include the neurotoxin responsible for tick paralysis or the spirochete responsible for Lyme disease. A foreign body granuloma is seen in persistent nodules in the skin where tick head parts remain.

Treatment

Removal of the tick is the treatment of choice. The preferred method of removal is the insertion of a blunt instrument, such as forceps or tweezers, between the tick head and the child's skin. Gentle outward pressure will cause the tick to back out. This method prevents any injury to the skin and the retention of tick parts within the skin. One should avoid all methods that may injure the skin, such as burning the tick, or using noxious substances on the skin.

Patient Education

Prevention is best for tick bites. Children and their dogs should be inspected routinely for ticks if they have been in wooded areas, and parents should be advised of the most common locations of tick bites and the preferred method of removal. It should be emphasized that most ticks do not carry Lyme disease.

Follow-up Visits

A follow-up visit 2 weeks after a bite to observe for signs of erythema chronicum migrans should be considered in areas endemic for Lyme disease.

SPIDERS

Clinical Features

Hemorrhagic, painful blisters may appear on the skin and evolve over the next few days into a cutaneous infarct with skin necrosis and a dry, gangrenous eschar (Fig 7–7). This reaction usually occurs on exposed areas of skin in a single lesion around the site of a spider bite. Systemic reactions, including nausea, vomiting, chills, malaise, syncope, and coma, may develop. Thrombo-

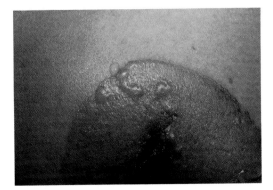

FIG 7–7.
Spider bite. Central necrosis and surrounding giant bullae.

cytopenia, hemolysis, and hemoglobinuria, which can result in renal failure, have been reported.

Differential Diagnosis

Spider bites must be differentiated from other forms of vascular infarction, such as vasculitis. In vasculitis, numerous lesions are present, whereas in spider bites a single lesion is seen. Other necrotizing infections, such as ecthyma gangrenosum, due to *Pseudomonas* infection, and the streptococcal gangrene syndrome, should be considered in the differential diagnosis. Lesions of herpes zoster, herpes simplex, cutaneous diphtheria, or anthrax may occasionally be confused with spider bite. In children who do not have a definite history of a spider bite, viral and bacterial cultures may be required.

Pathogenesis

The brown recluse spider is usually responsible for the lesion. This spider is prevalent in the midwestern United States, but it has occasionally been reported over many other areas of North America. The spider is small, 8 to 10 mm in diameter, and bears a violin-shaped band over the dorsal aspect of the thorax. It is often found in old buildings. A number of toxins have been found in the venom. Less often, black widow spiders are responsible for bites.

Treatment

High doses of oral corticosteroids may be useful in reducing or preventing the extent of tissue damage in this disease. Doses of 2 mg/kg/day of prednisone are usually recommended for a period of 5 days. Surgical removal of the necrotic area has been performed in some instances to prevent spread of the toxin. Hospitalization may be required in severe toxic reactions.

Patient Education

Emphasize that spiders of this type may hide in basements and that recognition of the small, thin-legged spider is important. Children should be kept from abandoned buildings.

Follow-up Visits

A daily follow-up visit, following initiation of treatment for the spider bite, is necessary to evaluate for the development of systemic symptoms and progression of the individual lesion. The child should be seen daily until healing is observed.

OTHER MITE INFESTATIONS

Clinical Features

Mites from nonhuman sources occasionally infest the skin of children. The canine scabies mite, usually carried on the fur of puppies with mange, may be temporarily transferred to the child. The puppy will have fur loss and crusted lesions. Also, harvest mites or chiggers, found in grasses, grains, or overgrowth of bushes, may similarly infest children. Grain mites found in stored seeds and grains and fowl mites found on chickens or domesticated birds, such as canaries, pigeons, or swallows, may also infest children. In each instance, the clinical lesions are characterized by urticarial papules, sometimes with hemorrhagic puncta, and, in intense responses, blister formation. Burrows are absent. The distribution on the child's skin is dependent on the location of the exposed skin. Characteristically, canine scabies produces lesions on the forearms, abdomen, and thighs. Harvest mites characteristically produce lesions on the legs and around the belt line. Grain mite lesions are on the exposed areas of the arms and legs, but may be quite generalized. Fowl mites produce lesions on exposed areas of skin.

Differential Diagnosis

Scabies and papular urticaria are the most important in the differential diagnosis. A history of exposure to the appropriate source is most important in the diagnosis of mite infestation. The

new puppy with hair loss and crusts on his skin, exposure to deep grasses and grain or stored grain, and association with birds are important historical information. Exposed skin infested with fowl mites may mimic a photoeruption.

Pathogenesis

In each case, the mites attach themselves to the skin to inject an irritating secretion and then fall off in a few days. Identifying the mites within skin lesions is very difficult. They do not persist on skin, however.

Treatment

Symptomatic relief with topical steroids or oral antihistamines, or both, is useful. Specific scabicides are not required.

Patient Education

Prophylaxis is an important part of patient education. Treatment of the infested puppy, the use of good insect repellents (such as diethyltoluamide), and staying away from those areas containing sources that are likely to produce the infestation should be emphasized. Parents and children should know that they cannot pass this eruption to others and that itching can be quite severe, lasting for several weeks after the initial exposure.

Follow-up Visits

A follow-up visit in 2 weeks to ascertain the institution of prophylaxis and the response to therapy is useful.

PEDICULOSES (LOUSE INFESTATIONS)

Clinical Features

Excoriated papules and pustules on the trunk and perineum are found in children and adolescents with body louse infestations. Often, only excoriations or their resultant hyperpigmented or hypopigmented scars are seen on the skin. The louse may be discovered by closely examining the seams of the underwear or the scalp hair. The gelatinous nits of the head louse appear as white, ovoid bodies tightly adherent to the hair shaft (Fig 7–8). Nocturnal pruritus is often severe with all human louse infestations. The prevalence of louse infestations is 34 times higher in whites than in blacks. The pubic (crab) louse may be seen crawling among the pubic hairs, or infestation with the

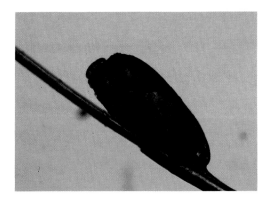

FIG 7–8.
Head lice. Photomicrograph of nit tightly adherent to one side of hair shaft. (Original magnification ×10.)

pubic louse may present as blue-black, crusted macules (maculae ceruleae) in the pubic area. Nits may also be seen attached to pubic hairs. The pubic louse may be seen in the eyelashes of newborns. Any "bug" seen crawling from the newborn's eye should be considered a pubic louse unless proved otherwise.

Differential Diagnosis

Scabies, dermatitis herpetiformis, neurotic excoriations, and other highly pruritic dermatoses may be confused with pediculoses. Parents with delusions of parasitosis may transfer their delusion to their children. In certain children, the retained external hair-root sheath may resemble head louse nits. Retained root sheaths may be easily removed by sliding them distally down the hair shaft, while the nit is tightly adherent to it. The blue-black, crusted macules of pubic lice may be confused with vasculitis, folliculitis, or impetigo.

Pathogenesis

The human louse, a six-legged insect, attaches itself to the skin, ingests blood, and produces skin lesions by mechanical puncture and perhaps by injecting toxic secretions. The body louse, which is 2 to 4 mm in length, is the longest of the lice that infest humans; the pubic louse is 1 to 2 mm in length. The female louse reproduces every 2 weeks, and each female louse may produce more than 80 offspring during her lifetime. The body louse produces more eggs during her lifetime than the pubic louse. Newly hatched lice mate with old, and hundreds of nits result every 2

weeks. The female louse attaches herself to a hair and slides along it laying eggs. If hair is not available, clothing fibers are used. Crowded living conditions are most conducive to the spread of lice, which can be transmitted either by person-to-person contact or by fomites, such as hairbrushes, caps, scarves, coats, or carpets. Sharing of clothing is a common source of transmission.

Treatment

The application of 1% gamma benzene hexachloride lotion to the affected skin area for 12 to 24 hours is effective in body lice infestation. For head lice or crab lice infestations, 1% gamma benzene hexachloride shampoo, applied for 5 minutes and then rinsed out, is usually sufficient. The shampoo is available in 60 or 480 mL bottles. An efficacious alternative is a 10-minute shampoo with 1% permethrin. These treatments will not, however, remove the gelatinous nits. The use of a warm, damp towel for 30 minutes on the scalp will loosen the nits and allow their mechanical removal with a fine-toothed comb. Retreatment in 7 days may be necessary. Topical malathion lotion 0.5% is effective, but toxicity is a concern. Measuring the distance of the nit closest to the scalp surface will provide a baseline measurement to help determine adequacy of treatment on follow-up. Boiling of clothing, bedding, and other possible fomites is ovicidal and lousicidal and necessary because nits may be attached to clothing.

Patient Education

It is tempting for parents to use pediculocides repeatedly in children with lice infestations. One should emphasize the hazards of central nervous system toxicity posed by such usage. All contacts should be identified and treated simultaneously. Students should be readmitted to school the morning after the first treatment. Schoolmates should be examined by the school nurse to determine if other children are infested.

Follow-up Visits

An office or visiting nurse follow-up to evaluate therapy 1 week after the initial visit is most helpful. If new eggs or nits are seen on the proximal hair shafts as close or closer to the scalp than the original measurement, retreatment is necessary. Nits will grow out with the hair shaft, and by 7 days after successful treatment they should be at least 6 to 7 mm from the scalp margin.

PAPULAR URTICARIA

Clinical Features

Pruritic erythematous papules, with or without an erythematous, urticarial flare, are characteristically arranged in clusters in papular urticaria (Fig 7–9). Such clusters are usually seen over the shoulders, upper arms, and buttocks. Papular urticaria occurs predominantly between the ages of 18 months and 7 years. In intense hypersensitivity, vesicles and bullae may be seen. Recurrent crops of these papules are the rule, with each crop lasting 2 to 10 days (Figs 7–9 and 7–10). Characteristically, the affected child is the only household member involved. The problem may persist from 3 to 9 months and most often begins in spring or summer.

Differential Diagnosis

Insect bites, viral exanthems, photoeruptions, acute parapsoriasis, and the early stages of other papulosquamous diseases (see Chapter 9) may be confused with papular urticaria.

Pathogenesis

The lesions represent delayed hypersensitivity reactions to a variety of biting or stinging arthropods. Dog and cat fleas are the usual offend-

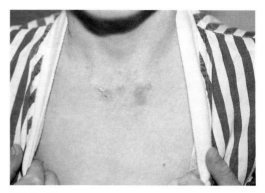

FIG 7–10.
Papular urticaria. Grouped lesions on lower area of neck where puppy was carried by child.

ers. Less commonly, mosquitoes, lice, scabies, fowl mites, and grain or grass mites are responsible. Epicutaneous testing with homogenized arthropods has reproduced the urticarial papule within 4 to 8 hours. The pathologic features of naturally occurring lesions are similar to those of a delayed-type (tuberculin) skin test.

Treatment

The logical treatment is removal of the offending insect. Dogs or cats should be treated for fleas or mites by a veterinarian. The child should be kept away from the pet. The use of fragrant lotions, such as Skin-So-Soft (Avon) may make the child less attractive to the insect. Fleas or mites living in carpets or furniture may be eliminated by treatment with a commercial insecticide such as Raid or Off. Window casings should be treated in the case of bird mites.

Symptomatic relief may sometimes be obtained with topical low-potency glucocorticosteroid creams (see Chapter 20) applied three times daily. Oral antihistamines are sometimes helpful.

Patient Education

When only one member of the household is affected, it is difficult to convince some parents of the cause. The extreme sensitivity of the affected person to the offending arthropod should be explained. Often, an obvious source is not evident from the initial history, and a thorough search should be made for the source. It is a great relief to both the parents and the child to learn that the sensitivity is transient.

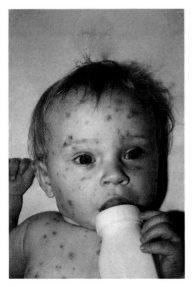

FIG 7–9.
Papular urticaria. Numerous central papules or edematous papules surrounded by an outer zone of urticaria.

Follow-up Visits

A visit within 2 weeks is useful in reviewing the possible sources and evaluating the response to therapeutic measures.

HELMINTHS: CUTANEOUS LARVA MIGRANS (CREEPING ERUPTION)

Clinical Features

Pruritic, serpiginous, erythematous lesions of the skin that advance at the rate of 1 cm/day represent the classic pattern seen in cutaneous larva migrans (Fig 7–11). Lesions are usually on the feet or hands and, occasionally, on the buttocks. Vesicles and bullae may be present along the tract, and pulsatile edema within the erythematous, serpiginous tract may be observed. A history of a child having played along the shorelines of the southeastern or eastern United States is usually obtained. A second clinical form involves strictly the perianal area, buttocks, and thighs, with serpiginous tracts that spread 5 to 10 cm/hr. The child may have a peripheral blood eosinophilia, with 10% to 35% eosinophils present.

Differential Diagnosis

The annular erythemas, including erythema chronicum migrans, urticaria, and even tinea infections, may be confused with cutaneous larva

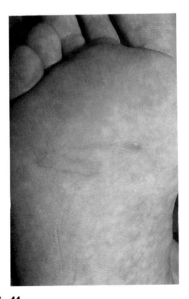

FIG 7–11.
Creeping eruption. Serpiginous red track on plantar surface of foot of a child with *A. braziliens* infestation.

migrans. The rapid progression and advancement of the border in cutaneous larva migrans and the presence of pulsations within the serpiginous tract are useful differentiating features.

Pathogenesis

Two larvae are responsible for the cutaneous lesions in cutaneous larva migrans. *Ancylostoma braziliens,* is the most common of these larvae and produces the clinical pattern involving the feet. Children playing along the shore of the southern United States are at the greatest risk. *A. braziliens* is the dog and cat hookworm. Ova of this organism are deposited in the soil or in the sandy beaches from dog and cat excretions and hatch into larvae that will penetrate bare skin. The larvae migrate 1 to 2 cm each day and produce the serpiginous lesions of the skin. Examination of stool samples does not reveal the presence of parasite eggs, and identification of the larvae within the tract is quite difficult because they are often found beyond the area of obvious inflammation. This parasite cannot complete its life cycle in humans, and the larvae disappear within 4 to 6 weeks after penetration of the skin. The second form of cutaneous larva migrans is caused by the larvae of *Strongyloides stercoralis*. These larvae usually penetrate the skin near the anus and spread onto the buttocks. They are able to leave the skin and may settle in the gastrointestinal tract; a stool sample examined for ova and parasites will identify the *Strongyloides* larvae or eggs.

Treatment

Topical thiabendazole 15% cream, applied three times a day for 5 to 7 days, is the treatment of choice for creeping eruption due to *A. braziliens.* Parents should be instructed to treat well beyond the area of obvious skin redness. Oral thiabendazole is also effective in a dose of 25 to 50 mg/kg given for 2 to 4 days, and it should be used for creeping eruption due to *S. stercoralis.*

Patient Education

Parents should understand that these infestations may be obtained from sandy beaches or sandboxes, and only in certain regions of North America. Moreover, they should know that the lesions are not contagious to other children and that usually one treatment protocol is curative.

Follow-up Visits

A visit at 4 to 5 days after initiation of therapy is useful to evaluate the response.

SWIMMERS' ITCH AND SEABATHER'S ERUPTION

Clinical Features

Pruritic papules appearing in areas not protected by the swimsuit are characteristic of swimmers' itch, which has occurred in those who swam in fresh-water lakes of the upper Great Lakes of North America. In seabather's eruption, the pruritic papules occur under the swimsuit-covered areas, after swimming in salt waters of the southern United States. The papules are persistent and may last for at least 2 weeks in both conditions.

Differential Diagnosis

Papular urticaria, insect bite reactions, and infestations due to scabies or other mites should be considered in the differential diagnosis. The strong historical and temporal association with swimming is a very useful differentiating point.

Pathogenesis

Parasitic flatworms have been implicated in swimmers' itch. Cercariae are released into the water from infected snails in freshwater lakes of the upper Great Lakes region. The parasites finish their cycle by penetrating the skin of warm-blooded hosts, but do not survive after penetration. The schistosomes usually come from the droppings of infested mammals and waterfowl and are then involved with the snail as intermediate host. Seabather's eruption is also thought to be due to cercariae, but the specific cercaria is not known.

Treatment

Since this is a self-limited disease, no specific anticercaria treatment need be introduced. Symptomatic treatment, such as the use of topical steroid preparations or oral antihistamines, or both, is usually recommended.

Patient Education

Parents and patients should have an explanation of the source of the itchy eruption and should know that it cannot be transmitted from the infested individual to other humans. They should also be told to recognize that this disease is self-limited and will disappear.

Follow-up Visits

Follow-up visits are usually unnecessary.

BIBLIOGRAPHY

Armoni M, Bibi H, Schlesinger M, et al: Pediculosis capitis: Why prefer a solution to a shampoo or spray? *Pediatr Dermatol* 1988; 5:273.

Bowerman JG, Gomez MP, Austin RD, et al: Comparative study of permethrin 1% creme rinse and lindane shampoo for the treatment of head lice. *Pediatr Infect Dis J* 1988; 6:252.

Helm K, Lane AT, McPhilmy J: Pseudoresistance to pediculocides in a case of pubic lice. *Pediatr Dermatol* 1988; 5:187.

Honig PJ: Bites and parasites. *Pediatr Clin North Am* 1983; 30:563.

Hurwitz S: Scabies in babies. *Am J Dis Child* 1973; 126:226.

Massie FS: Papular urticaria: Etiology, diagnosis and management. *Cutis* 1974; 13:980.

Rasmussen JE: The problem of lindane. *J Am Acad Dermatol* 1981; 5:807.

Sarov B, Neumann L, Herman Y, et al: Evaluation of an intervention program for head lice infestation in school children. *Pediatr Infect Dis J* 1988; 7:176.

Taplin D, Rivera A, Walker JG, et al: A comparative trial of three treatment schedules for the eradication of scabies. *J Am Acad Dermatol* 1983; 9:550.

8 _____ Viral Infections

Viruses may involve the skin either by dissemination to skin during a systemic viral infection (viral exanthem), sometimes accompanied by viral replication in skin, or by producing a virus-induced skin tumor. A number of viruses are epidermotropic and replicate within keratinocytes.

VIRAL EXANTHEMS: MORBILLIFORM ERUPTIONS

Any cutaneous eruption associated with an acute viral syndrome has been termed a *viral exanthem*. The exact incidence of viral exanthems is unknown, but herpes simplex alone accounts for a yearly incidence of 5.1 children affected per 1,000. Viral exanthems are seen frequently in general pediatric settings and are considered in the differential diagnosis of at least one child a week. A variety of different patterns are seen: a generalized maculopapular eruption that mimics measles (morbilliform), petechial eruptions, vesiculobullous eruptions, scarlet fever–like (scarlatiniform) eruptions, papulonodular eruptions, and oral erosions. It is important to recall that any viral exanthem, including morbilliform eruptions, may have a photodistribution. Morbilliform eruptions are the most common.

Measles (Rubeola)

Clinical Features
Classic Measles.—The features of classic measles include a severe prodrome followed by an exanthematous phase. After an incubation period of 9 to 14 days, a prodrome of high fever, cough, rhinitis, and conjunctivitis appears. The cough is described as "barking," and a diagnosis of bronchitis or croup is usually considered. The prodrome typically includes cervical lymphadenopathy and lasts 3 to 5 days. The preauricular lymph nodes are enlarged. The prodrome is then followed by a cutaneous eruption.

The exanthem begins on the forehead as blotchy erythema and progresses to involve the face, trunk, and extremities with multiple discrete macules and papules (Fig 8–1). The eruption is preceded by intense erythema of the mucous membranes, with 1 mm white centers, the so-called Koplik's spots (Fig 8–2). Koplik's spots are most prevalent on the buccal mucosa and gingiva, but may be found on other mucous membranes as well.

Bacterial otitis media, pneumonia, and encephalitis may complicate measles. Their exact incidence in measles is unknown. Severe pneumonias and encephalitis are the primary causes of death in children with both types of measles.

Atypical Measles.—In patients who have received killed measles vaccine, or in whom live measles vaccination has failed, a syndrome of high fever, abdominal pain, pulmonary consolidation, and an acral eruption consisting of vesicular, vesiculopustular, or purpuric lesions may occur (atypical measles) (Fig 8–3).

Differential Diagnosis
Classic Measles.—The severity of the prodrome, a high fever, and Koplik's spots in an acutely ill child are the most distinctive features differentiating measles from the other morbilliform eruptions (Tables 8–1 and 8–2). Viral isolation from mucosa, while difficult, will distinguish measles from other exanthems. Acute and convalescent sera, obtained 1 week and 3 weeks after the onset of the illness, will assist with a retrospective diagnosis.

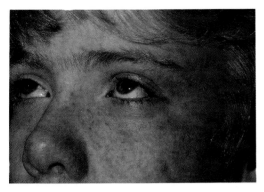

FIG 8–1.
Red macules and conjunctival erythema in a child with rubeola (measles).

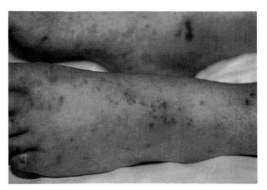

FIG 8–3.
Petechiae and palpable purpura on feet of an adolescent with atypical measles.

Atypical Measles.—Atypical measles may mimic meningococcemia and Rocky Mountain spotted fever, which are the main considerations in the differential diagnosis. Primarily acral petechiae may be the presenting symptom in echovirus 9 and other enterovirus infections. Other conditions to be considered in the differential diagnosis are listed in Table 8–3.

Pathogenesis

Despite the very active measles immunization program in the United States, outbreaks of measles continue to occur. Measles has not been eradicated because 35% of children are never immunized, and immunization fails in up to 15% of those immunized. Reimmunization is now recommended in view of the high rate of vaccine failures.

The cutaneous eruption is undoubtedly due to the measles virus, a paramyxovirus, since the virus has been detected within epidermal cells and endothelial cells of dermal blood vessels by electron microscopy and specific immunofluorescence. The measles virus induces increased nuclear volume within the epidermal cells, producing multinucleated epidermal giant cells (Warthin-Finkeldey cells). These cells may be demonstrated on exfoliative cytologic examination of the nasal or oral mucosa and differ from those induced by herpes simplex by the lack of epidermal cell separation (acantholysis).

TABLE 8–1.

Differential Diagnosis of Morbilliform Eruptions Due to Viruses

Common associations
Measles (rubeola)
Rubella
Roseola
Boston exanthem
Erythema infectiosum
Infectious mononucleosis
Pityriasis rosea (presumed viral)
Uncommon associations
Hepatitis
Mumps
Echoviruses 1, 2, 4, 5, 7, 9, 13, 14, 22, 25
Reoviruses 2, 3
Coxsackieviruses 1, 2, 3, 4, 5, 7
Respiratory syncytial virus
Cytomegalovirus
Adenoviruses 1, 2, 3, 4, 5, 7
Colorado tick fever
Dengue

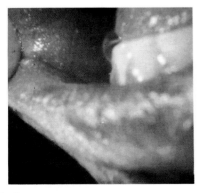

FIG 8–2.
Koplik's spots. Bright erythema of buccal mucosa with pinpoint white macules in a child with rubeola.

TABLE 8−2.

Differential Diagnosis of Morbilliform Eruptions

> Common viruses
> > Measles
> > Rubella
> > Roseola
> > Erythema infectiosum
> > Infectious mononucleosis
> > Pityriasis rosea
>
> Common bacteria
> > Scarlet fever
>
> Drug-induced eruptions
> > Ampicillin
> > Penicillin
> > Nonsteroidal antiinflammatory drugs
> > Salicylic acid
> > Barbiturates
> > Phenytoins
> > Phenothiazines
> > Thiazide diuretics
> > Isoniazid
>
> Papulosquamous disorders
> > Guttate psoriasis
> > Graft-vs.-host disease
>
> Reactive erythemas
> > Urticaria
> > Papular urticaria
> > Erythema multiforme

It is not certain how the altered immune response in atypical measles produces cutaneous lesions, but an immunologic mechanism, perhaps involving immune complexes, has been proposed.

Treatment

No specific treatment for measles or atypical measles is available. Supportive care with fever control by antipyretics or wet dressings and ensuring adequate fluid intake are important. If sec-

TABLE 8−3.

Morbilliform Viral Exanthems With Petechiae

> Echovirus 9
> Epstein-Barr virus
> Hepatitis
> Atypical measles
> Echoviruses 4, 7
> Coxsackievirus A9
> Respiratory syncytial virus
> Rubella
> Dengue

ondary bacterial otitis media or bacterial pneumonia occurs, antibiotic therapy should be instituted.

Patient Education

The high attack rate of measles should be emphasized, and the patient should be isolated during the contagious period (from the onset of respiratory symptoms through the third day of the cutaneous eruption). Unvaccinated normal infants and children should receive a preventive dose of immune serum globulin (0.25 mL/kg intramuscularly) as soon as possible after exposure, and 8 weeks later they should be vaccinated with live attenuated measles virus vaccine, provided the child is at least 15 months old. Unvaccinated infants and children with malignancies or immunodeficiencies or those receiving immunosuppressive therapy should be given 0.5 mL/kg of immune serum globulin intramuscularly to a maximum dose of 15 mL. Exposure to measles is not a contraindication to vaccination if given within 72 hours of exposure.

Follow-up Visits

Close contact should be maintained with the patient with rubeola to watch for bacterial superinfection, the development of severe pneumonia with pulmonary compromise, or encephalitis. Frequent visits may be required during the course of the illness.

Rubella

Clinical Features

Classic Rubella.—Classic rubella is a mild illness in most children. Rubella acquired postnatally in infants and children usually is accompanied by few or no prodromal symptoms. Up to 50% of rubella infections may be entirely asymptomatic. Mild lymphadenopathy may precede the cutaneous eruption by several days. The suboccipital and posterior auricular lymph nodes are usually prominently enlarged. A faint-pink, macular eruption appears first on the face and spreads to the trunk and proximal extremities. Within 48 hours, the face and trunk have cleared and the eruption involves the distal extremities. The child usually appears well. Rarely, petechiae or purpura may be seen. A monarthric arthritis may accompany the syndrome, particularly in adolescent girls. It may persist for several months. Fever is usually absent in patients with rubella.

Congenital Rubella.—Rubella acquired during the first trimester in pregnancy may result in the congenital rubella syndrome. This may be manifested by neonatal purpura and petechiae due to thrombocytopenia. Occasionally, jaundice due to rubella hepatitis occurs. Accompanying features include deafness, cataract, glaucoma congenital heart defects, and growth and psychomotor retardation, which may be subtle or severe. Any or all of these features may accompany the typical rubella exanthem. The exanthem may be recurrent during the first 5 years. In infants with congenital rubella, rubella virus may be recovered from peripheral leukocytes, stool, or urine for months to years after birth.

Differential Diagnosis
Classic Rubella.—In distinguishing classic rubella from rubeola (see Tables 8–1 and 8–2), the absence of fever with accompanying morbilliform eruption is helpful. The mild illness of rubella may be indistinguishable from enteroviral illnesses with exanthems. Culture of the virus from nasal mucosa will distinguish rubella from other exanthems.

Congenital Rubella.—Other microorganisms causing congenital infections responsible for producing neonatal purpura or hepatitis, or both should be considered in the differential diagnosis. These include *Toxoplasma,* enterovirus, herpes simplex virus, cytomegalovirus, and *Treponema pallidum.* Rarely, congenital lupus erythematosus, the Wiskott-Aldrich syndrome, and various platelet defects may mimic congenital rubella. The additional findings of cataracts, retinopathy, and heart disease should suggest congenital rubella.

Pathogenesis
Rubella virus, a rubivirus in the togavirus family, is an RNA virus that enters the bloodstream via the respiratory route. The method of production of the cutaneous eruption is unknown, but it is suspected to result from virus dissemination to skin.

Therapy
There is no specific treatment.

Patient Education
Exposure or potential exposure of susceptible women in the first trimester of pregnancy should be determined. If possible, the rubella patient should be kept isolated from pregnant women. In patients who acquire rubella postnatally, it is contagious from 7 days before the onset of the cutaneous eruption to 5 days after the onset. In congenital rubella, virus shedding usually ends by age 6 months, but may continue up to 5 or 6 years.

When a pregnant woman is exposed to rubella, a serum specimen should be obtained and tested for rubella hemagglutinin inhibition antibody. If antibody is present, there is no risk of infection. If no rubella antibody is detectable, a second blood specimen should be obtained 3 weeks later. If antibody is present, infection is presumed to have occurred, and termination of pregnancy may be considered. If termination of pregnancy is not an option, immune serum globulin should be given (20 mL intramuscularly).

Follow-up Visits
Follow-up visits are usually unnecessary in postnatally acquired rubella. In congenital rubella, a multidisciplinary approach, such as that offered by a birth defects clinic, is advisable.

Roseola (Exanthem Subitum)
Clinical Features
Roseola occurs predominantly in infants under 4 years of age. It is characterized by 3 days of sustained fever in an infant who otherwise appears well, following which the temperature falls (often to a subnormal level), and a pink, morbilliform, cutaneous eruption appears transiently and fades within 24 hours. A convulsion at the onset of fever is noted occasionally, but the exact incidence of febrile convulsions is unknown. Mild edema of the eyelids and posterior cervical lymphadenopathy are occasionally seen.

Differential Diagnosis
Roseola can be distinguished from other morbilliform eruptions (see Tables 8–1 and 8–2) by the distinctive history of 3 days of sustained fever in an infant followed by the appearance of a morbilliform eruption after the fever ends. It may be indistinguishable from echovirus 16 infections. Eruptions resulting from treatment with drugs may easily be confused with roseola in infants who received antibiotics for the febrile portion of the illness.

Pathogenesis

Roseola is a presumed viral infection because of its predilection to occur in epidemics in the springtime, its incubation period of 10 days, and the leukopenia that may develop during the course of the illness. In Japan, herpesvirus type 6 infection is thought to be the major causative agent for roseola, while in North America, children with echovirus 16 infections probably account for some cases of roseola.

Treatment

Fever can be controlled with wet dressings or tepid water sponge baths, supplemental fluids, and antipyretics.

Patient Education

Parents should be informed of the presumed viral nature of this disorder and told that there is no necessity for antibiotics. If the child is seen during the febrile state, it is worthwhile to document the morbilliform eruption by personally observing it.

Follow-up Visits

To be certain to exclude other infections that may mimic roseola, a follow-up visit 2 days later to ascertain the course of the illness is recommended.

Human Parvovirus B19 Infection (Erythema Infectiosum)

Clinical Features

The eruptions of erythema infectiosum (EI) (fifth disease) classically begin with an intense, confluent redness of both cheeks, the so-called slapped-cheek appearance (Fig 8–4), seen in 75% of patients. It may then spread to involve the arms (86%), legs (75%), chest (47%), and abdomen (45%) with a lacy, pink to dull red macular eruption (Fig 8–5); 25% of patients will have only the lacy eruption on their extremities. The original eruption lasts from 3 to 5 days. Stimulation of cutaneous vasodilation, however, will cause the eruption to "reappear" up to 4 months later. This may result from vigorous exercise, overheating of the skin, or sun exposure. Only 20% of affected children will have a mild fever. Occasionally, morbilliform, vesicular, or purpuric skin eruptions are seen. About 20% of infected children and adults are asymptomatic. During some outbreaks of EI, symmetric arthritis of hands, wrists,

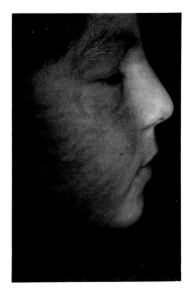

FIG 8–4.
Slapped-cheek appearance of a child with parvovirus B19 infection (erythema infectiosum).

or knees will be observed. Joint symptoms usually resolve in 1 to 2 months, but may be the presenting feature. In patients with chronic hemolytic anemias EI may be the cause of transient aplastic crises, and in immunosuppressed children may be responsible for red cell aplasia and severe anemia. It has recently been recognized that EI in pregnant women may result in fetal death.

Differential Diagnosis

Drug eruptions and the other morbilliform eruptions may be considered in the differential diagnosis (see Tables 8–1 and 8–2), but the lacy, mottled appearance of the eruption is characteristic. Occasionally, the more violaceous livedo retic-

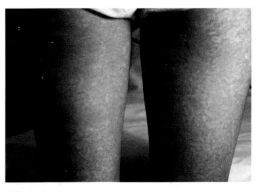

FIG 8–5.
Lacy pink eruption on thighs in erythema infectiosum.

ularis pattern of skin mottling associated with collagen vascular disease may be confused with EI, especially if associated with arthropathy. Diagnosis can be confirmed by analysis of serum obtained within 30 days of the onset of illness for the presence of IgM B19 antibodies.

Pathogenesis

Human parvovirus B19 is the causative agent of EI. The mechanism of the cutaneous features is unknown. The organism replicates in erythroid bone marrow cells, accounting for its role in red cell aplasia of immunodeficiency and transient aplastic crises in children with chronic hemolytic anemias.

Treatment

There is no specific treatment nor are there any specific control measures, although isolation of patients at risk for complications (pregnant women, immunosuppressed patients, patients with chronic hemolytic anemia) is recommended. The disease may no longer be contagious once the skin eruption occurs.

Patient Education

The patient or family should be informed of the dangers of B19 virus to pregnant women, immunosuppressed patients, and patients with chronic hemolytic anemia, (e.g., sickle cell disease). They should be advised to keep the infected child away from these individuals for 2 weeks, and good hand washing techniques in the affected family should be emphasized. They should also be told of the likely reappearance of the cutaneous eruption for up to 4 months.

Follow-up Visits

Follow-up visits are usually unnecessary unless arthritis or exposure of persons at risk is involved.

Echovirus 16 Infection (Boston Exanthem)

Clinical Features

Echovirus 16 infection in children is usually seen in epidemic form and may mimic roseola in that the cutaneous eruption may appear after the end of 2 or 3 days of fever. The eruption is characteristically morbilliform, but vesicles or punched-out erosions have occasionally been described. The morbilliform eruption lasts 1 to 5 days. Cervical, suboccipital, and postauricular lym-

phadenopathy are seen. Aseptic meningitis may occur, but it is usually seen in children without the cutaneous eruption.

Differential Diagnosis

Roseola should be considered in the differential diagnosis of morbilliform eruptions (see Tables 8–1 and 8–2). Roseola may mimic the Boston exanthem, but the fever and eruption in the latter often overlap. The identification of echovirus 16 in stools or throat washings helps to distinguish between these two disorders.

Pathogenesis

The incubation period is 3 to 5 days when the virus is spread by the enteric route. It is not known whether the virus appears within the cutaneous eruption. The mechanism that produces the cutaneous eruption is also unknown.

Treatment

Fever control is usually necessary, but no specific treatment exists.

Patient Education

It is important to emphasize that this eruption is not measles and that it is communicable via the enteric route. Good hand washing techniques in the family should be emphasized to help prevent spread.

Follow-up Visits

Follow-up visits are unnecessary.

Infectious Mononucleosis

Clinical Features

The annual incidence of infectious mononucleosis is approximately 50 per 100,000 children, with the highest incidence found among adolescents and young adults. The usual presenting symptoms and signs are fever (in 85%), sore throat with exudative tonsillitis (70%), fatigue (100%), and generalized lymphadenopathy (85%). Headache occurs in 45% of patients, and splenomegaly in 45%. Jaundice and hepatomegaly occur in up to 30% of patients. A pink, fleeting morbilliform eruption occurs in 15% of patients and may last 1 to 5 days. Treatment of children with infectious mononucleosis with ampicillin or penicillin for the sore throat results in an increase in incidence of morbilliform eruption in up to 80%. With antibiotic use, the eruption becomes bright red and more papular and may persist for 7 to 10 days (Fig 8–6).

The morbilliform eruption is the most characteristic seen with infectious mononucleosis, but occasionally other cutaneous eruptions may occur. Urticaria has been described as a prominent presenting feature, and petechial eruptions associated with thrombocytopenia may be seen occasionally. Palmar erythema has also been reported as a presenting symptom of infectious mononucleosis. Neurologic symptoms such as spatial and visual distortion or signs of encephalitis, meningitis, neuritis, or Guillain-Barré syndrome may accompany the cutaneous eruption.

The acute phase with fever and sore throat lasts 2 to 3 weeks. Extreme fatigue and lethargy may persist for 3 months, however. Rare complications include splenic rupture, thrombocytopenia, agranulocytosis, hemolytic anemia, orchitis, and cardiac involvement.

Laboratory studies are most useful in aiding with the diagnosis, with the detection of heterophil antibodies by Paul-Bunnell test as the most important diagnostic criterion. The laboratory findings most often encountered and their frequencies are as follows:

Finding	Percentage of Patients
Epstein-Barr virus antibody IgG or IgM	100
Lymphocytosis	92
Atypical mononuclear cells in peripheral blood film	92
Liver enzyme abnormalities	80
Hypergammaglobulinemia	80
Heterophil antibodies	75
Indirect Coombs' test	50
Thrombocytopenia	50
Hyperbilirubinemia	40

Differential Diagnosis

During the early phase of infectious mononucleosis, the possibility of streptococcal pharyngitis is usually considered, as are other causes of pharyngitis. Infectious mononucleosis can be distinguished from the other morbilliform eruptions (see Tables 8–1 and 8–2) by its prolonged course, the prominent symptom of excessive fatigue, and the laboratory findings. The petechial eruption must be differentiated from other causes of thrombocytopenic purpura in children, such as idiopathic thrombocytopenic purpura, lupus erythematosus, and malignancies. A similar syn-

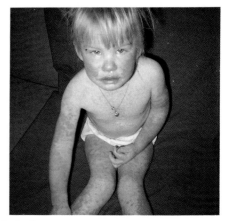

FIG 8–6.
Child with bright red morbilliform eruption due to infectious mononucleosis plus ampicillin.

drome may be produced by cytomegalovirus, another herpesvirus, but exudative tonsillitis and heterophil antibodies are not present. Isolation of Epstein-Barr virus (EBV) from oropharyngeal secretions will distinguish.

Pathogenesis

It is now accepted that EBV, a herpesvirus, is responsible for most cases of infectious mononucleosis. The incubation period is 4 to 8 weeks in adolescents but is usually shorter in prepubertal children. The period of communicability is uncertain, since most patients with infectious mononucleosis excrete small amounts of virus for many months after the onset of symptoms, and there are asymptomatic carriers of EBV.

Treatment

In mild cases, no treatment is required. In hemolytic anemia, thrombocytopenic purpura, airway interference, neurologic involvement, or in selected patients with toxemia and prolonged fever, systemic glucocorticosteroids may be given. Prednisone, 2 to 3 mg/kg/day for 3 days, is recommended for adolescents. Ampicillin or penicillin should not be administered in routine cases, because of the high frequency of drug rashes. Acylcovir has yet to be convincingly demonstrated to be efficacious in infectious mononucleosis, but the drug is active against EBV in vitro.

Patient Education

Concern that the spleen may rupture, which occurs in 0.5% of patients, should prompt avoidance of contact sports or other vigorous activity in which abdominal injury is likely. Neurologic complications occur in 1.5%, and patients should be warned about mental symptoms. They should also be apprised of the prolonged convalescence from this disorder and of the need to increase activities in a stepwise fashion.

Follow-up Visits

Weekly visits should be scheduled in patients with mild to moderate disease to ascertain the course of the disease and observe complications. In severe disease, daily visits or hospitalization may be necessary.

Hepatitis

Clinical Features

Although viral hepatitis is usually not associated with exanthems, it is a disease that should not be overlooked when searching for the cause of a viral exanthem. The exact incidence of cutaneous eruptions in hepatitis is not documented, but most are associated with hepatitis B. The incidence of morbilliform and urticarial eruptions in patients with the prodrome of hepatitis B is approximately equal. These eruptions are frequently associated with symmetric arthritis involving large joints that occurs in hepatitis B. Children infected with hepatitis A often have nonspecific symptoms of low-grade fever, irritability, and upper respiratory symptoms without cutaneous involvement or mild jaundice.

A variety of skin lesions have been associated with hepatitis B, including scarlatiniform eruptions and several eruptions with features of cutaneous vascular injury: urticaria, erythema marginatum, palpable purpura, and nodose lesions similar to those seen in periarteritis nodosa. Most of these have been reported in only a single patient with hepatitis. Papulonodular lesions of hepatitis have also been described over the extremities in the Gianotti-Crosti syndrome. The morbilliform eruption of hepatitis (Fig 8−7) characteristically precedes the icteric stage by 1 to 10 days.

It is important to identify patients whose blood is positive for hepatitis-associated antigen to prevent them from donating blood or blood products and to protect laboratory personnel. Enteric transmission of hepatitis can occur, and contact with patients' blood should be avoided. Isolat-

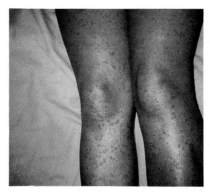

FIG 8−7.
Morbilliform eruption of legs in adolescent with preicteric hepatitis.

ing the patients from contact with persons at risk for severe hepatitis may be important. The incubation period is 6 weeks to 6 months.

Differential Diagnosis

The other viral exanthems, particularly rubella, should be considered (see Tables 8−1 and 8−2) during the prodromal phase of morbilliform and urticarial eruptions associated with arthritis. In hepatitis, however, the arthritis is usually symmetric, in contrast to rubella, in which it is often monarthric. A serum sickness reaction resulting from drugs and serum products may mimic the prodrome of hepatitis. Test results for hepatitis B surface antigen (HBsAg) are usually positive in the prodrome, but liver function test results may be normal. The eventual development of icterus, hepatic tenderness, and hepatic enlargement will allow a retrospective diagnosis of hepatitis. Diagnosis is usually made by the serologic test for HBsAg. In some acute cases, HBsAg has disappeared from sera, but the IgM anti-HBC (core antigen) test results will be positive.

Pathogenesis

Hepatitis B virus has been identified as a 42-nm, DNA-containing, double-shelled particle ultrastructurally. The morbilliform eruption is associated with HBsAg-positive hepatitis. Hepatitis antigen-antibody immune complexes have been identified in the sera and skin of patients with eruptions of the urticarial, anaphylactoid purpura, and periarteritis nodosa types. It is possible that the morbilliform and other eruptions may also be related to a circulating immune complex disease.

Treatment

Symptomatic treatment only is usually given. Bed rest and adequate diet are supportive measures. Exposed persons may be given large doses of hepatitis B immune serum globulin (HBIG), 0.06 mL/kg of body weight, within 24 hours of exposure and 1.0 mL of hepatitis B vaccine given intramuscularly within 7 days of exposure. The vaccine should be repeated 1 and 6 months afterward. For perinatal exposure, 0.5 mL of HBIG should be administered within 12 hours of birth, with 0.5 mL of vaccine given within 7 days and at 1 and 6 months.

Patient Education

It should be emphasized that hepatitis B can be transmitted not only through blood and blood products or contaminated needles but also by the enteric and possibly the oral route. The importance of personal hygienic measures such as hand washing in preventing spread should be emphasized.

Follow-up Visits

Patients should be seen weekly until the jaundice has disappeared. Although the course is benign in 95% of children, hepatitis is variable and may progress to liver failure. Patients' sera should be retested for HBsAg and antibodies to HBsAg 3 months later to detect possible chronic carriers.

Petechial Eruptions

Many viruses can produce petechial eruptions during the acute febrile phase of the viral illness. Petechiae are particularly characteristic of echoviruses and the herpes group of viruses.

Echovirus 9 Infection

Clinical Features

A great number of viral infections may present with petechial eruptions (see Table 8–3), but echovirus 9 characteristically presents with acral petechiae and may account for epidemics of petechial eruptions. Echovirus 9 infects preschool children primarily, and they present with a syndrome of fever, sore throat, abdominal pain, and vomiting. Aseptic meningitis may occur. The petechial eruption lasts 2 to 7 days. Complete recovery follows.

Differential Diagnosis

Atypical measles, Rocky Mountain spotted fever, and meningococcemia are the major considerations of serious diseases in the differential diagnosis (see Table 8–3). Other echoviruses (particularly 4 and 7) streptococcal infections, EBV, hepatitis, rubella, coxsackieviruses, dengue, and typhus may also be considered.

Pathogenesis

The mechanism of skin injury is unknown. An incubation period of 3 to 5 days is usual.

Treatment

There is no specific treatment. Symptomatic fever control is useful.

Patient Education

The contagious nature of the disease should be emphasized.

Follow-up Visits

Follow-up visits are unnecessary.

VIRAL EXANTHEMS: VESICULOBULLOUS ERUPTIONS

After dissemination to skin during a viremic phase, there may be productive viral infection of keratinocytes, resulting in vesicle formation. This is particularly characteristic of the herpes group of viruses.

Herpes Simplex

Clinical Features

Grouped vesicles on an erythematous base are the characteristic lesions of herpes simplex in the skin, regardless of the location. On mucous membranes the blister roof is easily shed, and the blister base (erosion) is seen. Herpesvirus infections may be primary or recurrent. Recurrent infections represent reactivation of latent herpes simplex virus (HSV). Several distinct clinical patterns are seen.

Gingivostomatitis.—In infants and children, 60% of herpes simplex infections appear as a gingivostomatitis (Fig 8–8), almost always due to herpes simplex virus type I (HSV-1). It primarily appears in infants less than 6 months of age,

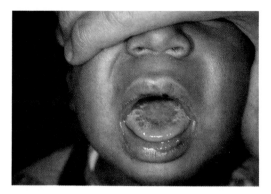

FIG 8–8.
Infant with primary herpes gingivostomatitis.

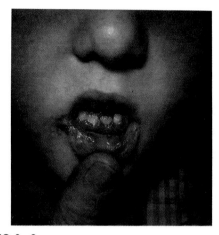

FIG 8–9.
Recurrent herpes labialis of lower lip and adjacent skin.

with pain in the mouth and throat on attempted swallowing, accompanied by fever and irritability. Erosions are extensive throughout the oral cavity, with moist crusts and foul breath. The child often is unable to eat. It lasts 7 to 14 days. Many infants are asymptomatic or suffer a mild pharyngitis on their first encounter with HSV-1.

Recurrent Herpes Simplex Virus Infection.—HSV after initial exposure may persist in nerve ganglia and be reactivated by a number of factors, including fever, ultraviolet light, trauma, and the menses. The mechanism of this reactivation of latent virus and its subsequent replication within epidermal cells are unknown. Nonetheless, once recurrent skin involvement appears, the disease is contagious and can be transmitted to other areas of skin or to other persons.

Sites of involvement vary, but the most common are the lips, eyes, cheeks, and hands. When specific skin locations are involved, the clinical appearance may vary. In all forms, however, grouped vesicles on an erythematous base are present. Regional lymphadenopathy may occur in all forms of herpes simplex.

Herpes Labialis.—Recurrent herpes simplex infection of the lip occurs in 20% of all infants and children infected with HSV, and accounts for the majority of all recurrent infections. It appears as grouped vesicles on one portion of the lip, usually the lower lip, and typically follows an acute febrile illness or intense sun exposure (Fig 8–9). The period from the appearance of the vesicles until complete healing averages 8 days. HSV-1 can be recovered from the vesicles during

the first 24 hours after onset. A prodrome of severe pain accompanies the lesions in 85% of patients.

Herpes Keratitis.—Although the cornea is involved in only 8% to 10% of children infected with HSV-1, this is a serious infection, leading to scarring and loss of vision. Any herpes simplex infection on the skin around the eye, whether or not accompanied by a red eye, should prompt a search for herpes keratitis. Dendritic ulceration of the cornea may be present and is an important characteristic. Ophthalmologic consultation should be obtained.

Herpes Hand and Finger Infections.— HSV-1 infection of the hand and finger occurs in 10% of infants and children, with perhaps a predilection for thumb suckers (Fig 8–10). Because it causes pain and erythema, it is often initially considered a pyoderma or cellulitis. A careful history will elicit the prodrome of pain, and careful examination will reveal thick-roofed blisters. Since the stratum corneum is thick on the palms and fingers, the vesicles appear deceptively deeper in the skin than in their epidermal location.

Herpes Facialis.—Recurrent episodes of grouped vesicles on the cheek or forehead are less common than other forms of HSV of the head and neck, but frequently they are confused with impetigo (Fig 8–11).

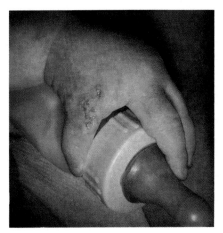

FIG 8–10.
Herpetic whitlow of thumb of baby caused by thumb sucking.

Herpes Progenitalis.—Herpes progenitalis, predominantly due to herpes simplex virus type II (HSV-2) infection, occurs almost exclusively in adolescents and young adults. Just as in HSV-1 gingivostomatitis, the symptoms may vary from none to severe widespread erosions, accompanied by fever, lymphadenopathy, severe pain, and lassitude. Recurrent herpes progenitalis characteristically presents with a prodrome of pain followed by the appearance of grouped vesicles on an erythematous base in a localized area of the genitalia. It is important to bear in mind that recurrent genital herpes is contagious and sexually transmitted. It is a common venereal disease among adolescents and young adults.

Neonatal Herpes Simplex.—Neonatal herpes simplex may develop in approximately 10% of infants born of parents with active HSV-2 infection. Signs may be present at birth, but grouped vesicles on an erythematous base may appear up to 7 days after birth (Fig 8–12). The disease may be mild, with primarily cutaneous manifestations, but central nervous system function may ultimately be impaired. More usual is a systemic illness with jaundice, progressive hepatosplenomegaly, dyspnea, hypothermia, and central nervous system symptoms. A severe encephalitis ensues, and death occurs in 48 to 96 hours.

Herpes Simplex Virus Infections in Immunodeficiency States.—In infants or children with immunodeficiency, on therapeutic immunosuppressive drugs, with severe protein-calorie malnutrition, or with cancer-associated immune deficiency, atypical forms of HSV infection occur. Grouped vesicles often become large bullae and lack an erythematous border. Deep erosions may occur even in the absence of inflammation. Purpura or hemorrhage appears within the bullous lesions. After 24 to 48 hours of local skin involvement, generalized skin involvement and visceral involvement may ensue. Herpes encephalitis or pneumonia may result in death.

Kaposi's Varicelliform Eruption (Eczema Herpeticum).—Infants and children with atopic dermatitis are susceptible to the development of generalized HSV infection characterized by high fever, lassitude, hundreds of skin vesicles, and sometimes death. Severe infections may develop in these patients, even when their dermatitis is in-

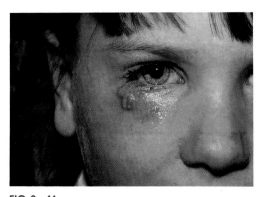

FIG 8–11.
Recurrent eruption of cheek in a child with herpes facialis.

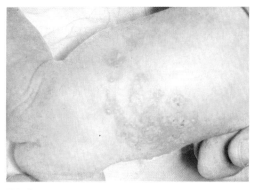

FIG 8–12.
Extensive blisters on trunk in neonatal herpes.

active (Fig 8–13). Rarely, disseminated HSV infection may develop in children with a variety of other skin problems, such as Darier's disease or burns.

Differential Diagnosis

A rapid clinical clue to HSV (or varicella-zoster virus) infection is the finding of epidermal giant cells on a Tzanck preparation (Fig 8–14; see Chapter 2 for technique). This finding correlates well with HSV cultures, but isolation of the virus is diagnostic. Other virus infections to be considered in the differential diagnosis of herpes simplex are listed in Table 8–4.

Gingivostomatitis.—Gingivostomatitis must be differentiated from aphthous ulcers, which are shallow, irregular, ragged, recurrent ulcerations on the oral mucosa. In erythema multiforme, in contrast to HSV gingivostomatitis, symmetric iris and target lesions are present on the skin. In herpangina, which is caused by enteroviruses, ulcers are limited to the anterior tonsillar pillars and have a linear arrangement; isolation of coxsackievirus A confirms the diagnosis. The Tzanck smear is most helpful in distinguishing HSV from the other causes of oral erosions.

Recurrent Herpes Simplex Virus Infection.—Recurrent skin infection due to HSV must be differentiated from herpes-zoster. Since both infections demonstrate epidermal giant cells on

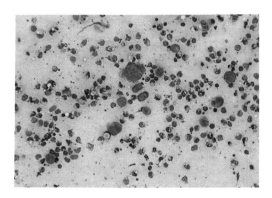

FIG 8–14.
Photomicrograph of smear of blister contents showing giant cells in herpes simplex infection. (Tzanck smear.)

Tzanck smear, viral culture is the only method for differentiating the two on first infection. The history of recurrent lesions in the same skin area suggests HSV rather than varicella-zoster virus.

Herpes Labialis.—Impetigo may mimic herpes labialis. Gram's stain and bacterial culture of the lesions will help distinguish the two.

Herpes Keratitis.—Herpes keratitis should be differentiated from bacterial conjunctivitis and epidemic adenovirus keratoconjunctivitis. The characteristic grouped vesicles on an erythematous base in periocular skin will help distinguish HSV from these infections. Furthermore, HSV is usually unilateral, whereas bacterial and adenovirus infections, although initially unilateral, often become bilateral.

TABLE 8–4.
Vesiculobullous Virus Infections

Common
Herpes simplex
Varicella-zoster
Hand-foot-and-mouth disease
(coxsackievirus A16)
Uncommon
Orf
Influenza
Coxsackieviruses A5, A9, A10
Echoviruses 4, 9, 11, 17, 25
Variola
Vaccinia

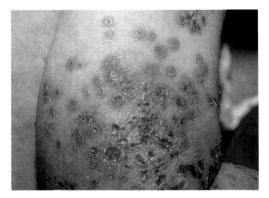

FIG 8–13.
Discrete ulcers and hundreds of erosions associated with dermatitis in infant with atopic dermatitis and widespread herpes simplex infection (Kaposi's varicelliform eruption, eczema herpeticum).

Herpes Hand and Finger Infections.—
HSV hand and finger infections are often confused with bacterial cellulitis. A Tzanck smear of
the vesicle base is a rapid method of distinguishing HSV from bacterial infection.

Herpes Facialis.—Impetigo may mimic facial herpes on the cheek or forehead. A Tzanck
smear will often distinguish the two.

Herpes Progenitalis.—Herpes progenitalis
may mimic other venereal diseases. Also, it is
not unusual to note more than one venereal
disease simultaneously in the sexually active person. A smear and culture for gonorrhea and a
serologic test for syphilis are most helpful in such
cases.

Neonatal Herpes Simplex.—Other congenital infections (e.g., toxoplasmosis, cytomegalovirus infection, congenital rubella, and coxsackievirus B infections) may mimic neonatal HSV. Vesicular skin lesions are not present in any of
these, however. In neonatal bacterial sepsis, isolated vesicular or pustulovesicular lesions may occur. They are not grouped as in HSV infection,
and Gram's stain and bacterial culture will distinguish them from herpes simplex.

Pathogenesis
HSV-1 and HSV-2 are complex DNA viruses
with an incubation period of 2 to 12 days. They
are epidermotropic viruses, and productive viral
infection occurs within keratinocytes. Active infection occurs despite high titers of specific antibody. This no doubt reflects the intracellular infection characteristic of these viruses in which antibody cannot interact with the active virus, which
is transferred from cell to cell. There are two possible outcomes of epidermal cellular infection:
productive and nonproductive infection. Productive infection is characterized by the biosynthesis
of infectious progeny and epidermal cell death,
producing the intraepidermal vesicle. Nonproductive infection results in the perpetuation of all or
part of the viral genome and survival of the epidermal cell, producing epidermal giant cells. It is
uncertain whether fusion of several epidermal
cells or nuclear division without cytoplasmic division is responsible for the epidermal giant cells
seen on Tzanck smear.

Treatment
Oral acyclovir capsules may be the specific
therapy of the future for localized cutaneous
herpes simplex infections. Intravenous acyclovir
has been safe and effective in children, but oral
dosages have not as yet been established. In severe primary herpes simplex infections, such as
herpes gingivostomatitis or Kaposi's varicelliform
eruption, acyclovir may be very useful. In localized forms of herpes simplex, such as those limited to a certain small area of skin, use of acyclovir ointment 5%, six times a day, may provide
some symptomatic relief and shorten the duration
of viral shedding. Neither topical nor systemic
acyclovir, however, will prevent recurrences of
herpes simplex, although it may prevent spread of
the lesion to adjacent skin sites or to family members or playmates. In patients experiencing frequent, severe recurrences, 6 months of acyclovir
prophylaxis may be considered.

In herpes keratitis, topical 5-iodo-2-deoxyuri-
dine ophthalmic ointment may be most efficacious. Similarly, topical adenine arabinoside (Vira-
A) is also useful for herpes simplex keratitis. Before initiation of treatment, consultation with an
ophthalmologist is recommended.

In neonatal herpes simplex infections and in
Kaposi's varicelliform eruption, intravenous acyclovir and adenine arabinoside have proved effective. Supportive measures, such as fever control,
maintenance of fluid and electrolyte balance, and
thermal regulation, are necessary. Infected patients shed virus and should be isolated.

Patient Education
Patients with local cutaneous infection
should be informed of the contagious nature of
the disease. Avoidance of precipitating factors may
be most useful (e.g., avoiding sun exposure or using sunscreens in sun-activated recurrent herpes
simplex virus and discontinuing sexual activity in
herpes progenitalis). In patients with atopic dermatitis or other skin diseases susceptible to disseminated HSV infections, optimal treatment of
the underlying skin disease and consistency of
care may be useful in preventing future episodes.

Follow-up Visits
Careful ophthalmologic follow-up (every 1 to
2 days) is required in herpes keratitis. Disseminated infections often require hospitalization and
intensive supportive therapy. Neonatal herpes

simplex virus requires careful developmental and neurologic examinations at 3-month intervals. Cutaneous herpes lesions may recur throughout childhood following neonatal herpes simplex.

Varicella-Zoster Virus Infections

Clinical Features

Varicella (Chickenpox).—Varicella is characterized by the abrupt onset of crops of skin lesions. Individual lesions begin as faint erythematous macules that progress to edematous papules and then to vesicles during a 24- to 48-hour period. The vesicles then develop moist crusts that dry and are shed, leaving a shallow erosion. Successive crops of lesions appear during the next 2 to 5 days, so that at any one time several stages of skin lesions can be observed concomitantly: macules, papules, vesicles, and crusted lesions (Fig 8–15). Lesions frequently involve mucous membranes, and isolated erosions may be seen in the conjunctiva, oral cavity, or nasal mucosa. Fever is usually low grade, and associated symptoms are mild. In a single family, varicella lesions may vary from fewer than ten in one child to hundreds in another. The total duration is 7 to 10 days. The disease is highly contagious from 1 to 2 days before the onset of the skin eruption to 5 to 6 days afterward.

Secondary bacterial infection of one to three of the many varicella lesions is common, producing the so-called bullous varicella. Often, this is the result of *Staphylococcus aureus* infection. Severe generalized varicella-zoster virus (VZV) infections may develop in immunosuppressed persons, with high fever, encephalitis, pneumonia, hepatitis, or disseminated intravascular coagulation.

Herpes Zoster.—In children who have previously had varicella, recurrent infection results in herpes zoster. Two to three groups of lesions appear within several adjacent dermatomes (Fig 8–16). They begin as macules and edematous papules and progress to grouped vesicles on an erythematous base. Rarely, dermatomal pain may precede the eruption in children, and postzoster neuralgia may also occur, but rarely. Almost all children, however, have a mild illness lasting 7 to 10 days. Pruritus may be severe. The thoracic segments are involved in 60% of children with herpes zoster, with the childhood distribution depicted in Figure 8–17. If the nose is involved, herpes zoster keratitis is likely to occur, and it may be as severe as herpes simplex virus keratitis. Ophthalmic zoster is also more likely to be associated with severe pain than is zoster of other skin regions in children. Herpes zoster involving the

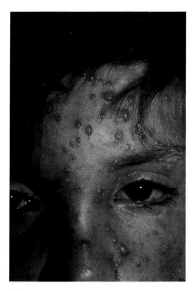

FIG 8–15.
Blisters, papules, and crusted lesion in a child with varicella.

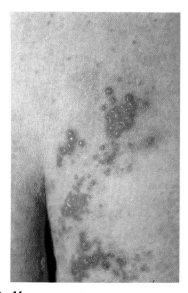

FIG 8–16.
Several groups of blisters occurring over adjacent thoracic dermatomes in a child with herpes zoster.

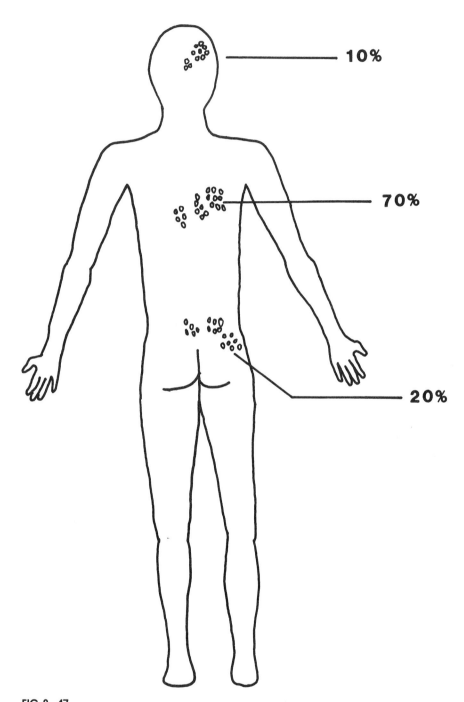

FIG 8–17.
Common distribution of herpes zoster in childhood: 10% cranial nerve involvement; 70% thoracic dermatome; 20% lumbosacral involvement.

skin around the eyes, nose, and forehead requires a careful ophthalmologic examination. Herpes zoster may be the initial finding in acquired immune deficiency (AIDS), but is rarely the presenting finding in childhood cancer. In immunosuppressed children, disseminated herpes zoster occurs 1 to 5 days after the dermatome infection begins. Even immunosuppressed children with disseminated herpes zoster recover without sequelae, but visceral involvement can occur. Involvement of the geniculate ganglion results in pain in the ear, vesicles on the pinnae, and facial palsy (Ramsay Hunt syndrome) (Fig 8–18) Motor paralysis of other nerves may follow herpes zoster.

Differential Diagnosis

Varicella.—Typical varicella is seldom confused with other illnesses (see Table 8–4). In hand-foot-and-mouth disease, vesicles are limited to acral areas, and vesicular forms of insect bite reactions (papular urticaria) usually have a typical history of bites. Acute parapsoriasis may mimic varicella in that it produces crops of lesions in different stages. True vesicles are less common in parapsoriasis, and papules with central purpura are more common. Rickettsialpox and dermatitis herpetiformis are rare in children, but may mimic varicella. A Tzanck smear of the vesicle base will

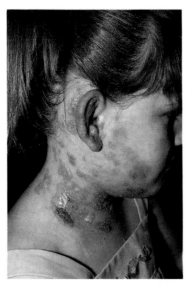

FIG 8–18.
Involvement of ear and adjacent skin associated with facial palsy in herpes zoster of geniculate ganglion (Ramsay Hunt syndrome).

differentiate varicella from these vesicular diseases. Occasionally, disseminated HSV infection will mimic varicella. Viral cultures may be necessary to distinguish between herpes simplex and varicella.

Herpes Zoster.—Local cutaneous HSV infections may also mimic herpes zoster in children. Usually, HSV involves one group of vesicles and herpes zoster involves three to four clusters of grouped vesicles. Viral culture may be required to distinguish the two. Impetigo is sometimes confused with herpes zoster, but honey-colored crusts, Gram's stain of lesions, and bacterial cultures will help distinguish it from herpes zoster.

Pathogenesis

VZV is a complex herpes group DNA virus that infects in much the same way as herpes simplex (see Herpes Simplex, Pathogenesis). The incubation period ranges from 10 to 27 days and averages 14 days. Productive infection occurs within keratinocytes, producing ballooning degeneration of cells and an intraepidermal blister form.

Treatment

In the healthy child varicella does not require specific therapy. Wet dressings, soothing baths, and oral antihistamines will give symptomatic relief of the pruritus in children. Zoster immune globulin, if given within 72 hours after exposure of an immunosuppressed host, may modify varicella. Secondary bacterial infection of varicella lesions should be treated with antistaphylococcal drugs, such as dicloxacillin, 12.5 to 25.0 mg/kg/day in four divided oral doses for 7 to 10 days.

Systemic antiviral agents, such as intravenous acyclovir, have been used for childhood VZV infections with success. Oral acyclovir has been successful in VZV in adults. In immunosuppressed children, children with ophthalmic zoster, or with the Ramsay Hunt syndrome, acyclovir may be a valuable therapeutic strategy. The role of varicella vaccine is unclear.

Patient Education

The highly contagious nature of varicella should be emphasized, and the child should be isolated until all lesions are crusted, which usually occurs 5 to 6 days after eruption of the lesions. Contact with the elderly, neonates, and immunocompromised children should be avoided.

Postvaricella scarring is always a concern for parents. What appear to be highly vascular purple-red scars return to normal skin color in 6 to 12 months and often leave little evidence of scarring. Patients should be advised to wait at least 1 year before seeking help for postvaricella scars.

Follow-up Visits

A visit in 48 hours to assess the development of secondary bacterial infection is useful in children with varicella. Children with disseminated zoster, ophthalmic zoster, or the Ramsay Hunt syndrome should be seen daily until symptoms improve.

Hand-Foot-and-Mouth Disease

Clinical Features

An abrupt onset of scattered papules that progress to oval or linear vesicles in an acral distribution should suggest hand-foot-and-mouth disease. The individual lesions are seen on the palms, fingertips, interdigital webs, and soles of the feet and are few in number (Figs 8–19 and 8–20). Scattered oral lesions may also be seen. Such children are not ill and characteristically are afebrile. During epidemics, incomplete forms may be seen. In some epidemics, skin lesions may

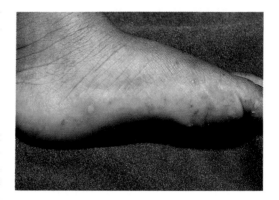

FIG 8–20.
Oval blisters on foot in a child with hand-foot-and-mouth syndrome.

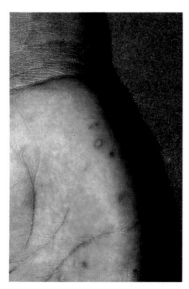

FIG 8–19.
Oval blisters on palm in a child with hand-foot-and-mouth disease (coxsackievirus A16 infection).

be more numerous and involve both proximal and distal extremities. Oral lesions appear as discrete, shallow, oval erosions.

Differential Diagnosis

In the early nonvesicular stage, rubella and the other morbilliform lesions must be considered (see Table 8–4), but the sparsity of lesions and the lack of truncal involvement make those diagnoses unlikely. In the vesicular stage, the disease may be confused with varicella, but the acral distribution of the lesions, the lack of pruritus, and the oval to linear nature of the individual vesicles will help differentiate hand-foot-and-mouth disease from varicella. Insect bites may also mimic hand-foot-and-mouth disease, particularly if they occur on acral-exposed skin. Isolation of coxsackievirus from throat washings or serologic evidence will distinguish.

Pathogenesis

Several coxsackievirus group A enteroviruses have been found to be responsible for hand-foot-and-mouth disease. The epidemic form is almost always due to coxsackievirus A16, but coxsackieviruses A5 and A10 have also been associated. The incubation period is 3 to 5 days, and the virus enters by the enteric route, with the eruption reflecting a viremic phase. The disease is contagious from 2 days before to 2 days after the onset of the eruption, but virus excretion in feces may persist for 2 weeks.

Treatment

No treatment is necessary.

Patient Education

Parents should be informed of the mild nature of the disease and of its differentiation from other viral exanthems. Good hygiene may limit household spread.

Follow-up Visits

Follow-up visits are unnecessary.

VIRAL EXANTHEMS: PAPULONODULAR EXANTHEMS

Papular Acrodermatitis (Gianotti-Crosti Syndrome)

Clinical Features

Groups of large, flat-topped, nonpruritic papules appear in acral areas in papular acrodermatitis. They involve the cheeks, buttocks, and limbs and are particularly prominent over the elbows and knees (Fig 8–21). The skin lesions are preceded by low-grade fever and mild upper respiratory symptoms. Of children described as having this syndrome, 85% are less than 3 years of age, although it may occur in school-age children. The eruption lasts 2 to 8 weeks. Generalized lymphadenopathy and hepatosplenomegaly develop in some children along with the cutaneous eruption. In such children, atypical lymphocytes are seen in

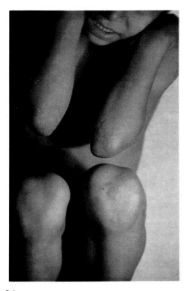

FIG 8–21.
Skin-colored papules of elbows and knees in Gianotti-Crosti syndrome.

peripheral blood films, and liver enzyme levels are elevated. Hepatitis-associated antigen can be detected in these children 10 days after the eruption appears. Icterus does not develop.

Differential Diagnosis

In irritant contact dermatitis, atopic dermatitis, and lichen planus, flat-topped acral papules that mimic papular acrodermatitis may be present, but they are usually associated with severe pruritus and a history of long-lasting itchy disease.

Pathogenesis

In the majority of infants with papular acrodermatitis in the United States, no associated virus has been identified. In Europe, 50% of patients with papular acrodermatitis have mild viral hepatitis B; HBsAg has been demonstrated in the lymph nodes in such children, with liver biopsy findings consistent with acute viral hepatitis. HBsAg antigenemia persists for 2 months in affected children and may last for several years. Japanese investigators have suggested that a particular subtype of hepatitis is associated with papular acrodermatitis, and that this subtype is usually not found in Japan or the United States but predominates in Europe.

Treatment

No treatment is needed. Lesions do not usually respond to topical steroids.

Patient Education

The prolonged nature of the eruption should be emphasized. In infants with hepatosplenomegaly or lymphadenopathy, or both, the importance of searching for viral hepatitis should be discussed with the parents, and modes of transmission of hepatitis B should be emphasized.

Follow-up Visits

A visit 2 weeks after the initial visit to determine whether the signs and symptoms of hepatitis have developed is recommended.

Human Immunodeficiency Virus Infections

Clinical Features

The cutaneous manifestations of human immunodeficiency virus (HIV) disease in children are predominantly the result of bacterial, fungal, and viral infections. Clinical findings of perinatally acquired HIV infection are noted at about 4 months but may occur as early as 3 months or as late as 21 months. The initial clinical manifestations are lymphadenopathy, chronic diarrhea, failure to thrive, and hepatosplenomegaly. The clinical disease, that is, AIDS, has many features of hereditary immunodeficiencies, such as severe combined immunodeficiency. Chronic cough, hypoxemia, and clubbing of fingers are the features of *Pneumocystis carinii* pneumonia, the most common infection in children with HIV infection. The first cutaneous sign of AIDS is persistent thrush, recalcitrant to antiyeast therapy. Esophageal involvement is frequent, and a resistant candidal diaper rash often accompanies the thrush. Thrush is common in infants less than 1 year old, and the other features of lymphadenopathy, failure to thrive and hepatosplenomegaly, are clues to the possibility of HIV infection.

A dermatitis that mimics seborrheic dermatitis is observed in half the children with HIV infection. It is not specific and there are no unique features. Severe herpetic gingivostomatitis may be seen or herpes zoster may be a presenting finding. Children with HIV infection may have hundreds of lesions of molluscum contagiosum, in contrast to 10 to 20 seen in normal children. Giant molluscum lesions may be seen. Recurrent pyodermas with *S. aureus* are frequent, and the children frequently develop severe cellulitis or bacterial sepsis from skin infections, which should remain localized. Dermatophyte infections of the nails, quite rare in infancy, may be found, and tinea faciei is also seen. Severe, crusted scabies with hundreds of mites, the so-called Norwegian scabies, is reported. Purpura as the result of thrombocytopenia or vasculitis may occur. Drug eruptions are far more frequent than expected, particularly with trimethoprim-sulfamethoxazole. A picture that mimics acrodermatitis enteropathica may be the result of nutritional zinc deficiency, and other cutaneous findings of malnutrition may be seen. Kaposi's sarcoma of skin has not been reported in children.

Differential Diagnosis

Virtually every skin infection known can be included in the differential diagnosis, but hereditary immune defects and malnutrition states will mimic HIV infection. An HIV serology, confirmed by Western blotting technique, is the most sensitive test to distinguish HIV infection, and it should be done on every infant or child suspected of having immunodeficiency or severe nutritional deficiency.

Pathogenesis

HIV is a retrovirus that selectively infects T lymphocytes, populations of lymphocytes that may be epidermotropic. It has been isolated from blood, tears, semen, saliva, vaginal secretions, cerebrospinal fluid, and breast milk. Eighty percent of infants are infected by transplacental passage from the mother. Older children are infected by sexual contact, and in hemophiliacs blood transfusions are a source of infection. If the infant's mother used intravenous drugs or was a prostitute, the likelihood of infection is high. HIV relentlessly destroys cell-mediated immunity, leaving the infected child at the mercy of a huge variety of opportunistic pathogens.

Treatment

Children are best treated at large medical centers experienced in management of AIDS. Treatments are directed at specific infections that are acquired. The antiviral drug zidovudine (Retrovir), formerly called azidothymidine (AZT) may suppress the disease.

Patient Education

Information about the transmission of AIDS and support groups for AIDS patients are essential. Patients should be informed about the susceptibility to a great variety of infections.

Follow-up Visits

Frequent visits are required and are determined by the nature of infections.

VIRUS-INDUCED TUMORS

Certain viruses do not destroy keratinocytes but induce proliferation, resulting in a benign tumor of skin.

Warts

Clinical Features

Warts are virus-induced epidermal tumors with a variety of clinical presentations, each of which can be correlated with one of the various subtypes of human papillomavirus (HPV) responsible for the infection. HPV, a small DNA virus, in-

TABLE 8–5.

Clinical Warts and Associated Human
Papillomavirus Type

Clinical Wart	HPV Type
Common wart	HPV-2a, b, c, d, e
Plantar (weight-bearing) wart	HPV-1a, b, c
	HPV-4
Flat wart	HPV-3a, b
	HPV-10a, b
Condyloma acuminatum	HPV-6a, b, c, d, e, f
	HPV-11a, b
	HPV-16

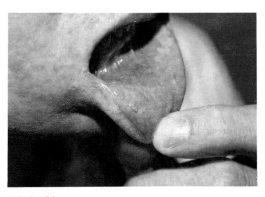

FIG 8–23.
Filiform wart of lip.

duces epidermal proliferation in all clinical forms of warts, producing the characteristic epidermal tumors. Table 8–5 lists the clinical types of warts with the corresponding HPV type thought to be responsible for them.

The common wart (verruca vulgaris) appears as a solitary papule with an irregular, scaly surface. Common warts may be found anywhere on the skin (Fig 8–22).

Filiform warts appear as thin projections from the skin surface on a narrow stalk. In children they are usually seen on the lips, nose, or eyelids (Fig 8–23).

Flat warts (verruca plana) are multiple, flat-topped, broad, skin-colored papules. They usually appear in groups and are found particularly on the face and extremities (Fig 8–24).

Plantar warts are common warts that occur in weight-bearing areas of the feet, where the papule is pushed into the skin in such a way that the verrucous surface appears level with the skin surface (Fig 8–25).

Venereal warts (condylomata acuminata),

multiple, confluent papules with an irregular surface, appear on the genital mucosa or adjacent skin, or both (Figs 8–26 and 8–27). Common warts also appear on genital skin; therefore, the finding of genital warts does not necessarily predict sexual transmission.

Periungual warts occur around the cuticles of several fingers or toes and are spread by trauma to the cuticle area (Fig 8–28).

The natural history of warts is variable, but most spontaneously resolve in 12 to 24 months. Most warts are asymptomatic, but in pressure- or weight-bearing areas they may be painful.

Differential Diagnosis

Common warts and filiform warts are so characteristic that they present no diagnostic problem. Plantar warts must be distinguished from calluses, which have a smooth rather than an irregular surface. Venereal warts must be distinguished from syphilitic lesions (condylomata

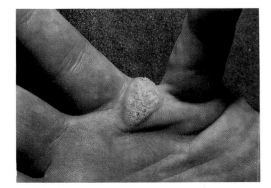

FIG 8–22.
Common wart of hand.

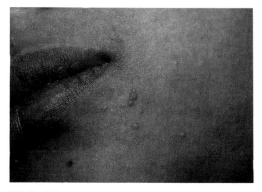

FIG 8–24.
Multiple flat warts (verruca plana) of face.

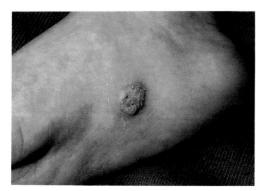

FIG 8–25.
Plantar (weight-bearing) wart.

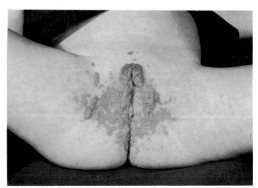

FIG 8–27.
Venereal warts in female infant.

lata), which appear as moist papules in genital areas. A serologic test for syphilis will readily distinguish the two. Flat warts are often overlooked and may be misdiagnosed as lichen planus, lichen nitidus, seborrheic keratosis, or birthmarks. The linear or grouped arrangement of flat warts is helpful in diagnosis, as is their occurrence along areas of skin trauma.

Pathogenesis

Immunity to warts is not well understood, but inducing inflammation around a single wart may result in regression of all others. The wart virus is located within the epidermal cell nucleus, which may be an immunologic privileged site where viral antigen has little opportunity to interact with antibody or white cells.

Treatment

All wart therapy is designed to be cytodestructive, that is, to destroy all the epidermal cells

within the wart tumor and, it is hoped, all the wart virus as well. Recurrence rate for all wart therapy is high, with the best results limiting recurrences to 15% of patients. Table 8–6 presents the recommended therapy for viral warts.

Cryotherapy.—A cryosurgery probe or copper bar cooled in liquid nitrogen may be used for cryotherapy, but a cotton swab with a loose, pointed tip is most commonly used. The cotton swab is dipped in a thermos containing liquid nitrogen ($-195°$ C), and the saturated swab is applied to the center of the wart until a white "ice ball" extending 1 to 3 mm beyond the margin of the wart is formed. The freeze is maintained 10 to 30 seconds. Warts greater than 7 mm in diameter should not be frozen, because scarring is likely to result. In 1 to 2 days, a blister, sometimes hemorrhagic, forms. Removing the blister roof in 1 week and refreezing may be necessary.

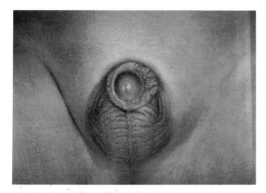

FIG 8–26.
Venereal warts (condylomata acuminata) of foreskin in infant.

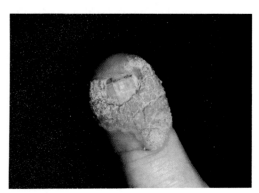

FIG 8–28.
Periungual warts.

TABLE 8–6.

Treatment of Viral Warts

| Type of Wart | Treatment | | Response Rate (%) |
	First Choice	Alternative	
Common	Cryotherapy	Salicylic acid paint	80–90
Periungual	Cantharidin	Salicylic acid paint	60
Flat	Retinoic acid	Salicylic acid paint	50
Filiform	Surgery		80
Plantar	Salicylic acid plaster	Salicylic acid paint	60
Venereal	Podophyllum	Cryotherapy	90

Salicylic Acid Paints.—Concentrations of salicylic acid above 20% result in the necrosis of epidermal cells when applied to the skin surface. Salicylic acid paints are applied once or twice a day for 2 to 4 weeks. On thick skin, such as that of the palms and soles, a preparation of salicylic acid 16.7% and lactic acid 16.7% in flexible collodion is used. Weaker concentrations, such as salicylic acid 20% in flexible collodion, may be used for flat warts. Redness around the base of the wart and itching herald the onset of wart regression.

Salicylic Acid Plasters.—Cotton plasters impregnated with salicylic acid 40% are applied to plantar warts. The plaster is cut to the size of the wart with scissors and firmly taped onto the skin, so that it may remain there for 3 to 5 days. Sweating solubilizes the acid out of the plaster, so that it may enter the skin. The plaster is removed every 3 to 5 days, the dead white epidermal tissue is removed gently, and a new plaster is taped in place. Three to six weeks of treatment may be necessary.

Retinoic Acid.—Retinoic acid is used as a 0.025% cream and is applied once or twice daily to flat warts. Resolution may occur in 2 to 4 weeks.

Cantharidin.—Cantharidin is a vesicant formed from the extract of whole frozen blister beetles and causes separation of epidermal cells. It is applied directly to periungual warts and covered with tape for 24 hours. A tender blister forms and is eventually sloughed off. Regulating the size of the blister is difficult.

Podophyllum.—Podophyllum is a metaphase inhibitor that is used in a 25% solution in alcohol and carefully applied to moist venereal warts. It must be washed off in 4 hours. Therapy may be repeated in 1 week. Podophyllum is most effective on warts on mucous surfaces. It is neurotoxic, causing an areflexic coma, and should never be applied to extensive areas of mucosa or given to patients for home use.

Surgery.—Filiform warts have a stalk of uninfected epidermis at their base. They may be excised by snipping the base with sharp scissors at skin level. Local hemostasis with pressure and gel foam or ferric subsulfate will be required. Excision of other warts results in a high recurrence rate (in 60% to 80%), and sharp scalpel surgery is generally contraindicated in warts. Scarring is a complication of surgical removal of warts.

Other Therapies.—X-ray treatment and electrocautery should not be used in children because of the high recurrence rate and high incidence of side effects. The great variety of unproved wart therapies generally should be avoided, particularly if they have a high likelihood of side effects.

Patient Education

The natural history of the wart should be emphasized. It may be best to leave many warts untreated.

Follow-up Visits

A visit 1 to 2 weeks after initiating therapy is needed to ascertain the need for retreatment.

Molluscum Contagiosum

Clinical Features

White or white-yellow papules with a central umbilication are seen in molluscum contagiosum (Fig 8–29). The lesions may vary in diameter

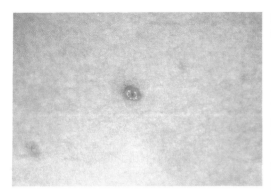

FIG 8–29.
Umbilicated dome-shaped papule characteristic of molluscum contagiosum.

from 1 to 15 mm, and a dermatitis often surrounds larger lesions (Fig 8–30). Genital grouped lesions may be seen in sexually active adolescents. Multiple lesions of molluscum contagiosum may be superimposed on the skin of children with atopic dermatitis. Hundreds of lesions of molluscum should raise the suspicion of AIDS. Extrusion of papule contents onto a microscope slide and Wright's stain will reveal the epidermal cytoplasmic viral inclusions.

Differential Diagnosis

Warts, closed comedones, and tiny epidermal cysts may mimic molluscum contagiosum. Careful inspection, however, will reveal the central umbilication characteristic of molluscum contagiosum, and microscopic examination will differentiate the disease from other skin papules. At first glance, molluscum may appear to be blisters, but palpation and careful inspection will reveal their solid nature.

Pathogenesis

Molluscum contagiosum is caused by a poxvirus that induces epidermal cell proliferation. Two types are recognized by restriction endonuclease analysis of viral DNA. Molluscum type 1 is believed responsible for common lesions on the extremities, head, and neck. Type 2 is most often associated with genital lesions. The incubation period is 2 to 7 weeks, and the child is contagious as long as active lesions are present.

Treatment

Removal of a papule is curative. In older children, the use of a sharp dermal curet to remove the entire papule is the treatment of choice. In infants and young children, this method is frightening and painful. In such children, a drop of cantharidin or trichloroacetic acid 25% applied with a wooden toothpick to the central umbilication and then neutralized with alcohol is less traumatic than excision. Recurrences are common, since it is often difficult to detect the pinpoint early lesions of molluscum.

Patient Education

The highly contagious nature of molluscum contagiosum should be emphasized. The lesions are benign, and patients should not be unduly concerned.

Follow-up Visits

A visit 1 to 2 weeks after initial therapy is advisable to determine the need for retreatment.

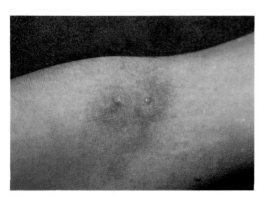

FIG 8–30.
Erythema and scaling surrounding resolving lesions of molluscum contagiosum (molluscum dermatitis).

BIBLIOGRAPHY

Balfour HH Jr, Englund JA: Antiviral drugs in pediatrics. *Am J Dis Child* 1989; 143:1307.

Bell LM, Naides SJ, Stoffman P, et al: Human parvovirus B19 infection among hospital staff members after contact with infected patients. *N Engl J Med* 1989; 321:485.

Bennett RS, Powell KB: Human papillomaviruses: Association between laryngeal papillomas and genital warts. *Pediatr Infect Dis J* 1987; 6:229.

Brodsky AL: Atypical measles. *JAMA* 1972; 222:1415.

Chadwick EG, Chadwick EG, Shulman ST: Advances in antiviral therapy: Acyclovir. *Pediatr Dermatol* 1984; 2:64.

Cherry JD: Newer viral exanthems. *Adv Pediatr* 1969; 16:233.

Dery P, Marks MI, Shapera R: Clinical manifestations of coxsackie virus infections in children. *Am J Dis Child* 1974; 128:464.

Donowitz LG: Practical infection control for human immunodeficiency virus infection in children. *Pediatr Infect Dis J* 1989; 8:133.

Douglass MC, Koblenzer PJ, Moroz B, et al: Management of warts in children. *Pediatr Dermatol* 1987; 4:36.

Gilchrest B, Baden HP: Photodistribution of viral exanthems. *Pediatrics* 1974; 54:136.

Glover MT, Atherton DJ: Congenital infection with herpes simplex type 1. *Pediatr Dermatol* 1987; 4:336.

Hall C: The return of the Boston exanthem. *Am J Dis Child* 1977; 131:323.

Hayman JM Jr, Read WA: Some clinical observations on an outbreak of jaundice following yellow fever vaccination. *Am J Med Sci* 1945; 209:281.

Highet AS: Viral warts. *Semin Dermatol* 1988; 7:53.

Huff JC: Herpes zoster. *Curr Probl Dermatol* 1988; 1:8.

Huff JC, Bean B, Laskin O, et al: Therapy of herpes zoster with acyclovir. *Am J Med* 1988; 85:84–89.

Ishimaru Y, Ishimaru H, Toda G, et al: An epidemic of infantile papular acrodermatitis (Gianotti's disease) in Japan associated with hepatitis-B surface antigen subtype ayw. *Lancet* 1976; 1:707.

Kawasaki T, Kosaki F, Okawa S, et al: A new infantile acute febrile mucocutaneous lymph node syndrome prevailing in Japan. *Pediatrics* 1974; 54:271.

Kerdel FA, Penneys NS: Cutaneous manifestations of AIDS in adults and infants. *Curr Probl Dermatol* 1989; 1:101.

Kibrick S: Herpes simplex infection at term: What to do with mother, newborn, and nursery personnel. *JAMA* 1980; 243:157.

Koch WC, Adler SF: Human parvovirus B 19 in women of childbearing age and within families. *Pediatr Infect Dis J* 1989; 8:83.

Kohl S: The neonatal human's immune response to herpes simplex viral infection: A critical review. *Pediatr Infect Dis J* 1989; 8:67.

Koskiniemi M, Happonen J-M, Jarvenpaa A-L, et al: Neonatal herpes simplex virus infection: A report of 43 patients. *Pediatr Infect Dis J* 1989; 8:30.

Krabbe S, Hesse J, Udall P, et al: Primary Epstein-Barr virus infection in early childhood. *Arch, Dis Child SG149.* 1981; 56:49–52.

MMWR: Risks associated with human parvovirus B19 infection. *Arch Dermatol* 1989; 125:475.

Niederman JC, Miller G, Pearson HA, et al: Infectious mononucleosis: Epstein-Barr virus shedding in saliva and the oropharynx. *N Engl J Med* 1976; 294:1355.

Novelli VM, Brunell PA, Geiser CF, et al: Herpes zoster in children with acute lymphocytic leukemia. *Am J Dis Child* 1988; 142:71.

Olding-Stenkvist E, Bjorvatn B: Rapid detection of measles virus in skin rashes by immunofluorescence. *J Infect Dis* 1976; 134:463.

Pattison JR: Diseases caused by the human parvovirus B19. *Arch Dis Child* 1988; 63:1426.

Porter CD, Blake NW, Archard LC, et al: Molluscum contagiosum virus types in genital and nongenital lesions. *Br J Dermatol* 1989; 120:37.

Prose NS, Mendez H, Menikoff H, et al: Pediatric human immunodeficiency virus infection and its cutaneous manifestations. *Pediatr Dermatol* 1987; 4:67.

Report of the Committee on Infectious Diseases. 21st ed. Chicago: American Academy of Pediatrics, 1988.

Rubenstein D, Esterly NB, Fretzin D: The Gianotti-Crosti syndrome. *Pediatrics* 1978; 61:433.

Segool R, Lejtenyi C, Taussig LM: Articular and cutaneous prodromal manifestations of viral hepatitis. *J Pediatr* 1975; 87:709.

Tindall JP, Callaway JL: Hand, foot and mouth disease: It's more common than you think. *Am J Dis Child* 1972; 124:372.

Trepo CC, Thivolet J, Prince AM: Australia antigen and polyarteritis nodosa. Am J Dis Child 1972; 123:390.

Tunnessen WW Jr: Cutaneous infections. *Pediatr Clin North Am* 1983; 30:515.

9 _____ Papulosquamous Disorders

Children with papulosquamous disorders have skin lesions characterized by red or violaceous macules that progress to papules and develop scales. The exact prevalence of this group of diseases is unknown. Psoriasis has a yearly prevalence of 3.1 per 1,000 children. Pityriasis rosea accounts for a further increase in prevalence of papulosquamous eruptions in childhood. Thus, papulosquamous disorders are common in children and should be readily recognized by those caring for them.

PSORIASIS

Clinical Features

Psoriasis is thought to be a hereditary disorder that requires an interplay of genetic and environmental factors for full clinical expression. Psoriasis is a clinical diagnosis, based on the presence of thick, silvery scales on at least some lesions, the characteristic distribution and nail involvement, and presence of the isomorphic phenomenon. The eruption consists of erythematous macular or papular lesions that develop a thick, silvery scale (Fig 9–1). Discrete, scaly papules (guttate lesions) may be seen, or groups of papules may coalesce to form raised, sharply marginated erythematous plaques. The sites of predilection for psoriasis include the scalp, ears, eyebrows, elbows, knees, gluteal crease (Fig 9–2), genitalia, and nails. Complete examination of the entire cutaneous surface is necessary because lesions may be few in number. The most common clinical picture of psoriasis in childhood is involvement of the elbows, knees, and scalp by a few plaques. Sixty-six percent of children have this form.

Guttate psoriasis, the term given to the form of psoriasis with multiple discrete papules, begins on the trunk as multiple erythematous macules that mimic a viral exanthem (Fig 9–3). Guttate psoriasis was the form of psoriasis seen in 34% of children in one study. As noted, the lesions progress to papules that develop a silvery scale. These droplike papules (gutta, Latin for drop); they are seen predominantly on the trunk and proximal extremities. Guttate psoriasis may follow a sore throat, particularly streptococcal pharyngitis, by 2 to 3 weeks. Follicular accentuation of the skin lesions may be seen. Children with guttate psoriasis should be evaluated for pharyngeal or rectal streptococcal infection.

The isomorphic (Koebner's) phenomenon, in which psoriatic lesions develop in sites of skin trauma several days after the traumatic event, is a useful diagnostic feature of psoriasis. It occurs in a linear fashion along a scratch, but may also be precipitated by lacerations, abrasions, sunburn, insect bites, or pressure (Fig 9–4).

Scalp involvement with psoriasis results in accumulation of thick scales covering the entire scalp area, with thickened scales along the frontal hairline and behind the ears (Fig 9–5). The scalp is involved in 82% of children with psoriasis. Hair loss does not occur.

Involvement of the palms and soles is uncommon in children, but psoriasis may appear as fissured, painful, symmetric plaques or multiple small, sterile pustules.

Genital involvement (perineal area, penis, inguinal folds, labia) occurs in 44% of children with psoriasis. Gluteal cleft involvement is common (see Fig 9–2), as is involvement of the penis (Fig 9–6).

Nail signs in psoriasis (Table 9–1) include multiple tiny pits on the surface of the nails (pitting); yellowing of the distal area of the nail

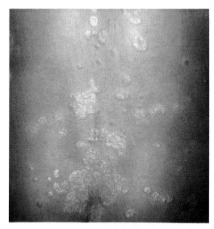

FIG 9–1.
Papules and plaques, some of which are covered with thick, silvery scales, on back of a child with psoriasis.

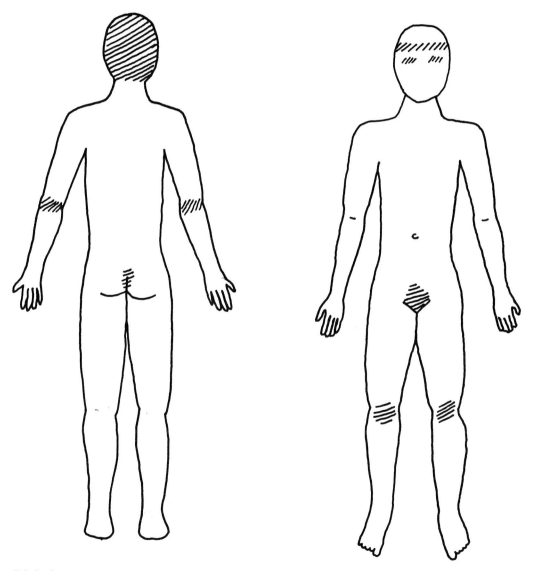

FIG 9–2.
Distribution of psoriasis vulgaris in childhood.

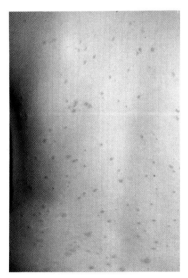

FIG 9–3.
Dozens of discrete, red papules scattered on back of a child with acute guttate psoriasis following a streptococcal throat infection.

caused by separation of the nail plate from the nail bed (onycholysis); thickening of the distal area of the nail (distal hyperkeratosis); or thickening, crumbling, and destruction of the entire nail (Fig 9–7). All 20 nails may be involved, and rarely, nail changes may be the presenting feature of psoriasis in children. Nail changes are seen in 15% of children with psoriasis, but absence of nail involvement does not exclude the diagnosis.

Erythroderma with thousands of pinpoint pustules, which eventuates in sheets of desquama-

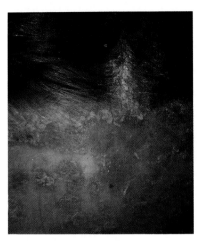

FIG 9–5.
Thick scales covering scalp, with red plaques on forehead of a child with psoriasis.

tion, is called pustular psoriasis. It is quite rare in childhood, but may result from treatment of psoriasis with systemic steroids (Fig 9–8).

Itching is a variable feature in psoriasis; most children do not complain of it. Scratching of lesions may induce the isomorphic phenomenon and make individual lesions worse. Arthritis is seldom seen in children with psoriasis.

Differential Diagnosis

Conditions to be considered in the differential diagnosis are listed in Table 9–2. Lichen planus with involvement of the elbows and knees can mimic psoriasis. The silvery scale and red color of psoriatic plaques distinguish them from

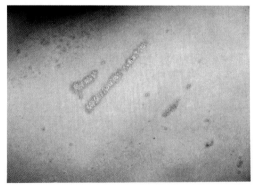

FIG 9–4.
Psoriasis appearing within line of a previous scratch demonstrating the isomorphic (Koebner) phenomenon.

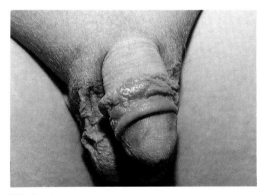

FIG 9–6.
Scaly plaque on foreskin and red plaque on glans penis in a child with psoriasis.

TABLE 9–1.

Nail Signs in Psoriasis

> Pitting of the nail surface
> Distal onycholysis
> Distal hyperkeratosis
> Hyperkeratosis and crumbling of entire nail

the purple papules of lichen planus, however. Whitish plaques of the oral mucosa are seen in lichen planus, but not in psoriasis. The isomorphic phenomenon is also seen in lichen planus, but the papules are purple in color.

In contrast to psoriasis, linear epidermal nevi are present from birth. Flat warts occurring along a line of skin trauma do not have a scaly surface. Lichen striatus appears as a solitary lesion progressing down an extremity. Scaly macules on the elbows and knees, seen in childhood dermatomyositis, may be confused with psoriasis. The presence of a malar photoeruption and muscle weakness and pain will help distinguish. Chronic cutaneous lupus erythematosus (LE) lesions may mimic psoriasis, but the scale is thin, not thick, and central atrophy is present. Guttate psoriasis is most often confused with pityriasis rosea. The large herald patch of pityriasis rosea is lacking in guttate psoriasis, and the overlying scale in pityriasis rosea is thin and central rather than thick and diffuse as in psoriasis. Early guttate lesions are not scaly and may be confused with a morbilliform viral exanthem, urticaria, a drug eruption, or secondary syphilis. Scaling in the scalp in psoriasis is nongreasy, in contrast to the seborrheic dermatitis of adolescents. In atopic dermatitis of the scalp, the scales are mild, thin, and dry in contrast to the thick scales of psoriasis.

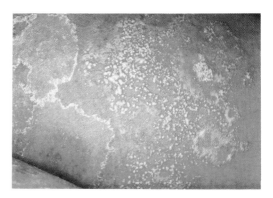

FIG 9–8.

Pinpoint pustules, erythema, and sheets of desquamation in a child with pustular psoriasis.

Nail pitting occurs in alopecia areata, but the pits are broader, more shallow, and fewer in number than in psoriasis. Onycholysis and hyperkeratosis of the nails occur in lichen planus, but synechiae from the cuticle to the fingertip and narrowing of the nail are seen. Fungal involvement of the nail is seen rarely in childhood, and usually only one or two nails are involved, in contrast to psoriasis. All 20 nails are affected in ectodermal dysplasia and its variants, but alopecia, dental disorders, and other features are usually present to distinguish them from psoriasis.

Genital psoriasis must be differentiated from candidal intertriginous infections by potassium hydroxide (KOH) examination and fungal culture.

Pathogenesis

In most families with psoriasis, inheritance is apparently autosomal dominant, but environmental factors influence the expression of psoriasis

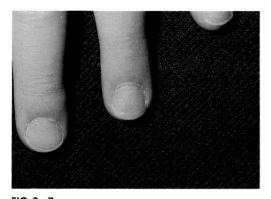

FIG 9–7.

Nail pitting in a child with psoriasis.

TABLE 9–2.

Differential Diagnosis of Papulosquamous Disorders

> Psoriasis
> Pityriasis rosea
> Secondary syphilis
> Parapsoriasis
> Lichen planus
> Lupus erythematosus
> Dermatomyositis
> Dermatophyte infections
> Seborrheic dermatitis
> Lichen striatus
> Linear epidermal nevi
> Warts

significantly. The histocompatibility antigens HLA-B13 and HLA-B17 are increased in psoriasis but apparently are not closely linked to the genes responsible for psoriasis.

The classic pathologic features of psoriasis seen on skin biopsy denote inflammation associated with features of epidermal proliferation. The epidermis is thickened, with elongation of the rete ridges to the same level (regular acanthosis), increased epidermal mitosis, parakeratosis (nuclei retained in the stratum corneum), thinning of the granular layer, and microabscesses of neutrophils within the epidermis and the stratum corneum. In the dermis, the dermal papillae are clubbed, and there is vasodilation of dermal blood vessels, with a lymphocytic infiltrate around them. Increased numbers of epidermal cells enter the mitotic cellular pool; the epidermal turnover time in psoriasis is three to four times faster than that of normal skin.

The factors responsible for increased epidermal turnover are unknown. In many ways, the psoriatic epidermis mimics skin healing from a wound. In children, the association with streptococcal infection is intriguing, and there is some experimental evidence to suggest that psoriasis patients, particularly children with guttate psoriasis, have greater lymphocyte activation by specific streptococcal antigens than do children without psoriasis. Studies on the inflammatory events before epidermal stimulation may help elucidate the mechanism of psoriasis.

Treatment

Most therapies are designed to retard epidermal proliferation, but they have some antiinflammatory effects as well. It is not certain which of these effects produces the most successful therapeutic results.

Ultraviolet light (UVL), such as sunbathing or artificial UVL sources, is effective in the management of psoriasis. Sunbathing daily alone may help psoriasis by interfering with epidermal cell division. One should caution the patient about sunburn, however, as Koebner's phenomenon may occur. Lubrication of the skin surface with mineral oil or petrolatum before exposure to UVL will produce uniform penetration of UVL by reducing the reflection of light from the disrupted skin surface.

In severe, generalized psoriasis, in-hospital therapy with crude coal tar ointment 1% and UVL (290 to 320 nm ultraviolet B [UVB]) therapy daily

for 14 to 21 days often produce prolonged remission.

For the scalp, softening the scales with salicylic acid 3% in mineral oil or olive oil, massaged in and left on overnight, is useful. Then the scalp can be shampooed with a tar shampoo and the scales mechanically removed with a comb and brush. This is repeated daily until the scales are gone.

Topical steroids will temporarily improve psoriasis, with the most benefit obtained from moderate- to strong-potency glucocorticosteroids. The maximal benefit is obtained with 2 to 3 weeks of daily therapy, and remissions are shorter than with phototherapy. Topical steroid therapy may be followed with phototherapy to maintain the remission.

Children with guttate psoriasis and evidence of streptococcal infection should be treated with antibiotics to eliminate the infection.

Systemic steroids are contraindicated in childhood psoriasis because psoriatic erythroderma may follow withdrawal, resulting in fever, hypoalbuminuria, and other metabolic changes associated with generalized skin involvement.

Anthralin is a tricyclic hydrocarbon that is efficacious in the management of psoriasis. The so-called "short-contact" protocols are particularly useful. Anthralin 1% ointment is applied once daily to the psoriatic lesions for 20 minutes, followed by neutralizing with a neutral soap, such as Dove, thoroughly washing off all the anthralin. Anthralin stains the skin and clothing a brown color. Most patients require 3 to 8 weeks of daily anthralin therapy to clear.

Photochemotherapy with methoxsalen and long-wave UVL (320 to 400 nm ultraviolet A [UVA]), so-called PUVA therapy, is reserved for children who have failed on standard therapies.

Oral retinoids are efficacious in severe psoriasis, but their effects on growing bones prohibit their long-term use in childhood. Experience in treating children with oral retinoids is quite limited. Antimetabolites such as methotrexate inhibit the formation of epidermal DNA. They are reserved for the most severe, disabling forms of psoriasis because of their significant side effects. The use of antimetabolites in children should be avoided if possible.

Patient Education

Children with psoriasis have a chronic disease, and education is a crucial aspect of overall care. Childhood-onset psoriasis tends to increase in severity in adult life. One should emphasize that good remission and good control of psoriasis can be achieved, but that sometimes childhood psoriasis is difficult to treat. Adolescents in particular need considerable emotional support. The occurrence of exacerbations at times of emotional stress is well recognized.

Patients should understand that trauma to the skin will induce psoriasis, but severe restriction of activities is unwarranted. Not scratching psoriasis lesions should be stressed.

Staphylococcus aureus can be cultured in large numbers from the skin surface in patients with psoriasis. Occlusive dressings should be avoided, since they enhance the overgrowth of skin bacteria. Hospitalized children with psoriasis will shed bacteria continually into the room air.

Follow-up Visits

Patients should be seen every 2 weeks during therapy to evaluate their response and to provide supportive care. Dermatology nurse specialists or psoriatic day care centers are ideal for this type of specialized care.

PITYRIASIS ROSEA

Clinical Features

Pityriasis rosea is most commonly seen in adolescents and children. It may be preceded by a prodrome of pharyngitis, lymphadenopathy, headache, and malaise, but in most children no history of constitutional symptoms is given. An annular, scaly, erythematous lesion (the herald patch) precedes the appearance of the remainder of the lesions by 1 to 30 days (Fig 9–9). The herald patch is present in 80% of children. It is usually on the trunk, but may appear on the face or extremities. The herald patch, unlike the other lesions, shows central clearing and may mimic tinea corporis.

The lesions consist of multiple erythematous macules progressing to small, red papules appearing over the trunk. The papules enlarge and become oval. The long axes of the oval lesions tend to be parallel to each other and to follow the lines of skin stress (Fig 9–10). A thin scale develops in the center of the oval lesions. In black skin, lesions over the proximal extremities, inguinal and axillary areas, and neck often predominate, with few lesions appearing on the trunk (Fig 9–11).

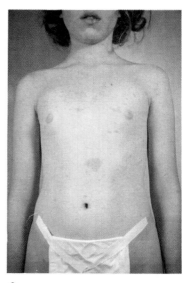

FIG 9–9.
Pityriasis rosea. Herald patch, which is larger than other papules, is seen on epigastric skin.

Despite the different distribution, the course is similar. The lesions last 4 to 8 weeks. Mild itching is common during the first week of the generalized eruption, but the lesions are asymptomatic thereafter.

Differential Diagnosis

The herald patch is often confused with tinea corporis before the appearance of the generalized eruption. The generalized papular eruption may mimic urticaria, the viral exanthems, morbilliform drug eruptions, or guttate psoriasis (see Table 9–2), but the presence of the herald patch is a useful distinguishing feature. As the lesions become more oval, secondary syphilis should be considered. Although secondary syphilis is usually characterized by lesions of the oral and genital mucosa and ham-colored macules on the palms and soles, every adolescent with pityriasis rosea should have a VDRL (Venereal Disease Research Laboratories) test to exclude secondary syphilis. The oval lesions may also be confused with guttate parapsoriasis.

Pathogenesis

Since epidemics occur in a susceptible age group, pityriasis rosea has long been considered to be an infectious process. No viral or other microbial agent has been discovered in pityriasis ro-

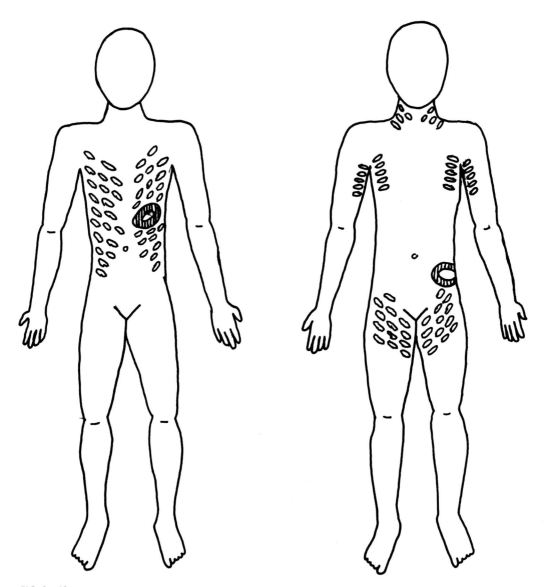

FIG 9–10.
Distribution of pityriasis rosea in white *(left panel)* and in black *(right panel)* children. Herald patch is indicated by circle.

sea, however. Pathologic changes consist only of mild inflammation, with edema of the epidermis and dermis and a mild perivascular accumulation of lymphocytes. Focal areas of parakeratosis are seen.

Treatment

Most children and adolescents require no therapy. A single dose of UVL, either natural sun-light exposure to redness or one minimal erythema dose of sunlamp exposure, will stop the itching and hasten the disappearance of the lesions. Oral antihistamines are rarely necessary.

Patient Education

The long duration of the lesions should be explained, with assurance that they will disappear, leaving normal-appearing skin.

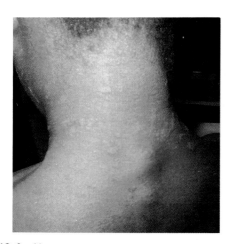

FIG 9–11.
Pityriasis rosea in black child reveals oval plaques with central scale seen on neck.

Follow-up Visits

Follow-up visits are usually unnecessary except for follow-up on syphilis serology.

SECONDARY SYPHILIS

Clinical Features

Secondary syphilis is characterized by discrete, pink macules or pink papules with a fine scale, distributed on the trunk and associated with lymphadenopathy (see also Chapter 5). Skin lesions erupt 3 to 6 weeks after the appearance of the chancre. Serologic tests for syphilis are always positive at the time of the secondary cutaneous eruption. A list of the cutaneous signs of secondary syphilis is presented in Table 9–3. The major signs include maculopapular lesions, condylomata lata, and mucous patches. Condylomata lata are moist, warty papules seen in the perineum and other intertriginous areas, such as under the breast and in the interdigital webs and axillae. Mucous patches are papular lesions seen most often on the tongue as red papules lacking tongue papillae. On the buccal mucosa, palate, tonsils, vaginal mucosa, glans penis, and coronal sulcus, they appear as papules with a central erosion.

The maculopapular lesions, condylomata lata, and mucous patches contain hundreds of spirochetes and are infectious. Generalized lymphadenopathy accompanies these features in 85% of cases; low-grade fever, lethargy, and arthralgias accompany the eruptions in 50% of cases.

TABLE 9–3.
Cutaneous Signs of Secondary Syphilis

Major
Papular lesions
Condylomata lata
Mucous patches
Minor
Annular
Nodular
Pustular crusted lesions
Alopecia
Keratotic macules of palms and soles
Usually associated with generalized lymphadenopathy

Minor variants of secondary syphilis include annular lesions of the face, neck, and genitalia, most commonly seen in blacks; acral nodules that are few in number; sterile pustules and crusted lesions that mimic ecthyma; a "motheaten" alopecia of the eyebrows and scalp hair; and keratotic, ham-colored macules of the palms and soles.

Untreated secondary syphilis may progress to nephrotic syndrome, cranial nerve palsies, meningism, osteolytic lesions, syphilitic hepatitis, or neurosyphilis.

Differential Diagnosis

It is well known that syphilis can mimic a wide variety of cutaneous conditions (see Table 9–2), but, most commonly, pityriasis rosea. The generalized eruptions may be differentiated from pityriasis rosea by the involvement of the palms and soles, lymphadenopathy, mucous patches, and a positive VDRL flocculation test.

Condylomata lata must be distinguished from venereal warts by the VDRL flocculation test or dark-field microscopic examination.

Mucous patches may be confused with geographic tongue, aphthous stomatitis, angular cheilitis, or other mucocutaneous syndromes.

For discussions of pathogenesis, treatment, patient education, and follow-up visits, see Chapter 5.

PARAPSORIASIS

Clinical Features

Parapsoriasis, an uncommon disorder, may be seen in two distinct childhood forms: acute parapsoriasis (Mucha-Habermann disease) and guttate parapsoriasis (pityriasis lichenoides chronica). Both forms may occur in the same patient, or one form may progress to the other. Thus, they are considered two forms of the same disease. In acute parapsoriasis, the eruption consists of recurrent crops of red papules 2 to 4 mm in diameter (Fig 9–12). The papules have central petechiae and progress to crusting (Fig 9–13). Lesions in different stages are seen, particularly on the trunk. They heal, leaving depressed scars. The eruption lasts approximately 9 months and is occasionally associated with low-grade fever.

In guttate parapsoriasis, salmon-colored, oval papules with central thin scales are seen primarily in the perineal area, thighs, and trunk (Fig 9–14). They are few in number, but may persist for 2 to 3 years. Both forms are seldom associated with itching.

Differential Diagnosis

Acute parapsoriasis mimics varicella, and acute parapsoriasis should come to mind when examining a child with "prolonged varicella." Occasionally, insect bites or necrotizing vasculitis is confused with acute parapsoriasis. In acute parapsoriasis, at least some lesions have a purpuric center, which helps to distinguish it from varicella or insect bites. The presence of lesions in many different stages is useful in separating acute parapsoriasis from vasculitis. A skin biopsy will distinguish.

The guttate form mimics pityriasis rosea, and thus "prolonged pityriasis rosea" should suggest the diagnosis of guttate parapsoriasis. Dry skin dermatitis, secondary syphilis, guttate psoriasis,

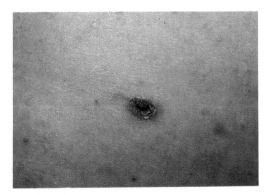

FIG 9–13.
Characteristic red papule with central crust in acute parapsoriasis.

and tinea corporis sometimes make correct diagnosis difficult (see Table 9–2). The long duration and sparse number of lesions help in making the diagnosis.

Pathogenesis

Acute parapsoriasis is a vascular injury, with extravasation of erythrocytes, a superficial perivascular lymphohistiocytic infiltrate, and necrosis of the overlying epidermis. Focal parakeratosis is also seen. In contrast to necrotizing vasculitis, no fibrinoid necrosis of the vessel walls is seen, neutrophils are not present, and nuclear fragments

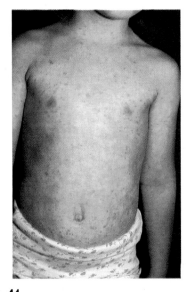

FIG 9–14.
Chronic parapsoriasis. Discrete, oval salmon-colored papules with a thin scale seen on child's trunk.

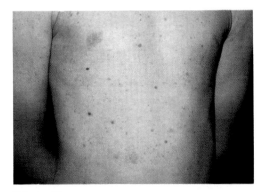

FIG 9–12.
Acute parapsoriasis. Red papules with central purpura or crusts and vesicles scattered over a 10-year-old child's trunk.

are not found around vessels. The mechanism of the disease remains unknown.

The histologic findings in guttate parapsoriasis are similar to those of pityriasis rosea. The mechanism of the disease is unknown.

Treatment

Treatment with oral erythromycin at 40 mg/kg/day for 1 to 2 months may benefit some children. For children who fail erythromycin therapy, a conservative approach is recommended, with therapy much like that for psoriasis; UVB phototherapy may control the disease. Topical steroids do not affect the disease, and claims for efficacy from high-dose tetracycline or low-dose methotrexate therapy cannot be substantiated.

Patient Education

The prolonged course of these disorders should be emphasized.

Follow-up Visits

A single visit in 1 month is useful to reevaluate the child's disease state and to determine response to phototherapy.

LICHEN PLANUS

Clinical Features

Lichen planus is a chronic papular skin disorder characterized by the appearance of purple, flat-topped papules. The list in Table 9–4 is helpful in recalling the major features. The classic polygonal purple papules occur on the wrist and extensor surfaces of the forearm (Fig 9–15). On the knees, feet, and lower legs, thick scaling is found over thickened, purple plaques (hypertrophic lichen planus) (Fig 9–16). Bullae or erosions may be seen on the feet or the head and neck. The shaft of the penis is commonly involved (Fig 9–17). Lichen planus may be inherited as autosomal dominant.

TABLE 9–4.

"P's" of Lichen Planus

Planar (flat topped)
Pruritic (itchy)
Purple
Polygonal (angulated borders)
Papules
Penile

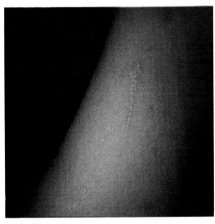

FIG 9–15.
Lichen planus. Linear purple papules seen along line of previous scratch in a child with lichen planus. Lichen planus, like psoriasis, may have the isomorphic phenomenon.

Oral lesions are seen most commonly on the buccal mucosa as white, thickened papules in a lacy pattern (Fig 9–18). Erosions or thickening of the tongue or gingivae may be seen.

In the scalp, a circumscribed area of hair loss with replacement of follicles by scarring rarely occurs.

The nail changes of lichen planus are rare in children, but total destruction of all 20 nails with synechiae formation is seen. The nail is narrowed, with an overgrowth of fibrous tissue from the proximal nail fold across the nail plate to the tip of the digit. A few children with lichen planus

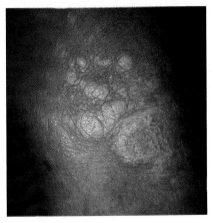

FIG 9–16.
Thick, scaly, purple plaques on knee in a child with lichen planus.

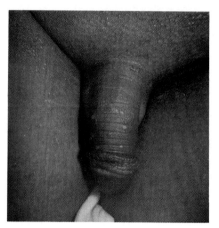

FIG 9–17.
Linear purple papules on penis in a child with lichen planus.

have only nail involvement when first seen by the physician. It is often diagnosed as 20-nail dystrophy of childhood until a nail biopsy is done or other mucocutaneous lesions of lichen planus develop.

Itching is severe in lichen planus, and the isomorphic phenomenon occurs commonly with the appearance of lichen planus papules along an area of skin trauma. Localized forms also occur in children. The natural history of lichen planus is

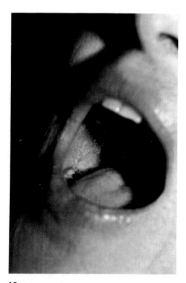

FIG 9–18.
Lacy white thickening of buccal mucosa in an adolescent, demonstrating mucosal involvement in lichen planus.

that it resolves in 9 to 18 months, leaving hyperpigmented areas in sites where lesions occurred.

A variant of lichen planus, called lichen nitidus, has histologic features identical to those of lichen planus, yet is more focal in nature. It demonstrates tiny (1 to 2 mm) hypopigmented, flat-topped papules occurring in clusters, usually on the trunk (Fig 9–19). The papules do not itch. Lesions of lichen nitidus have been found in 25% of children with lichen planus.

Differential Diagnosis

The characteristic purple color, with flat-topped papules with angulated borders, distinguishes lichen planus from the other papulosquamous disorders (see Table 9–2). The hypertrophic lesions on the lower legs mimic psoriasis. Erosive lesions in the mouth mimic aphthous stomatitis and herpes simplex, and the white, lacy appearance of the buccal mucosa may be confused with premalignant leukoplakia or the white sponge nevus. A skin biopsy may be required to confirm the diagnosis of lichen planus.

A variety of drugs (including thiazide diuretics, atabrine, chloroquine, quinine, quinidine, and gold) can produce an eruption identical to lichen planus, but these agents are rarely used in children.

Lichen nitidus may mimic keratosis pilaris, but the inspissated, dry, scaly follicular plugs of keratosis pilaris are not seen, and lichen nitidus lesions are smooth topped.

Pathogenesis

Lichen planus results from an acute injury to the basal cells of the epidermis to the extent that

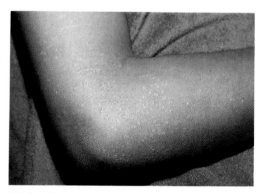

FIG 9–19.
Hundreds of discrete, pinpoint, white, flat-topped papules on leg of a child with lichen nitidus.

liquefaction degeneration of basal cells occurs and the dermoepidermal junction is obscured. In bullous lichen planus, the epidermis separates from the dermis. Amorphous colloid bodies representing degenerating basal cells, combined with immunoreactants such as IgA, IgG, IgM, complement, and fibrin, are seen in the basal layer or just beneath it. The damaged basal cells have decreased ability to divide. Thus, there are features of prolonged retention of cells in the epidermis, with acanthosis, hyperkeratosis, and a thickened granular layer. The exact mechanism of the epidermal basal cell injury is unknown, but it is thought to be due to inflammatory injury by mononuclear cells that interact with the basement membrane.

In lichen nitidus, the same pathologic changes occur, but are limited to a single dermal papilla.

Treatment

Topical glucocorticosteroids are effective in controlling the itching and resolution of the lesions. They are used twice daily, and 4 to 8 weeks of therapy are often required for remission. In children with severe generalized lichen planus, prompt relief from prednisone, 1 to 2 mg/kg/day in a single morning dose, can be expected in 2 weeks, although the lichen planus may return as the steroids are reduced. Oral lesions are usually asymptomatic. When painful, they will respond to steroid gels or topical isotretinoin gel applied to the mucosa. Lichen nitidus need not be treated.

Patient Education

Patients should be informed of the prolonged nature of lichen planus and the tendency for hyperpigmentation to occur after healing.

Follow-up Visits

Follow-up visits every 2 to 4 weeks are needed to monitor the course of the disease and the response to therapy.

LUPUS ERYTHEMATOSUS

Clinical Features

Lupus erythematosus (LE) occurs eight times more often in females than in males. In approximately 15% of all patients with LE, the onset is between the ages of 9 and 15 years.

A cutaneous eruption is present in 80% of

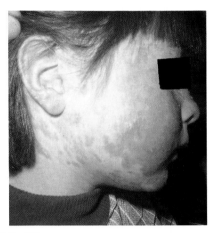

FIG 9–20.
Bright red, scaly plaques on cheek of a boy with acute systemic lupus erythematosus.

adolescents with LE, and in 25% it is the presenting sign. The most frequent cutaneous sign is the erythematous maculopapular eruption, with a "butterfly" distribution, on the cheeks and nose (Fig 9–20). It is covered by a fine scale and occurs in one third of the patients. The next most common sign is the discoid lesion, a chronic, persistent skin change that progresses to scarring and pigmentary changes; in black patients, severe hypopigmentation may be seen. Discoid lesions are seen most frequently on the face and hands, ears, and scalp, where scarring hair loss results (Fig 9–21). More transient annular papulosquamous

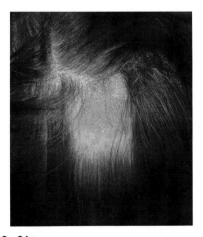

FIG 9–21.
Scarring hair loss with redness and scaling of underlying scalp in an 8-year-old girl with discoid lupus erythematosus.

lesions limited to sun-exposed areas of skin are observed in subacute cutaneous LE (Fig 9–22).

Other kinds of skin involvement may occur in adolescents with LE, including telangiectatic erythema on the thenar and hypothenar eminences of the palms and the pulps of the fingers and diffuse erythema and telangiectasia of the cuticle, with erythematous, scaly macules occurring on the dorsa of the fingers between the knuckles (Fig 9–23). Mottling of the extensor surfaces of the extremities, the so-called livedo reticularis, occasionally occurs. Features of cutaneous vasculitis, such as subcutaneous nodules, splinter nail hemorrhages, purpuric acral infarcts, palpable purpura, and distal gangrene, may be seen. Raynaud's phenomenon, a two-phase color change of the digit upon cold exposure with pallor and cyanosis, occurs in 35% of adolescents. Rarely, persistent, tender, red-purple nodules on the cheeks, proximal extremities, or trunk, which represent LE panniculitis, will be seen in children (Fig 9–24). A distinct history of sun sensitivity may not be obtained in children with LE, and careful questioning may be required to uncover photosensitivity.

Diagnosis depends on a constellation of clinical, pathologic, and serologic findings. Use of the American Rheumatism Association (ARA's) criteria for LE is recommended.

The neonatal LE syndrome is characterized by congenital heart block or annular papulosquamous skin lesions, or both (Fig 9–25). Although affected infants do not meet ARA criteria for LE, the association with maternal LE or Sjögren's syndrome and the clinical skin lesions, skin pathology, and distinctive pattern of autoanti-

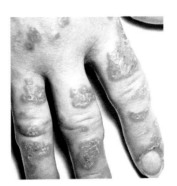

FIG 9–23.
Scaly plaques between knuckles in systemic lupus erythematosus. Compare with Fig 9–28.

bodies similar to those found in subacute cutaneous LE permit the use of LE as the diagnosis in this neonatal syndrome. The skin lesions fade by 6 to 7 months of age, but the heart block will persist.

The most useful serologic test in the diagnosis of LE is the fluorescent antinuclear antibody (ANA) test, which is positive in more than 90% of children with LE. Sensitivity is improved if human rather than rodent tissue substrates are used. Autoantibodies in LE are directed against a variety of nuclear components. The most specific is that directed against the nuclear acidic chromosomal proteins, such as the Sm antigen. It is very specific, but is found in only 30% of patients. In addition to screening with a fluorescent ANA test, in some children in whom LE is suspected, an ANA profile in which immunodiffusion tests are done against soluble nuclear antigens may be performed. This is especially useful in detecting anti-

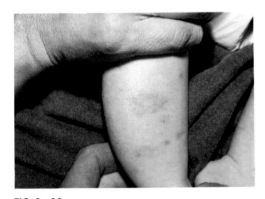

FIG 9–22.
Scaly, annular red patches on leg of an infant with subacute cutaneous lupus.

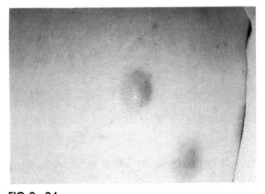

FIG 9–24.
Red-purple nodules on upper arm of girl with lupus profundus (panniculitis).

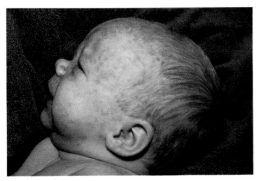

FIG 9–25.
Neonatal lupus syndrome. Four-week-old female infant with dozens of scaly, annular, red macules on forehead and cheeks.

bodies to SS-A (Ro), which is a diagnostic marker for neonatal LE syndrome.

Depressed complement levels, especially the C4 level, are useful for detecting active vasculitis, particularly in the central nervous system and kidney. Direct immunofluorescence of skin biopsy specimens of involved skin is positive for granular deposits of IgG or C3 at the dermoepidermal junction in 90% of patients. IgG deposits over basal keratinocytes are observed in subacute cutaneous and neonatal LE.

The initial evaluation of patients with suspected LE should include the tests listed in Table 9–5.

In general, patients with discoid cutaneous lesions, subacute cutaneous LE, or lupus panniculitis have a low incidence of disease in other organs, whereas those with the butterfly maculopapular eruption or vasculitis lesions are likely to have renal, central nervous system, or other vital organ involvement.

Differential Diagnosis

Childhood dermatomyositis and LE may have similar cutaneous features at initial presentation. The photosensitive butterfly eruption may be seen in children with dermatomyositis or drug-induced photosensitivity, such as that caused by the phenothiazines or thiazide diuretics. A butterfly eruption may also be seen in polymorphous light eruption. Skin biopsy and immunofluorescence are useful in distinguishing LE from these. The eruption may be scaly enough to consider psoriasis, lichen planus, or other papulosquamous disorders (see Table 9–2). Dermatophyte facial in-

TABLE 9–5.

Initial Laboratory Evaluation of Lupus Erythematosus

Skin biopsy, formalin fixed for routine histologic study
Skin biopsy, frozen section, for immunofluorescence
Serum for ANA test and ANA profile
Serum for total hemolytic complement and
    complement components
Urinalysis
Complete blood count with differential and platelet
    count

fection (tinea faciei) must be excluded by KOH examination of the scales.

Biopsy is necessary to differentiate discoid lesions of the face from psoriasis and lichen planus and the discoid lesions of the scalp from other causes of circumscribed alopecia.

Drug-induced LE syndromes rarely cause cutaneous eruptions, but sometimes may mimic LE. The drugs likely to produce LE syndromes are listed in Table 9–6. The livedo reticularis pattern is seen in dermatomyositis, scleroderma, and other collagen vascular diseases, as is Raynaud's phenomenon, palmar erythema, and cuticular telangiectasia.

Careful examination of the dorsa of the hands may help distinguish LE from dermatomyositis. In LE, scaly erythematous macules are seen between the knuckles on the dorsum of the hand, while in dermatomyositis, scaly macules or papules are seen on the knuckle pads. (Compare Fig 9–23 with Fig 9–28.)

The annular papulosquamous lesions of subacute cutaneous LE may mimic tinea corporis or pityriasis rosea, but a skin biopsy will distinguish.

The red-purple nodules of LE panniculitis

TABLE 9–6.

Drugs Responsible for Inducing Lupus
Erythematosus–Like Syndromes

High risk
Hydralazine
Procainamide
D-Penicillamine
Practolol
Moderate risk
Isoniazid
Phenytoin
Ethosuximide
Propylthiouracil
Trimethadione

may be confused with vascular tumors or cutaneous lymphomas or leukemias.

Pathogenesis

LE is associated with circulating immune complexes, which may account for many of the vasculitis features in the joints, kidneys, and central nervous system. In the skin, there is an injury to epidermal basal cells with liquefaction degeneration, which may lead to dermoepidermal separation. A patchy accumulation of lymphocytes around dermal blood vessels and hair follicles is seen. These findings are found in acute, subacute, chronic (discoid), and neonatal skin lesions. In addition, discoid LE shows epidermal atrophy and follicular plugs of scale. Usually, no evidence of necrotizing vasculitis is found in the skin, although antigen-antibody complexes have been eluted from the skin. In LE panniculitis, there is usually a dense lymphocytic infiltrate around subcutaneous vessels between fat lobules without the superficial skin injury observed in other forms of cutaneous LE.

The exact mechanism of skin injury and photosensitivity is unknown. A possible association with viruses or virus-induced tissue injury is suggested from animal models of LE-like diseases.

Treatment

It is beyond the scope of this book to discuss the treatment of systemic LE. The chronic cutaneous lesions respond to potent topical fluorinated glucocorticosteroids applied twice daily. In the discoid LE form, response is slow, over many months. Although chloroquine has been demonstrated to be efficacious in discoid LE, particularly that associated with arthritis, it produces a cardiomyopathy in prepubertal children, which precludes its use. In older adolescents, chloroquine, 200 mg twice daily, may be efficacious. Prior visual screening should be obtained by ophthalmologic consultation and regular 3-month eye examinations.

In children and adolescents with systemic involvement, skin lesions clear with immunosuppressive agents in the doses used to treat renal disease. Sometimes skin lesions require additional topical therapy with potent or superpotent topical steroids for control.

Photoprotection should be a mainstay of therapy for cutaneous LE even when photosensitivity is uncertain. Protective clothing and regular use of sunscreens are recommended.

Patient Education

Sun sensitivity should be discussed and the use of photoprotective agents strongly emphasized. Daily use of a sunscreen of at least SPF 30 is advised. In addition, it is advisable for the patient to avoid sun exposure between the hours of 10:00 AM and 4:00 PM. During this time, 60% of UVL reaches the earth's surface. The patient should be advised to wear a hat to protect the face. Severe sunburn has resulted in systemic exacerbations of LE. Cosmetic coverings are helpful, both as sunscreens and for disguising unsightly skin lesions.

Follow-up Visits

After the initial visit, a visit in 1 week is useful for the evaluation of laboratory evidence, which may indicate potential systemic involvement. Often, adolescents presenting with acute symptoms, such as fever, acute arthralgias, or renal disease, must be hospitalized. It is important to remember that in 5% to 10% of those presenting with cutaneous lesions only, the disease may progress to involvement of internal organs. Thus, reevaluation every 3 months is recommended.

DERMATOMYOSITIS

Clinical Features

The onset of most cases of childhood dermatomyositis is between 4 and 12 years. The presenting symptom of childhood dermatomyositis often is a photosensitive facial rash involving the malar areas and the upper eyelids (Fig 9–26). Periorbital edema and a violaceous hue to the eyelids are seen. On the elbows and knees, erythe-

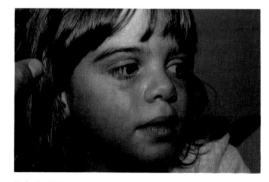

FIG 9–26.
Dermatomyositis. Purple-red discoloration of eyelids and cheeks in a "butterfly" distribution that mimics lupus.

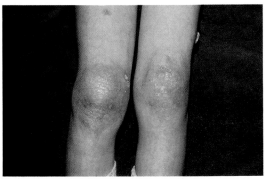

FIG 9-27.
Dermatomyositis. Scaly, rosy-colored plaques on knees, mimicing psoriasis.

matous plaques with a fine scale are observed (Fig 9–27), and flat-topped, red papules are present on the knuckles (Gottron's papules) (Fig 9–28). Cuticular or eyelid margin telangiectasia is seen. A livedo reticularis pattern on the extremities may be prominent. The skin changes may precede, occur simultaneously with, or follow signs of muscle disease. Occasionally, the cutaneous features are present for months before muscle symptoms are noted. Children with dermatomyositis appear ill, with low-grade fever, malaise, and anorexia.

Weakness, with or without pain in the proximal muscles, is the most frequent symptom. Inability to run and to climb stairs, easy fatiguability during play, and inability to comb hair or reach

upward may be presenting symptoms. Dysphagia from pharyngeal muscle weakness is found in 10% of patients.

As the disease slowly progresses, muscle weakness may be so profound as to make the child bedridden. Calcinosis of skin and muscle eventually develops in 40% of children and becomes a major problem. Skin calcinosis is seen as crusted papules or plaques around joints or as nonhealing sores. Muscle calcification may result in contractures or severe muscular pain.

Muscle enzymes, particularly creatine phosphokinase, aspartate aminotransferase, and aldolase, may be elevated. Muscle biopsy or electromyography may assist in the diagnosis. Skin biopsy findings are not diagnostic.

Differential Diagnosis

LE is most often confused with dermatomyositis because of the facial photosensitive eruption. Examination of the dorsa of the hands (see Lupus Erythematosus) will help differentiate, as will muscle signs and symptoms. The scaly plaques on elbows and knees are often confused with psoriasis. In dermatomyositis, the scale is thin, not thick, there are associated muscle findings, and the child appears ill in contrast to psoriasis.

The livedo reticularis pattern may also be found in periarteritis nodosa and LE; and the cuticular telangiectasias are found in a number of collagen vascular diseases.

Pathogenesis

The mechanism of cutaneous injury is unknown. Skin biopsy specimens show edema of the papillary dermis with a sparse perivascular mononuclear cell infiltrate, and immunofluorescent studies are usually nonspecific. A skin biopsy may be most useful for detection of calcification.

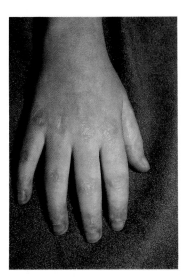

FIG 9-28.
Dermatomyositis. Scaly, red papules on knuckles (Gottron's papules) in childhood dermatomyositis. Compare with Fig 9–23.

Children with dermatomyositis may have autoantibodies to muscle proteins (such as Jo-1, PM/SCL, or Mi) and may have positive ANA test results. Of interest is the dermatomyositis syndrome produced by enteroviruses in children with congenital immunodeficiencies. Whether dermatomyositis is a viral disease is yet unproved.

Treatment

Systemic steroids and steroid-sparing drugs such as azathioprine are the primary modes of therapy in dermatomyositis. Skin lesions usually are controlled by systemic therapy, but occasionally potent or superpotent topical steroids will be required in addition. Low-dose coumarin may be useful in preventing or reversing cutaneous calcification.

Patient Education

It should be emphasized that a multidiscipline approach to care for children with dermatomyositis is required. Children should be treated in settings where muscle disease specialists, dermatologists, and rheumatologists can coordinate the care and where physical therapy and nutritional support are available. Parents must recognize the serious and disabling nature of the condition and must be prepared for long-term therapy. They must be apprised of the potential complications of the disease and the long-term immunosuppressive therapy.

Follow-up Visits

If not hospitalized, the child should be seen weekly until good control of the disease is achieved.

LICHEN STRIATUS

Clinical Features

Lichen striatus is a disorder peculiar to childhood, characterized by linear, shiny, hypopigmented papules limited to one extremity (Fig 9–29). It does not follow vascular or neural structures. It is most common in children 2 to 12 years of age. Although the lesions begin as pink or dull-red papules, they quickly become hypopigmented. Characteristically, they begin on a buttock and spread down the leg, or begin on the shoulder and progress down the arm. They may first be noticed distally, however. The lesions last 3 to 9 months and then spontaneously disappear.

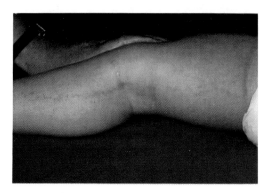

FIG 9–29.
Lichen striatus. Linear red, scaly papules extending down flexor surface of a child.

Differential Diagnosis

The linear lesions are so characteristic that they are seldom confused with other lesions. Koebner's phenomenon, seen in lichen planus, lichen nitidus, or psoriasis, may be confused with lichen striatus, but lesions will be present in other areas in these diseases. Epidermal birthmarks may be confused, but they are irregular on the surface rather than shiny and are present from birth, rather than acquired later in life. Porokeratosis of Mibelli may be confused, but it does not transcend an entire extremity. A skin biopsy will distinguish but is usually not required.

Pathogenesis

A chronic dermatitis is seen on histologic examination of stained sections of tissue, but the mechanism of the disease is unknown.

Treatment

Treatment is unnecessary.

Patient Education

The benign nature and the complete resolution of these lesions should be emphasized.

Follow-up Visits

A follow-up visit in 4 weeks is useful to examine for skin lesions in other areas and to rule out other papulosquamous conditions.

POROKERATOSIS OF MIBELLI

Clinical Features

Porokeratosis of Mibelli may appear as a segmental single lesion or group of lesions that may mimic lichen striatus or an epidermal nevus (Fig 9–30). The condition occurs more frequently in males and has a predilection for the face, neck, forearms, and hands, although the buttocks and feet may also occasionally be involved. Individual lesions appear as craterlike areas on the skin, with a scaly, irregular, oval border. The crateriform area may measure from 5 to 50 mm in diameter, and several craters may be grouped together. The most important diagnostic feature of porokeratosis of Mibelli is the appearance of a scaly border in which a double row of scales surmounted by a furrow is observed. Diagnosis is made by biopsy of the border of the lesion.

Differential Diagnosis

Porokeratosis of Mibelli may be confused with lichen striatus or epidermal nevi. In contrast to lichen striatus, however, lesions are often segmental and do not completely extend down an extremity. In contrast to epidermal nevi, they are never present at birth but develop later in childhood and do not have as verrucous a surface. Biopsy is often useful in distinguishing among these possibilities.

Pathogenesis

The characteristic biopsy finding demonstrates focal areas of parakeratosis within the epidermis and, if proper sectioning of the double ridge has been obtained, a pair of focal parakeratotic columns with a normal or slightly thinned epidermis sandwiched between them. Sparse or moderate inflammation may be seen beneath the parakeratotic columns. It is believed that this represents hyperplastic clones of sweat duct keratinocytes, perhaps transformed by a papillomavirus. This would explain its generalized nature in immunosuppressed patients or those with chronically sun-damaged skin.

Treatment

The lesions of porokeratosis of Mibelli may produce some concern in the parents about cosmetic appearance, but no satisfactory therapy has been developed. Progressive growth may occur over 2 to 3 years, and in some cases spontaneous resolution has been reported. Topical keratolytic agents have not been of use in therapy; topical 5-fluorouracil solution has been reported to be efficacious, although it should be used cautiously in children. Some promising results have been obtained with combinations of topical tretinoin and 5-fluorouracil.

Patient Education

The parents must be told that the cause is unknown and that the likelihood of spontaneous remission within a few years is high. They must be warned against rushing into cosmetic surgery for improvement because the scarring after surgery may be worse than the lesion itself. The advantages of a conservative approach to such lesions should be emphasized.

Follow-up Visits

A follow-up visit in 6 to 12 months may be useful to determine the course of the lesion in the child.

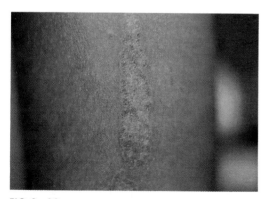

FIG 9–30.
Porokeratosis of Mibelli. Linear, scaly plaque with moatlike border in a 9-year-old child.

BIBLIOGRAPHY

Anderson TF: Pediatric phototherapy. *Pediatr Clin North Am* 1983; 30:701.

Arndt FA, Paul BS, Stern RS, et al: Treatment of pityriasis rosea with ultraviolet radiation. *Arch Dermatol* 1983; 119:381.

Aronson IK, Zeitz HJ, Variakojis D: Panniculitis in childhood. *Pediatr Dermatol* 1988; 5:216.

Atherton DJ, Kahana M, Russell-Jones R: Naevoid psoriasis. *Br J Dermatol* 1989; 120:843.

Bencini PL, Crosti C, Sala F: Porokeratosis: Immunosuppression and exposure to sunlight. *Br J Dermatol* 1987; 116:113.

Bjornberg A, Hellgren L: Pityriasis rosea. A statistical, clinical and laboratory investigation of 826 patients and matched healthy controls. *Acta Derm Venereol* [Suppl] (Stockh) 1962; 42:1.

Black MM, Marks R: The inflammatory reaction in pityriasis lichenoides. *Br J Dermatol* 1972; 87:533.

Braathen LR, Botten G, Bjerkedal T: Psoriasis in Norway. *Acta Derm Venereol* [Suppl] (Stockh) 1989; 142:1.

Lee LA, David KM: Cutaneous lupus erythematosus. *Curr Probl Dermatol* 1989; 1:161.

Kwee DJ, Dufresne RJ, Ellis DL: Childhood bullous lichen planus. *Pediatr Dermatol* 1987; 4:325.

Lee LA, Weston WL: Neonatal lupus erythematosus. *Semin Dermatol* 1988; 7:66.

Lowe NJ: Psoriasis. *Semin Dermatol* 1988; 7:43.

Menter MA, Whiting DA, McWilliams J: Resistant childhood psoriasis: An analysis of patients seen in a day-care center. *Pediatr Dermatol* 1984; 2:8.

Miller LC, Michael AF, Youngki K: Childhood dermatomyositis: Clinical course and long term follow-up. *Clin Pediatr* 1987; 26:561.

Otsuka F: Porokeratosis has neoplastic clones in the epidermis: Microfluorimetric analysis of DNA content of epidermal cell nuclei. *J Invest Dermatol* 1989; 92:231S.

Perlman SG: Psoriatic arthritis in children. *Pediatr Dermatol* 1984; 1:283.

Plotz PH, Dalakas M, Leff RL, et al: Current concepts in the idiopathic inflammatory myopathies: Polymyositis, dermatomyositis and related disorders. *Ann Intern Med* 1989; 111:143.

Rosinka D, Wolska H, Jablonska S, et al: Etretinate in severe psoriasis of children. *Pediatr Dermatol* 1988; 5:266.

Toda K, Okamoto H, Horio IT: Lichen striatus. *Int J Dermatol* 1986; 25:584.

Truhan AP, Hebert AA, Esterly NB: Pityriasis lichenoides in children: Therapeutic response to erythromycin. *J Am Acad Dermatol* 1986; 15:66.

Weston WL, Harmon C, Peebles C, et al: A serological marker for neonatal lupus erythematosus. *Br J Dermatol* 1982; 107:377.

10 _____ Sun Sensitivity

Sun exposure in children may result in sunburn or abnormal reactions in the skin. Abnormal reactions occur in the skin areas predominantly exposed to sunlight: the face and extensor surfaces of the arms and hands. Sun sensitivity is suspected when the distribution of the cutaneous eruption is limited to these areas. Three diseases account for the majority of cases of sun sensitivity in children: polymorphous light eruption, erythropoietic protoporphyria, and lupus erythematosus (see Chapter 9). These conditions should be considered in every child with sun sensitivity.

SUNBURN

An expected result of excessive sun exposure is sunburn. Sunburn readily occurs in fair-skinned children, who have less melanin protection than darker skinned children. Intense sun exposure can produce sunburn in children with dark skin as well, however, any child who seeks medical assistance because of sunburn should be questioned about exposure to agents that make patients sun sensitive.

Clinical Features

Erythema and skin tenderness begin 30 minutes to 4 hours after sun exposure, depending on the intensity of the exposure and the degree of the child's natural protection against the sun (Table 10–1; Fig 10–1,). On the face, sunburn is usually most prominent on the nose and cheeks, with sun-protected areas under the nose, the chin, and upper eyelids uninvolved (Fig 10–2). On the extremities and trunk, protective clothing may produce sharp borders between burned and non-burned areas (Figs 10–1 and 10–3). After intense sun exposure, edema and blistering occur (see Fig 10–3). Some 2 to 7 days after intense sun exposure, five to ten cell layers of epidermis are shed in one piece as a white scale (desquamation). With acute sunburn, sleep is often disturbed because of the tenderness of the skin. Extensive sunburn causes a reduction in the sweating rate and may contribute to collapse from heat stroke. Sunburn over large areas of the body in a child may result in fever, headache, and fatigue.

Differential Diagnosis

It is occasionally difficult to determine in children what constitutes overexposure to sunlight (Table 10–2). In such a case, one should consider the presence of a photosensitizing agent that would induce a sunburn reaction in an unusually short period of time (5 minutes to ½ hour of sun exposure). Agents that cause photosensitivity are listed in Chapter 18. Most have been associated with photosensitivity in adults, but they may also cause photosensitivity in children. Burning pain in the skin following 5 minutes of sun exposure should suggest erythropoietic protoporphyria. In contrast, sunburn alone requires at least 30 minutes to produce symptoms. Rapid onset of sunburn and persistent sunburn reactions may be early clues to xeroderma pigmentosum (XP). In lupus erythematosus (LE), the eruption occurs 1 to 7 days after sun exposure and is characterized by scaling and erythema, which are present for several weeks. It is important to recall that many viral exanthems appear primarily in sun-exposed areas (see Chapter 8). The laboratory evaluation of photosensitivity, listed in Table 10–3, should be considered when involved in the differential diagnosis of sun sensitivity.

TABLE 10–1.

Skin Types and Sun Sensitivity

Skin Type	Description
I	Fair skin; always burns, never tans
II	Fair skin; usually burns, sometimes tans
III	Lightly pigmented; usually tans, sometimes burns
IV	Pigmented; always tans, never burns
V	Moderately pigmented; never burns
VI	Heavily pigmented (black) skin

TABLE 10–2.

Differential Diagnosis of Sun Sensitivity

Polymorphous light eruption
Erythropoietic protoporphyria
Lupus erythematosus
Dermatomyositis
Photosensitizing drugs (see Table 10–3)
Viral exanthems
Sunburn
Xeroderma pigmentosum
Hepatoerythrocytic porphyria

TABLE 10–3.

Laboratory Evaluation of Photosensitivity

Skin biopsy
Red blood cell fluorescence
Red blood cell protoporphyrin levels
Antinuclear antibody and antinuclear antibody profile

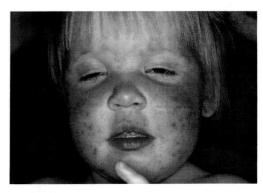

FIG 10–2.
Sunburn of infant's face. Note protection of upper eyelids, nasolabial folds, beneath nose, under hair.

Pathogenesis

The tanning or burning ultraviolet rays from the sun represent radiation. This form of radiation generates toxic oxygen species and injures the skin. The skin will protect itself against ultraviolet radiation by tanning. Ultraviolet radiation effects are cumulative as well, with many types of cutaneous cells retaining the additive effects of years of radiation exposure. Long-term effects are expressed as fine wrinkling, scaly, red patches (actinic keratoses), and, ultimately, skin cancer formation.

In acute ultraviolet injury, the skin changes noted reflect immediate effects of radiation. The first changes noted after prolonged sun exposure are vasodilation of the dermal blood vessels. There is evidence to implicate several eicosanoids as mediators of the pain and erythema of sunburn. Metabolic changes then occur within epi-

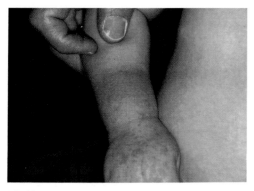

FIG 10–1.
Acute sunburn in an infant. Note sharp line of demarcation between uninvolved arm protected by clothing and unprotected skin. Note red papules of sweat duct obstruction.

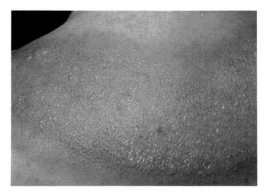

FIG 10–3.
Acute sunburn with vesiculation of back of neck. Note sharp demarcation of area protected by clothing.

dermal cells. Individual epidermal cells within the midepidermis demonstrate clumping of monofilaments and abnormalities of cytoplasmic and nuclear shape, producing the rounded, so-called sunburn cell. Such cells lose their epidermal cell attachments; with increased sun exposure, a large number of these cells appear within the epidermis and produce an intraepidermal separation and blister cavity.

Treatment

The pain and erythema of sunburn can be relieved by the use of wet dressings or cool compresses. Inhibitors of prostaglandin synthesis, such as aspirin and indomethacin, may modify sunburn if given soon after sun exposure. There is no convincing evidence that systemic or topical glucocorticosteroids are beneficial in the treatment of sunburn. Topical anesthetics such as benzocaine are sensitizing, transient in their relief of pain, and not recommended.

Patient Education

Infants and children should be protected against sun exposure. Infants younger than 6 months should not be subjected to prolonged sun exposure for more than 15 minutes because of the decreased sweating rate and the likelihood of heat stroke. For those older than 6 months, clothing and umbrellas are good sun protection. Sunscreen agents with SPF (sun protection factor) 15 or greater are recommended (Tables 10–4 to 10–6). These creams or lotions should be applied to the skin the night before and the morning of sun exposure. Regular daily use throughout the spring and summer months is the best method of protection. Sun blocks, such as zinc oxide pastes or titanium dioxide, are less cosmetically acceptable but are good sun-protective agents. Sun avoidance, such as planning outdoor

TABLE 10–4.

Sunscreen SPF

$$SPF = \frac{MED \text{ of sunscreened skin}}{MED \text{ of unprotected skin}}$$

MED = minimal erythema dose, that is, the amount of UVB energy required to produce minimal erythema to human skin.

TABLE 10–5.

Recommendations for Sunscreen Use in Children

Use a sunscreen with UVB SPF of 15 or greater.
Select a waterproof preparation.
Apply at least ½ hour before sun exposure.
Reapply every 1 to 2 hours.
UVA sunscreens may be required in special situations.

TABLE 10–6.

Types of Available Sunscreens

UVB
  PABA (p-aminobenzoic acid)
  PABA esters
  Benzophenones
  Cinnamates
  Salicylates
  Combinations of ingredients
UVB plus UVA
  Parsol 1789
  Physical agents that block light

activities before 10:00 AM and after 4:00 PM, is advisable for infants and toddlers.

Follow-up Visits

Follow-up visits are unnecessary.

POLYMORPHOUS LIGHT ERUPTION

Clinical Features

Polymorphous light eruption comprises a group of related sun-sensitive conditions that are sometimes separated by distinct clinical patterns. Four major types are reported (Table 10–7).

Hutchinson's summer prurigo (actinic prurigo) and photodermatitis of North American Indians have many overlapping features. They begin as a dermatitis predominantly occurring on the face and extensor surface of the forearms of school-age children. Actinic prurigo has been described in the United Kingdom and northern Europe, and the related form is seen in the Plains Indians of North America. Both characteristically start in the early spring, when sufficient sunlight energy reaches the earth's surface. Onset is by age 5 years in 35% of children, and by age 10 years in 70%; the eruption develops during adolescence in the remainder. The initial eruption consists of

TABLE 10–7.

Types of Polymorphous Light Eruption

Actinic prurigo
Photodermatitis of North American Indians
Juvenile spring eruption (hydroa aestivale)
Hydroa vacciniforme

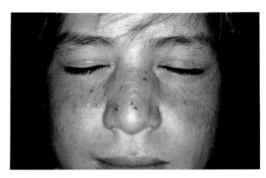

FIG 10–5.
Chronic polymorphous light eruption with lichenification by midsummer.

an itchy, acute facial or forearm dermatitis with edematous papules (Fig 10–4) and vesicles. As the spring progresses, the dermatitis becomes subacute, with crusting on the surface and epidermal thickening or lichenification (Fig 10–5). Papular lesions may predominate on the face. In summer the eruption may spontaneously clear, to recur again the next spring. Some very sun–sensitive children will have the eruption throughout the year. It is characteristic that several patches of skin are involved, with uninvolved areas of skin in between. In North American Indians, the disease differs in two respects: (1) a chronic cheilitis of the lower lip is frequently observed (Fig 10–6) that may be related to living in regions of intense sunlight and (2) a family history of the disease is often obtained. Overlap between atopic dermatitis that gets worse with summer heat is frequent in both actinic prurigo and photodermatitis of North American Indians.

Juvenile spring eruption (hydroa aestivale) is described in European children. It characteristically begins as 2- to 3-mm discrete papules or vesicles on the ears and cheeks of fair-skinned chil-

dren. The episode lasts 1 week and reappears the next spring (Fig 10–7).

Hydroa vacciniforme is characterized by a few discrete, deep-seated vesicles on the ears or nose that heal with scarring (Fig 10–8). They are frequently persistent, lasting up to 4 weeks, and more episodes may occur with further sun exposure. The eye may be affected with keratitis, and uveitis is observed. This is the rarest of all forms of polymorphous light eruption.

It is unclear how these clinical patterns are interrelated, but, until pathologic or biochemical tests can distinguish, they are catalogued under the broad term *polymorphous light eruption.*

Biopsy of early lesions shows an acute der-

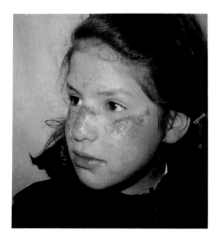

FIG 10–4.
Polymorphous light eruption. Photodermatitis of a North American Indian child, with vesicles and crusting of face at springtime onset.

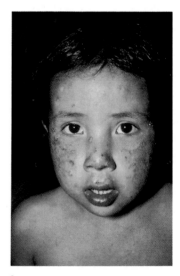

FIG 10–6.
Involvement of lower lip with redness, edema, and fissures in polymorphous light eruption.

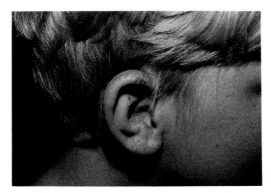

FIG 10-7.
Vesicles and crusts on tops of ears in child with juvenile spring eruption.

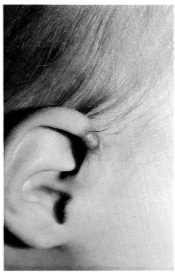

FIG 10-8.
Deep-seated vesicle on ear of child with hydroa vacciniforme.

matitis, while biopsy of papular, crusted, and lichenified forms shows a chronic dermatitis.

In American Plains Indians and Spanish Americans living in Western North America, polymorphous light eruption occurs as an autosomal dominant condition. Females predominate 2:1. Non-Indian children may also have polymorphous light eruption, but the hereditary pattern is not defined. As in any dermatitis, itching may be severe, and scratching, resulting in secondary bacterial infection, may occur.

Differential Diagnosis

Atopic dermatitis, in addition to other photosensitive states, may mimic polymorphous light eruption (see Table 10-2). During hot weather, sweating in children with atopic dermatitis may induce itching and a dermatitis on the face and sun-exposed areas. A family history of allergies and the finding of flexural dermatitis in addition to the photodermatitis are useful differentiating features. Acute sensitivity to airborne substances may also lead to the appearance of a contact dermatitis, predominantly on sun-exposed areas. In airborne contact dermatitis, the upper eyelids are usually involved, in contrast to polymorphous light eruption. LE, erythropoietic protoporphyria, dermatophyte infections of the face, and sunburn are likely to be confused. Laboratory tests listed in Table 10-3 should be considered. Photodermatitis due to drugs characteristically produces a diffuse involvement of sun-exposed areas, rather than the patchy areas of dermatitis seen with polymorphous light eruption.

Erythropoietic protoporphyria and XP have an onset in early infancy rather than childhood,

and they may have symptoms out of proportion to skin changes. They usually do not develop dermatitis-like changes.

Pathogenesis

The mechanism of any form of polymorphous light eruption is unknown. Repeated daily exposure to wavelengths of light in the sunburn range (UVB, 290 to 320 nm) will reproduce the dermatitis in 3 to 14 days (see Fig 10-7). The biochemical change responsible for initiating the dermatitis following sun exposure is unknown. Twenty percent of children may be sensitive to long-wave ultraviolet light (UVA 320 to 400 nm), especially those children with the hydroa vacciniforme type of dermatitis.

Treatment

Treatment of polymorphous light eruption involves the use of topical glucocorticosteroids in an ointment base applied twice daily for the dermatitis. In addition, wet dressings in the form of a face mask made of a damp washcloth, with eye, nose, and mouth holes, will serve to enhance the steroid effect on the face. This may be used for 2 to 3 days.

Sun avoidance is crucial in such patients and should be the mainstay of any treatment program. The child should restrict outdoor activities to the hours before 10 A.M. and after 4 P.M. Further photoprotection with a wide-brimmed hat or sunscreens of SPF greater than 30 may be necessary (see Table 10–6).

Children with polymorphous light eruption who are sensitive to the UVA spectrum of light are best treated with beta carotene capsules, 40 to 120 mg/day. Approximately 20% of all children with polymorphous light eruption will respond to beta carotene.

In cases of severe polymorphous light eruption, treatment with a psoralen may be considered. Although it appears contradictory to treat a photosensitive disorder with a photosensitizing agent, low-dose oral psoralen will induce melanin pigmentation and epidermal thickening, increasing the natural protection to sunlight. Oral trimethoxypsoralen, 10 mg/day, has been successful in treating North American Indians who have polymorphous light eruption. Secondary bacterial infection is best treated with systemic antibiotics.

Patient Education

The concept of sun sensitivity must be understood by patients and their parents. Sun protection methods should be carefully explained and reexplained at each visit. Many parents are reluctant to accept sun avoidance or to restrict their children's activities at school or play.

Follow-up Visits

A visit 1 week after initial therapy is useful to assess the therapeutic response. Visits at 4-week intervals thereafter are advised until the condition has cleared.

ERYTHROPOIETIC PROTOPORPHYRIA

Clinical Features

Erythropoietic protoporphyria is an inherited disorder of porphyrin metabolism. Most children show an autosomal dominant pattern of inheritance. The preschool child experiences burning, stinging, or itching sensations in the skin. Often, this occurs after a sun exposure of only 1 to 10 minutes. Despite the severe discomfort the child suffers, no skin lesions are found. The child soon learns to stay indoors. Intense sun exposure may result in facial edema, erythema, or urticaria, followed by petechiae. These occur primarily on the face. Less often, vesiculation and crusting of the face appear (Fig 10–9).

More commonly, however, acute skin

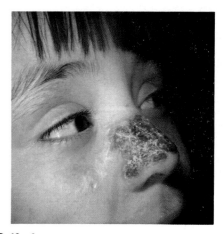

FIG 10–9.
Crusting of nose after acute sun exposure in erythropoietic protoporphyria. Note depressed scars on cheek from prior episode.

changes do not occur, and chronic changes are apparent. Chronic changes usually do not appear until late childhood. Slightly thickened, skin-colored papules appear over the dorsa of the hands, nose, and cheeks. Pitted scars on the face and perioral linear skin-colored papules may result from previous vesicular injury.

Skin biopsy specimens from sun-exposed skin show thickening of the small blood vessels of the papillary dermis, with a perivascular deposit of periodic acid–Schiff (PAS)–positive material. Direct immunofluorescence of such lesions demonstrates deposit of immunoglobulins, mostly IgG, around superficial dermal blood vessels. Of children with erythropoietic protoporphyria, 5% may suffer cholelithiasis with porphyrin stones in the gallbladder and varying degrees of liver injury. Nine deaths from hepatic failure and erythropoietic protoporphyria have been reported in children and adolescents. A mild anemia may also occur.

The diagnosis can be confirmed by laboratory tests. Heparinized blood diluted 1:10 in unpreserved saline can be examined with a fluorescence microscope for coral-red fluorescence of red blood cells. It is important that the blood be withdrawn in a light-protected tube, since light exposure may allow protoporphyrin to be converted to a nonfluorescent metabolite. In normal children, less than 1% of red cells fluoresce, while in those with erythropoietic protoporphyria, from 5% to 30% of the total erythrocytes fluoresce. Quantitative red blood cell protoporphyrins are also useful. Most hospital and commercial laboratories have great difficulty with the quantitative protoporphyrin assay. If required, 5 to 7 mL of heparinized blood in a tube protected from the light by aluminum foil, or two to three drops of blood on a filter paper (the same paper used for phenylketonuria testing), may be submitted to M. B. Poh-Fitzpatrick MD, Department of Dermatology, New York Medical College, Valhalla, NY 10595, where a reliable evaluation for erythropoietic protoporphyria will be carried out.

Differential Diagnosis

Most other photosensitive states (see Table 10–2), such as polymorphous light eruption, LE, sunburn, and drug photosensitivity, can be excluded by the striking history of cutaneous burning seen in children with erythropoietic protoporphyria, by a positive family history, and by laboratory studies. Occasionally, the family is unable to relate the symptoms to exposure to sunlight, and airborne allergens are suspected. This is particularly true if facial edema or urticaria is a major feature. A careful history, however, will reveal the role of sun exposure.

Pathogenesis

Abnormally elevated tissue levels of protoporphyrin IX, a normal precursor of heme, are found in erythropoietic protoporphyria. Excessive protoporphyrin IX has been found in the circulating erythrocytes, plasma, liver, and bone marrow of children with erythropoietic protoporphyria. Protoporphyrin IX absorbs light at 400 nm and becomes a molecule with an altered energy state. The molecule then transfers energy to molecular oxygen; toxic oxygen products are thought to be responsible for the injury to the vascular membranes, and perhaps to the lysosomal membranes, with subsequent inflammation.

Ultraviolet light producing 400-nm wavelengths is found in sunlight, reflected sunlight, sunlight traveling through window glass, and fluorescent lighting. Thus, a child could develop symptoms indoors or through window glass.

Treatment

Oral administration of beta carotene is the treatment of choice. In children, a dosage of 40 to 120 mg/day will raise serum carotene levels to 600 to 800 µg/100 mL, the desired therapeutic range. The child becomes carotenemic, but sun tolerance is greatly increased. Children who pre-

viously refused to go outdoors may play for 3 to 4 hours outside without symptoms.

Conventional sun protection methods have been uniformly unsuccessful because of the poor ability of sunscreens to protect in the 400 nm UVL range and the small amount of light necessary to induce symptoms.

Patient Education

The hereditary nature of the disease should be discussed with the patient and the parents, and all family members should be screened by protoporphyrin level determinations. Liver function tests may be performed on family members as well. It must be emphasized that photosensitivity can occur with fluorescent lamps, such as those in overhead lighting in school.

Follow-up Visits

During the initiation of therapy, a visit every 2 to 3 weeks is useful to ascertain the response and to adjust the therapeutic dosage of beta carotene. After 4 weeks, serum carotene levels may be used to monitor for the correct dosage. After an effective therapeutic response is achieved, visits every 6 months to examine the patient for possible liver involvement are valuable.

PHYTOPHOTODERMATITIS

Clinical Features

Redness and blisters that occur in bizarre shapes, such as linear streaks, and that leave intense hyperpigmentation are characteristic of phytophotodermatitis (Fig 10–10). Exposure to plants in the spring and summer months from outdoor activities is the usual history. Some children present with only the hyperpigmented streaks and with macules of unusual shapes without a distinct history of erythema or blistering. Exposure to limes or certain perfumes may also produce the syndrome.

Differential Diagnosis

The linear streaks of blisters may be confused with acute allergic contact dermatitis from plants such as poison ivy, while the hyperpigmented macules can be confused with incontinentia pigmenti because of the linear arrangement or irregular café au lait spots. The bizarre shapes and simultaneous onset of phytophotodermatitis lesions help differentiate.

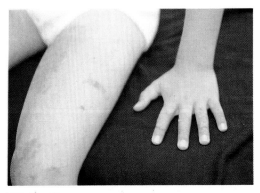

FIG 10–10.
Phytophotodermatitis. Linear and bizarre shapes of hyperpigmentation in 8-year-old boy from fight with brother; they were hitting each other with plants found along a lakeshore.

Pathogenesis

Plants that contain the furocoumarin psoralen are responsible. This includes the celery family and certain grasses and limes. The plants produce the psoralen transiently, usually after a rainy week. The child gets the psoralen onto the skin from the plant touching the skin (the epicutaneous application of the photosensitizer). The psoralen, when exposed to sunlight, produces a photodermatitis with blister formation, followed by intense stimulation of melanin production. The resultant hyperpigmentation may last for months.

Treatment

The acute dermatitis phase is treated as an acute allergic contact dermatitis with moderate-potency topical steroid ointments twice daily for 2 weeks. The hyperpigmentation phase usually is not treated, but bleaching creams may be considered if cosmetically important areas are involved.

Patient Education

Patients and parents should be advised that once hyperpigmentation occurs, it may persist for 6 to 12 months. They should be told of the nature of the photosensitizing chemical from plants and should avoid play in the area where the plants were contacted.

Follow-up Visits

A follow-up visit in 4 weeks to evaluate the progress of the condition is recommended.

XERODERMA PIGMENTOSUM

Clinical Features

XP is an autosomal recessive disorder of sun sensitivity in which ten different forms have been recognized. Onset of skin lesions by 18 months of age is characteristic, with early sunburn reactions from minimal sun exposure and numerous freckles as the predominant findings. An important clue is that the sunburn may persist for several weeks rather than resolve within a week. Telangiectasia of the sun-exposed areas and cutaneous atrophy develop within a few years of the other cutaneous findings. Actinic keratoses, which appear as persistent red, scaly, rough macules in sun-exposed skin, are found next, and the child's skin appears prematurely aged. In dark-skinned children, these findings may be difficult to appreciate. Skin cancers may develop by the age of 6 to 8 years, with basal cell carcinomas, squamous cell carcinomas, and malignant melanomas reported before puberty. Skin-colored or pigmented papules should be regarded as suspicious of skin cancers, and biopsy should be done promptly. The majority of precancerous and cancerous skin lesions occur on the head and neck. Early death from metastatic skin cancers is reported, with 10% of patients dead before puberty. Up to 20% of affected patients have ocular or neurologic disease, or both. Photophobia may be a prominent symptom, and decreased vision is observed. Mild to severe mental retardation is found, as well as hearing loss and areflexia. Most cases of mental retardation are found in children with the De Sanctis-Cacchione type of XP. Diagnosis and classification of suspected XP are accomplished by examination of abnormal DNA repair by patient's cells following ultraviolet light exposure.*

Differential Diagnosis

The early freckling should be differentiated from lentigines observed in the multiple lentigines syndromes and the LEOPARD and NAME syndromes. Freckling is earlier in onset, macular, and tan, whereas lentigines are slightly raised and brown. Ordinary freckles usually begin at the age of 3 to 5 years rather than before 2 years in children with XP and are not accompanied by skin

*To arrange for the test in North America, inquiries should be made to James Cleaver, PhD, Laboratory of Radiobiology, University of California, San Francisco, 3rd and Parnassus Ave., San Francisco, CA 94143; phone (415)476-4563.

changes that make the child appear old. Actinic keratoses and skin cancers in prepubertal children may be seen in the basal cell nevus syndrome or Bazex's syndrome, but not at an age as young as in children who have XP. Diagnosis is confirmed by skin biopsy showing severe actinic skin damage at an early age. Confirmation is made by culture of skin cells with evaluation of DNA repair.

Pathogenesis

Enzymes involved in several steps of DNA repair may be abnormal. Thus far, at least ten different defects in DNA repair can be found by the fusion of cultured cells from different patient groups with each other to determine if normal DNA repair is restored. Molecular biology techniques will eventually precisely define the specific defects in DNA repair. Failure to repair ultraviolet DNA damage results in carcinogenesis, and XP patients are an important model in the ultimate understanding of sun-induced cancers.

Treatment

Sun avoidance is essential to minimize skin damage and skin cancer formation. Children with XP should avoid sunlight, wear protective clothing, and use sunscreens with SPF of 30 or greater each day. Biopsy of any suspect skin lesion is necessary. Referral to a center with experience in management of this condition is recommended. Dermatologic, ophthalmologic, and neurologic consultations should be obtained.

Patient Education

The autosomal recessive inheritance of this disease should be emphasized. Twenty percent of reported patients have parents who are cousins. A great deal of effort at stressing the critical role of sunlight in producing skin cancers is required. The need for frequent evaluations must be emphasized because many skin cancers are preventable or cured if detected early and removed.

Follow-up Visits

A cutaneous examination every 3 months is necessary, preferably at a center with experience in XP. At the follow-up visit, careful examination for skin cancers should be done, with biopsy of any suspect lesions. An evaluation of the child's sun protection program should be performed at each visit.

BIBLIOGRAPHY

Bundino S, Topi GC, Zina MA, et al: Hepatoerythropoietic porphyria. *Pediatr Dermatol* 1987; 4:229.

DeLeo VA, Poh-Fitzpatrick M, Mathews-Roth M, et al: Erythropoietic protoporphyria: Ten years experience. *Am J Med* 1976; 60:8.

Ferguson J: Polymorphous light eruption. *Curr Probl Dermatol* 1990; 2:65.

Harber LC, Bickers DR: *Photosensitivity Diseases.* Philadelphia. WB Saunders, 1989.

Kraemer KH, Lee MM, Scotto J: Xeroderma pigmentosum. Cutaneous, ocular and neurologic abnormalities in 830 published cases. *Arch Dermatol* 1987; 123:241.

Menni S, Piccinno R, Baietta S, et al: Sutton's summer prurigo: A morphologic variant of atopic dermatitis. *Pediatr Dermatol* 1987; 4:205.

Norris PG, Morris J, McGibbon DM, et al: Polymorphic light eruption: An immunopathological study of evolving lesions. *Br J Dermatol* 1989; 120:173.

Poh-Fitzpatrick M, Ramsay CA, Frain-Bell W, et al: Photodermatitis in infants and children. *Pediatr Dermatol* 1988; 5:189.

Sonnex TS, Hawk JLM: Hydroa vacciniforme: A review of ten cases. *Br J Dermatol* 1988; 118:101.

Stern RS, Weinstein MS, Baker SG: Risk reduction for nonmelanoma skin cancer with childhood sunscreen use. *Arch Dermatol* 1986; 122:537.

11 _____ Bullous Diseases and Mucocutaneous Syndromes

Blister formation in the skin of children usually brings to mind an acute dermatitis, viral infection, or bullous impetigo. A large variety of noninfectious blistering skin diseases may be seen, however. These may be spontaneously occurring blisters or trauma-produced blisters (mechanobullous disorders). A history of trauma-induced blisters is important in distinguishing the mechanobullous disorders from spontaneously appearing blisters. Blisters on the palms and soles often have a thick roof of stratum corneum and appear deceptively deep in tissue when they are within the epidermis or at the dermoepidermal junction. In contrast, blisters on mucous membranes shed their roofs quickly, so that only blister bases (erosions) are seen.

SPONTANEOUS VESICULOBULLOUS ERUPTIONS

Viral blisters (see Chapter 8), bullous impetigo (see Chapter 5), chemical or thermal burns, papular urticaria, and acute dermatitis (see Chapter 4) are the most common forms of blisters that appear spontaneously. The injury in thermal burns is similar to that in sunburn. Erythema multiforme, Stevens-Johnson syndrome, and toxic epidermal necrolysis (TEN) are uncommon, but serious, blistering mucocutaneous syndromes in children. Miliaria, aphthous ulcers, and geographic tongue are common more benign forms of spontaneous vesiculobullous diseases, while linear IgA dermatosis and dermatitis herpetiformis are quite uncommon. Bullous mastocytosis, an uncommon blistering condition, is discussed in Chapter 13. Kawasaki disease is included in this chapter, although not truly a bullous disease, because it mimics the major mucocutaneous syndromes.

ERYTHEMA MULTIFORME, STEVENS-JOHNSON SYNDROME, AND TOXIC EPIDERMAL NECROLYSIS

Clinical Features

Erythema multiforme (EM) is divided into two distinct syndromes: EM minor and EM major (Stevens-Johnson syndrome). Because cutaneous features and etiologies of EM major and TEN may be indistinguishable, they are considered together.

EM minor is a syndrome characterized by the acute onset of oval or round, fixed, erythematous skin lesions appearing symmetrically on the skin. Each lesion remains at the same site at least 7 days, and often for 2 or 3 weeks (Fig 11–1). The lesions progress for several days to form concentric zones of color change where the central zone becomes dusky. These colored lesions are called "target" or "iris" lesions (Fig 11–2). Occasionally, the central dusky zone will develop a blister. Prodromal symptoms in EM minor are conspicuously absent. EM minor lesions are frequently recurrent and preceded by a lesion of herpes labialis (Fig 11–3). Skin lesions initially involve the dorsal surface of the hands and the extensor aspects of the extremities. The palms and soles are frequently involved; the flexor aspects of the extremities are involved less frequently. The isomorphic (or Koebner's) phenomenon has been reported in erythema multiforme (Fig 11–4). Systemic symptoms and signs are absent in EM minor. Usually there are no mucosal lesions, but when present, only the oral mucosa is involved and lesions are few (5 to 10), in contrast to hundreds on the skin (Fig 11–5). EM minor lasts on average 3 weeks. It is most common in adolescents.

EM major (Stevens-Johnson syndrome), in contrast to EM minor, has a distinct prodrome

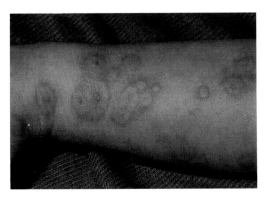

FIG 11—1.
Early fixed papules of erythema multiforme minor on dorsum of hand of child.

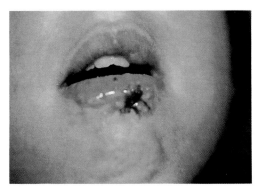

FIG 11—3.
Herpes simplex labialis lesion in child with recurrent erythema multiforme (EM) minor. Lip lesion cultured HSV and preceded episode of EM minor by 5 days.

lasting 1 to 14 days and is characterized by fever, headache, sore throat, malaise, and sometimes cough, vomiting, and diarrhea. Mucosal involvement is severe and always at least two mucosal surfaces are involved (Figs 11–6 and 11–7). The initial cutaneous lesions mimic those found in EM minor but progress rapidly from central blisters to severe epidermal necrosis with loss of the epidermis, leaving a denuded skin. Large sheets of epidermis may be lost (Fig 11–8). TEN has similar cutaneous findings in the absence of mucosal involvement. Although lesions first begin on the extremities in a pattern similar to that noted in EM minor, extensive truncal and facial involvement soon follows. The mouth is affected in every case of EM major. Hemorrhagic crusts often appear on the lips (Fig 11–9). Mucous membrane involvement often precipitates hospitalization in

children because of severe limitation of the ability to eat. Redness, swelling, bullae, or denuded erosions may be seen on the conjunctivae, with pain and photophobia. Genital involvement is less common. The course of disease is more prolonged and is accompanied by systemic symptoms of fever, dehydration, cough, and lymphadenopathy. The child is often sick for 3 or 4 weeks. EM major is more likely to occur in children aged 2 to 10 years, younger than the children in whom EM minor occurs. Complications tend to be se-

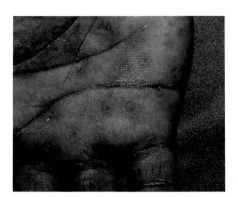

FIG 11—2.
"Target" or "iris" lesions of erythema multiforme minor on child's palm. Note concentric zones of color change, with red border and dusky center.

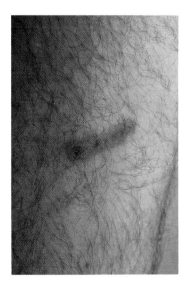

FIG 11—4.
Isomorphic (Koebner) phenomenon in adolescent with erythema multiforme minor. "Target" lesions appear along a scratch.

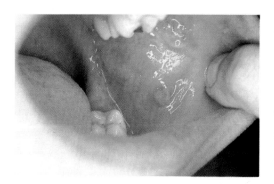

FIG 11–5.
Oral involvement in erythema multiforme minor. A few erosions are present in buccal mucosa.

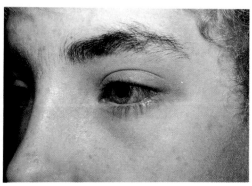

FIG 11–7.
Eye involvement in erythema multiforme major. Erythema of bulbar and palpebral conjunctivae.

vere, with pseudomembrane formation of mucosa, leading to mucosal scarring and loss of function. Fluid and electrolyte imbalance, renal and respiratory complications, and secondary bacterial infections complicate the illness.

Differential Diagnosis

Acute urticaria is most often confused with erythema multiforme. This confusion results from the fact that urticaria may frequently have lesions with concentric color changes with a pale edematous center and an erythematous border. Urticarial lesions are transient, however, usually lasting 24 hours or less, whereas erythema multiforme lesions are fixed and stay at the same site for at least 7 days. Further, the first concentric zone of color change seen in EM minor is not pale in the center, as seen in urticaria, but is a dusky blue.

Urticarial lesions will clear with subcutaneous epinephrine; EM minor will not. Skin biopsy will also distinguish erythema multiforme from urticaria.

Oral mucous lesions that are confused with erythema multiforme include aphthous ulcers, bullous pemphigoid, pemphigus, and epidermolysis bullosa. Exfoliative cytologic study of the blister base will demonstrate epidermal giant cells of herpes simplex.

EM major and TEN must be distinguished from the staphylococcal scalded skin syndrome and acute graft-vs.-host disease by skin biopsy. EM major and TEN show full-thickness epidermal necrosis and subepidermal rather than intraepidermal blister formation (Fig 11–10). In graft-vs.-host disease there are satellite cell necrosis in the epidermis and severe injury to cutaneous vessels not seen in EM major.

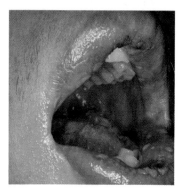

FIG 11–6.
Early oral involvement in erythema multiforme major. Dozens of erosions and early crust formation. Compare with Fig 11–5.

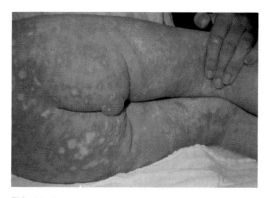

FIG 11–8.
Bulla formation and extensive purpura with islands of uninvolved skin in erythema multiforme major.

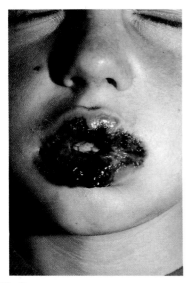

FIG 11–9.
Hemorrhagic crusts on lips of child with erythema multiforme major.

Pathogenesis

EM minor is thought to be due to a herpes simplex virus (HSV) specific host response to HSV antigens expressed on keratinocytes within the target lesion. There is compelling evidence to show that HSV antigens and DNA are present within the skin lesions even when a distinctive preceding HSV episode is not observed. Children who have recurrent lesions may have recurrent HSV preceding most, but not all, EM minor episodes.

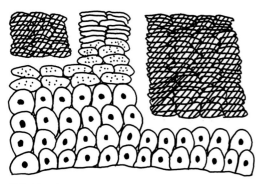

FIG 11–10.
Pathologic differentiation of scalded skin syndrome *(left)* and erythema multiforme (EM) major *(right)*. Dark areas of epidermal necrosis are superficial in scalded skin syndrome, almost full thickness in EM major.

In EM major, there is increasing evidence that a toxic injury to keratinocytes and mucosal epithelium occurs. Most cases of EM major and TEN are related to drug ingestion, with nonsteroidal anti-inflammatory agents, sulfonamides, and anticonvulsant drugs the most often incriminated. Because the skin is a large organ involved in drug detoxification, toxicity is thought to be related to the accumulation of arene oxides in keratinocytes as the result of cytochrome P-450 action on the parent drug. The detoxification of arene oxides, which bind to keratinocyte RNAs, depends on epoxide hydrolases, which may be genetically decreased in children susceptible to EM major or TEN. In a few cases, infections with *Mycoplasma pneumoniae* or HSV have been associated with EM major. The mechanism of epithelial damage with those infectious agents is not known.

Treatment

For EM minor, symptomatic relief may be obtained from wet compresses or oral antihistamines. There is no evidence to support the use of systemic steroids in EM minor. In patients with recurrent episodes of EM minor, prophylaxis with oral acyclovir may be considered.

Patients with EM major or TEN require treatment as for burns, preferably in a burn unit. The offending drug must be discontinued. Careful attention to fluid and electrolyte balance, fever control, and prevention of secondary bacterial infection of the denuded skin is required. Ophthalmologic consultation should be obtained and efforts to prevent conjunctival scarring initiated. There is no evidence that systemic steroids are of benefit.

Patient Education

Patients should be informed of the role of HSV in EM minor, and children with recurrent episodes should attempt to reduce sun exposure or other factors that might precipitate the antecedent HSV infection. With EM major, the drugs thought to be associated should be avoided, and patients should be informed that they may be genetically susceptible to development of the condition.

Follow-up Visits

A visit in 24 to 48 hours is wise early in the disease to determine the progress of EM minor. For hospitalized EM major patients, follow-up should be directed by their complications.

KAWASAKI DISEASE (MUCOCUTANEOUS LYMPH NODE SYNDROME)

Clinical Features

The child presents with a high fever of abrupt onset that lasts longer than 5 days and is accompanied by conjunctival injection (Fig 11–11). One of three oral changes occurs: (1) erythema, fissures, redness, and crusting of the lips (Fig. 11–12), (2) diffuse erythema of the oropharynx, or (3) strawberry tongue. One of four changes is seen in the extremities: (1) prominent edema and induration of the hands and feet (Fig 11–13), (2) erythema of the palms and soles, (3) desquamation beginning at the tips of the digits and spreading proximally in transverse nail grooves (Fig 11–14), or (4) an erythematous eruption that is polymorphous at one point in time but mostly scarlatiniform and generalized. Lymph node masses larger than 1.5 cm, particularly in the cervical lymph nodes, may be noted. Kawasaki disease is often a diagnosis of exclusion, so that other forms of acute febrile syndromes must be considered first. Laboratory tests in Kawasaki disease are nonspecific, including test results showing an increased sedimentation rate of red cells, elevated nonspecific acute-phase reactants, a mild anemia, and a thrombocytosis that can be quite striking.

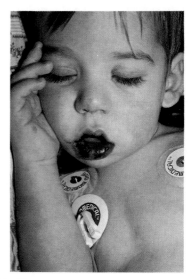

FIG 11–12.
Hemorrhagic crusts on lower lip in toddler with Kawasaki disease.

Aneurysms of the coronary artery occur in 10% to 20% of patients with Kawasaki disease, and 2% of all patients will die from thrombosis of the aneurysms of coronary vessels. Coronary aneurysms, when present, may be detected by echocardiography, but coronary angiography may be required. Although there is some evidence that coronary aneurysms may heal spontaneously, careful cardiac monitoring and involvement of a pediatric cardiologist are recommended.

Kawasaki disease was originally described in Japan, but cases have been reported from virtually all areas of the world.

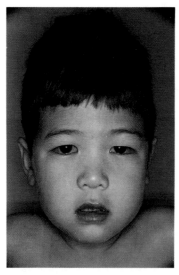

FIG 11–11.
Red, swollen lips and injected conjunctivae in toddler with Kawasaki disease.

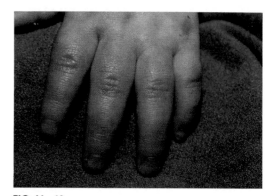

FIG 11–13.
Red, edematous hand in infant with Kawasaki disease.

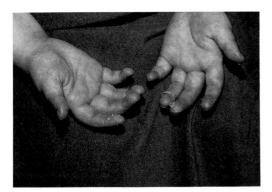

FIG 11–14.
Peeling of fingertips from distal tip toward palm in infant with Kawasaki disease.

Differential Diagnosis

Many diseases with fever and mucocutaneous symptoms can be confused. The most common conditions that mimic Kawasaki disease are Stevens-Johnson syndrome, toxic shock syndrome, staphylococcal scarlet fever, and acute infections such as leptospirosis. By rigidly adhering to the United States Communicable Disease Center criteria for Kawasaki disease, these diseases can be differentiated. Cultures can be helpful in differentiating toxic shock syndrome and staphylococcal scarlet fever from Kawasaki disease.

Pathogenesis

The pathogenesis is unknown, although the clustering of cases and close grouping have implicated an infectious agent. It is believed that microorganisms, perhaps carried by fomites, may have a role in the disease.

Treatment

Intravenous gamma globulin, if given within 10 days of the onset of fever along with low-dose salicylate therapy, has been recommended to prevent aneurysms. Early studies suggest that this is helpful, although a definitive study has not been performed. High-dose steroids are contraindicated and may increase the prevalence of heart disease in this syndrome. Careful cardiac monitoring for arrhythmias is required. Involvement of a pediatric cardiologist is recommended.

Patient Education

Patients should be informed that Kawasaki disease is probably the result of a yet unknown infectious agent. They should be further advised

of the seriousness of the heart disease, which may eventually prompt the need for careful monitoring of cardiac signs and symptoms.

Follow-up Visits

Frequently the child is hospitalized and regular hospital follow-up examinations are performed. Management as an outpatient should be done only when good cardiac consultation and follow-up care are available.

APHTHOUS ULCERS

Clinical Features

Recurrent, shallow erosions of the gums, tongue, palate, lips, and buccal mucosa are seen in aphthous ulcers (Fig 11–15). The erosions are 1 to 10 mm in diameter and have a gray-yellow base (Fig 11–16). Burning and tenderness may occur. Healing occurs in 7 to 10 days, without scarring. Recurrences are usually irregular, several months apart, and consist of two to four lesions. In a more severe form, recurrences with numerous lesions are frequent, so that the child is seldom free from discomfort.

Differential Diagnosis

Aphthous ulcers must be distinguished from herpes simplex and other viral oral ulcerations

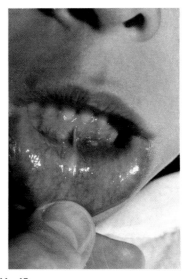

FIG 11–15.
Red border surrounding shallow aphthous ulcer in child's mouth.

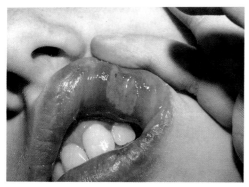

FIG 11–16.
Large aphthous ulcer with gray center.

and from EM minor. Exfoliative cytologic study of the erosion will identify the epidermal giant cells of herpes simplex, and viral culture will distinguish the disorder from herpes simplex, coxsackieviruses A5, A10, and A16, and other enteroviruses. Oral erosions may be the presenting symptom of EM minor, but the symmetric target skin lesions will suggest the disorder.

Pathogenesis

The mechanism of aphthous ulcers is unknown. Several studies have demonstrated lymphocytotoxic activity against oral epithelium, suggesting an autoimmune phenomenon. Biopsy shows ulceration of the epidermis and a mixed inflammatory infiltrate. Recent studies suggest that HSV antigens may be present in oral epithelial cells within aphthous ulcer lesions, even though virus cannot be cultured. The cytotoxic response that produces the injury to oral epithelium may therefore be herpes specific.

Treatment

Treatment is symptomatic. Mild attacks may respond to liquid antacids or half-strength peroxide mouth rinses. Severe lesions may require topical steroids, such as triamcinolone acetonide in a base that adheres to mucous surfaces. Oral prednisone, 1 to 2 mg/kg/day for 3 to 5 days, may be necessary for severe involvement that impairs eating. Antiviral agents against herpes simplex may prove useful in future therapy of this disease.

Patient Education

The recurrent nature of this disorder should be discussed and the lack of effective therapy emphasized.

Follow-up Visits

Follow-up visits are necessary only when attacks occur.

GEOGRAPHIC TONGUE

Clinical Features

Children under the age of 4 years are most commonly affected by geographic tongue, a benign inflammatory disorder. Multiple annular, smooth patches that mimic blister bases on the tongue have a gray, slightly elevated border (Fig 11–17). There are usually no symptoms, but occasionally a child will complain of tenderness. The pattern of involvement changes from day to day, and spontaneous remission occurs.

Differential Diagnosis

Diagnosis is usually easy, since the migratory pattern occurs exclusively in geographic tongue. Malnutrition states usually produce uniform redness of the tongue, with swelling and surface changes. Aphthous ulcers, EM minor, and viral ulcers do not migrate from day to day, and, once established, they remain fixed for at least 3 to 5 days.

Pathogenesis

Pathologic changes in the annular border of the lesion of the tongue are surprisingly similar to those in psoriasis. There are microabscesses in the epithelium and epithelial thickening, but the pathogenesis is unknown. Although the smooth area looks like an erosion clinically, there is no pathologic evidence of blister formation.

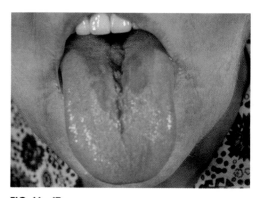

FIG 11–17.
Geographic tongue.

Treatment

Treatment is unnecessary.

Patient Education

The benign nature of this disorder should be discussed and emphasized.

Follow-up Visits

Follow-up visits are unnecessary.

LINEAR IMMUNOGLOBULIN A DERMATOSIS (BENIGN CHRONIC BULLOUS DISEASE OF CHILDHOOD)

Clinical Features

Oval or sausage-shaped bullae located on the groin, perineum, and buttocks of children are indicative of linear immunoglobulin A (IgA) dermatosis (Fig 11–18). Itching is usually absent or mild. Lesions form sausage-shaped bullae or assume annular or ringlike configurations, with blisters forming the outer border of the ring. In addition to the groin and buttock areas, lesions may be present on the lower extremities (Fig 11–19), the lower portion of the upper extremities, and occasionally the face (Fig 11–20). In contrast to dermatitis herpetiformis, this disease is not associated with gluten-sensitive enteropathy or with HLA types B5 and DRw3. Diagnosis is made by biopsy of normal skin adjacent to a blister and immunofluorescent staining, which demonstrate linear IgA deposits at the dermoepidermal junction and on keratinocytes. Some authorities believe

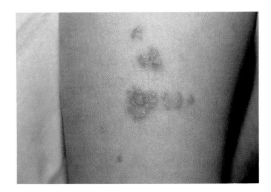

FIG 11–19.
Rosette of blisters on leg of child with linear IgA dermatosis.

that this is the most common nonhereditary blistering disease of childhood.

Differential Diagnosis

Differential diagnosis should include bullous pemphigoid, dermatitis herpetiformis, bullous impetigo, and scabies. Bacterial culture should help differentiate bullous impetigo, and direct microscopic examination for scabies mites will help distinguish scabies. A biopsy for immunofluorescence will differentiate dermatitis herpetiformis, bullous pemphigoid, and linear IgA dermatosis. The deposits are linear and within the basement membrane zone in linear IgA dermatosis, and granular and beneath the basement membrane zone in dermatitis herpetiformis. In bullous pemphigoid, linear deposits are of the IgG class, not IgA.

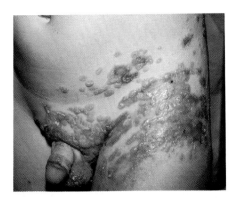

FIG 11–18.
Numerous sausage-shaped blisters; blisters around edge of a red plaque; moist crusts and erosions on lower aspect of abdomen, thigh, and genital skin of toddler with linear IgA dermatosis.

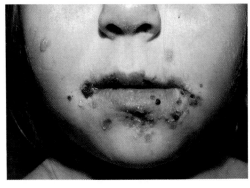

FIG 11–20.
Moist crusts and blisters in perioral distribution in child with linear IgA dermatosis.

Pathogenesis

In linear IgA dermatosis, IgA antibody binds to structures presumably secreted by keratinocytes that appear in the lamina lucida of the basement membrane zone. This location of antibody binding is similar to that seen in bullous pemphigoid. In contrast, in dermatitis herpetiformis, the IgA deposits are granular or globular and below the basement membrane zone, frequently along young collagen fibers and fibrils in the papillary dermis. Occasionally, the serum of an affected child with linear IgA dermatosis will demonstrate a circulating IgA that binds to basement membrane zone antigens in skin sections. The precipitating event is not known.

Treatment

Sulfapyridine, 500 mg three or four times daily, or dapsone, 25 mg twice daily, often produces rapid clearing of the skin lesions in linear IgA dermatosis. By 7 days of treatment no new lesions appear, and by 14 days the skin is often clear. The mechanism of action of these drugs is unknown, but at least some of the effect is related to antineutrophil activity of the drugs. In some children, after 8 to 12 months of therapy, spontaneous remission may occur and the drug can be withdrawn. In a few children, sulfapyridine or dapsone does not control the disease by itself, and the addition of small doses of oral prednisone may be required. Doses of prednisone in the range of 0.5 to 1.0 mg/kg/day may be added to sulfapyridine or dapsone.

Patient Education

Frequently, affected children have been treated for many misdiagnoses by the time the correct one is made, and parents are very frustrated and upset. Considerable time should be spent informing the parents that linear IgA dermatosis easily mimics other conditions, and that it is only a newly recognized disease. The patient should be cautioned about side effects of sulfapyridine or dapsone therapy, and a complete blood count and liver function tests, as well as a glucose-6-phosphate dehydrogenase determination, should be done before therapy is started.

Follow-up Visits

Weekly follow-up visits are necessary while the disease is being controlled with therapy. Two weeks after a visit, a repeat complete blood count and liver function tests are advisable. Measure-ment of serum sulfapyridine levels may be useful in determining the therapeutic dosage of that drug if it is used.

DERMATITIS HERPETIFORMIS

Clinical Features

Dermatitis herpetiformis is a benign disease characterized by recurrent crops of intensely pruritic grouped vesicles or bullae found on the extensor surfaces of the limbs, sacral area, and shoulders (Fig 11–21). It may begin as urticarial lesions or annular erythema (Fig 11–22). Large bullae are found in children, and the intense itching stimulates scratching to such degree that erosions and excoriations are seen rather than intact blisters. Dermatitis herpetiformis should be considered in any patient with severely pruritic skin lesions.

Mucous membrane lesions are unusual and occur in only 15% of patients. It is not clear whether spontaneous remissions occur in dermatitis herpetiformis. In most children with chronic bullous disease of childhood, the clinical features are similar to those of dermatitis herpetiformis.

Gluten-sensitive enteropathy has been associated with dermatitis herpetiformis in adolescent and young adult patients, and the incidence of HLA antigen B8 and B lymphocyte antigens BI and WI is high in both diseases, providing a hereditary linkage of the two diseases. In addition, dermatitis herpetiformis patients have partial villous atrophy of the jejunum, asymptomatic steatorrhea, and disaccharidase deficiency; they gain some relief with a gluten-free diet.

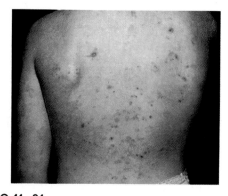

FIG 11–21.
Blisters and excoriated blisters on shoulders and back of child with dermatitis herpetiformis.

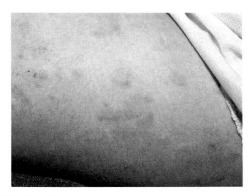

FIG 11–22.
Urticarial papules preceding blister formation in a child with dermatitis herpetiformis.

The diagnosis is made by examination of frozen sections of skin biopsy specimens taken adjacent to vesicles or from urticarial lesions that demonstrate granular IgA deposits in the tops of dermal papillae by direct immunofluorescence.

Differential Diagnosis

Differential diagnosis should include neurotic excoriations, bullous pemphigoid, bullous impetigo, scabies, and erythema multiforme (Table 11–1). Neurotic excoriations mimic dermatitis herpetiformis and may be distinguished by the absence of specific immunofluorescence. In bullous pemphigoid, linear C3 or IgG deposition is seen on immunofluorescence, rather than granular IgA. A circulating IgG directed against the basement membrane zone is also seen. Erythema multiforme lacks dermoepidermal immunofluorescence and shows epidermal necrosis on skin biopsy. Bacterial culture will distinguish bullous impetigo, and scabies will yield mites or eggs on skin scrapings.

Pathogenesis

Early lesions are characterized by accumulations of neutrophilic abscesses and fibrin bands "stuffed" into dermal papillae. Edema fluid collects at the tip of the dermal papillae, and a blister forms. Uninvolved skin adjacent to urticarial or vesicular lesions contains globular or granular deposits of IgA along the dermoepidermal junction. In 15% of the patients, these granular deposits appear linear, as has been described in chronic bullous disease of childhood. C3 and other complement components may be found along the dermoepidermal junction.

TABLE 11–1.
Differential Diagnosis of Spontaneous Vesiculobullous Disease

Commonly seen
  Acute dermatitis
  Bullous impetigo
  Viral vesicles (HSV, VZV)
  Thermal or chemical burns
  Miliaria
Uncommon disorders
  Erythema multiforme
  Stevens-Johnson syndrome
  Linear IgA dermatosis (benign chronic bullous
    disease of childhood)
  Papular urticaria
  Bullous mastocytosis
  Dermatitis herpetiformis
  Bullous pemphigoid
  Lupus erythematosus
  Lichen planus
  Polymorphous light eruption
  Pemphigus
  Incontinentia pigmenti
  Bullous ichthyosiform erythroderma

Currently, most investigators regard dermatitis herpetiformis as a hereditary disorder.

Treatment

Sulfapyridine, 500 mg four times daily, or dapsone, 50 mg twice daily, provides rapid and dramatic relief in children with dermatitis herpetiformis. Pruritus resolves within 72 hours, and skin lesions clear in 7 to 14 days. The mechanism of action of these drugs is unknown, but believed to be due in part to the antineutrophil effect. Since sulfapyridine is variably absorbed from the gastrointestinal tract, blood levels 2 hours after administration are useful in determining the therapeutic dosage. Often, these agents can be reduced or withdrawn once control is achieved. In children not responding to therapy, a gluten-free diet for 8 to 12 months may bring the disease under control if used in combination with sulfapyridine or dapsone.

Before starting sulfapyridine or dapsone, liver function tests and a complete blood count should be obtained.

Patient Education

The hereditary nature of the disease and its persistence should be stressed, with the likelihood that long-term therapy will be required. The correct dosage of medication that is prescribed should also be stressed, and the side effects of such drugs should be carefully explained. Before dapsone is started, the patient should be screened for glucose-6-phosphate dehydrogenase deficiency.

Follow-up Visits

Weekly follow-up visits are necessary while the disease is being controlled, with monthly visits thereafter. Two weeks after therapy is initiated, a repeat complete blood count and liver function test should be obtained. Measurement of serum sulfapyridine levels is useful in determining the therapeutic dosage when that drug is used.

MILIARIA

Clinical Features

There are two forms of miliaria: miliaria crystallina and miliaria rubra. Miliaria crystallina occurs in newborn infants or in areas of sunburn, and miliaria rubra (heat rash) occurs primarily in infants in hot, humid weather or with airtight occlusion of the skin.

Miliaria crystallina is characterized by clear, thin-walled vesicles, which are 1 to 2 mm in diameter, without erythema (Fig 11–23). The vesicles rupture within 24 to 48 hours and leave a white scale. They are seen on the head, neck, and upper part of the trunk in newborn infants and within areas of sunburn in older children.

The characteristic finding in miliaria rubra

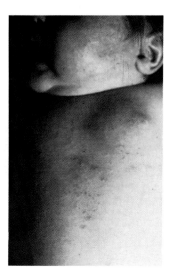

FIG 11–24.
Red pinpoint papules on chest of infant with miliaria rubra.

consists of 2 to 4 mm papules and papulovesicles surrounded by erythema (Fig 11–24). Lesions are seen in flexural areas, such as the neck, groin, and axillae, following excessive sweating. The face and upper part of the chest may be involved. Miliaria rubra may appear in a localized skin area where airtight occlusion has occurred, for example, in an immobile or comatose child lying on a plastic bed cover.

Both forms of miliaria may be secondarily infected by *Staphylococcus aureus,* producing pustules in the sweat pores (periporitis staphylogenes). If continued sweating occurs, repeated daily episodes of miliaria result. Allowing the skin to cool and dry produces mild desquamation and healing in a few days.

Differential Diagnosis

Table 11–1 presents the conditions to be considered in the differential diagnosis of miliaria. Miliaria crystallina can be distinguished from viral infections of the skin or from acute dermatitis by the lack of erythema and negative exfoliative cytologic findings. On smear of the vesicle contents in miliaria crystallina, neither inflammatory cells nor epidermal giant cells are seen.

Miliaria rubra may be confused with neonatal acne, viral exanthems, or drug eruptions, but it is so characteristic that it is seldom misdiagnosed.

FIG 11–23.
Pinpoint, clear vesicles in infant with miliaria crystallina.

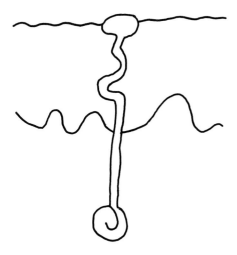 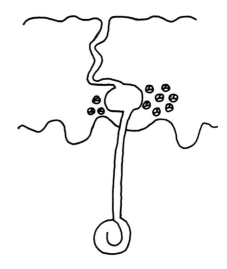

FIG 11–25.
Superficial sweat duct obstruction in miliaria crystallina *(left)* does not result in inflammation, in contrast to midepidermal sweat duct obstruction in miliaria rubra *(right).*

Pathogenesis

Occlusion of sweat ducts following sweating, with rupture of the sweat duct as it spirals through the epidermis, is seen in miliaria. In miliaria crystallina, ductal rupture occurs within the stratum corneum, while in miliaria rubra it occurs in the lower epidermis, with attraction of inflammatory cells to the area of rupture (Fig 11–25). Induction of sweating, overheating, and mechanical occlusion of the sweat pores are essential to the production of miliaria.

Treatment

The treatment of choice consists of avoidance of further sweating and allowing the skin surface to dry and cool. If pustule formation occurs and secondary staphylococcal infection appears, systemic antibiotics should be administered. Cooling lotions and other agents used for miliaria are not effective unless sweating is reduced.

Patient Education

The role of overheating and sweating should be emphasized. The parent who overdresses the infant or child should be duly informed. Avoidance of plastic occlusive dressings and cooling of the skin must be stressed.

Follow-up Visits

Follow-up visits are unnecessary.

MECHANOBULLOUS DISEASE

Trauma or friction on the skin surface will induce blister formation in this group of diseases, and virtually all blisters and erosions seen clinically will be associated with skin trauma. One should think of friction blisters and the forms of epidermolysis bullosa.

Friction Blisters

Clinical Features

These blisters occur on the soles of the feet after prolonged walking and on palmar surfaces because of excessive friction on the hands. Hemorrhage into the blisters is uncommon, and they heal without scars.

Differential Diagnosis

Friction blisters differ from epidermolysis bullosa states (see next section) by the difficulty in inducing blister formation (Table 11–2). Friction blisters are produced by major skin surface trauma, whereas minor or trivial skin trauma will produce blisters in epidermolysis bullosa.

Pathogenesis

Friction produces a blister cavity within the epidermis, shearing apart the cells of the midepidermis.

TABLE 11–2.

Differential Diagnosis of Mechanobullous Disease

Friction blisters
Recurrent bullous eruption of hands and feet (Weber-Cockayne disease)
Epidermolysis bullosa simplex (generalized and superficialis types)
Epidermolysis bullosa dystrophica, recessive and dominant types
Epidermolysis bullosa letalis (fatal and nonfatal types)
Porphyria cutanea tarda

Treatment and Follow-up Visits

Treatment and follow-up visits are unnecessary.

Patient Education

Friction may be reduced by padding shoes, wearing protective gloves, or painting the palms and soles with tincture of benzoin.

Epidermolysis Bullosa

At least 17 distinct hereditary types of epidermolysis bullosa have been described (Table 11–3). They may generally be divided into scarring and nonscarring forms. The disease is quite uncommon, with the incidence estimated at 1 in 50,000 births. Correct diagnosis in the immediate newborn period may be difficult, particularly in the instance of junctional bullous dermatosis (epidermolysis bullosa letalis), in which the baby may have few or no blisters in the first 30 days of life but may develop severe blisters in the second or third month, and may eventually even die of the illness. In contrast, in the generalized form of epidermolysis bullosa simplex, many blisters may be present at birth, suggesting epidermolysis bullosa of a dystrophic type, but few lesions appear after the first month of life. In all 17 described forms of epidermolysis bullosa, the evolution of individual lesions during the first month of life may confuse the clinician. Extreme care must be taken in obtaining and interpreting skin biopsy specimens from newborn infants to distinguish among the mechanobullous diseases. Shave or ellipse biopsy of the edge of a blister that is less than 12 hours old is preferred. Both light and electron microscopic examination should be done.

Clinical Features (Nonscarring Forms)

Recurrent Bullous Eruption of the Hands and Feet (Weber-Cockayne Disease).— The usual onset of recurrent bullous eruption of the hands and feet (Weber-Cockayne disease) is in late childhood or adolescence, when blistering

TABLE 11–3.

Classification of Epidermolysis Bullosa (EB)

Nonscarring	Heredity	Type
Intraepidermal separation	AD	EB simplex, generalized (Koebner)
	AD	EB simplex, localized (recurrent bullous eruption of hands and feet (Weber-Cockayne disease)
	AD	EB simplex superficialis
	AD	EB simplex (Ogna)
	AD	EB simplex (Dowling-Meara)
	AD	EB simplex with mottled pigmentation
Junctional separation	AR	Junctional bullous dermatosis, lethal type (Herlitz)
	AR	Junctional bullous dermatosis, nonlethal type
	AR	Localized atrophic EB
	AR	Inverse localized atrophic EB
	AR	Generalized atrophic benign EB
	AR	Cicatricial junctional EB
Subepidermal separation	AR	Dystrophic EB, recessive
	AD	Dystrophic EB, dominant
	AD	Albopapuloid EB (Pasini)
	AR	Dystrophic EB, localized
	AR	Dystrophic EB, inverse

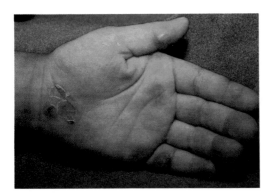

FIG 11–26.
Hand of child with recurrent bullous eruption of hands and feet, Weber-Cockayne variety of epidermolysis bullosa simplex. Minor trauma of play-induced palmar blisters.

of the hands and feet follows minor trauma (Fig 11–26). In warm weather, blistering may be so severe that the shoes cannot be worn. Blisters heal without scars. The condition is inherited as an autosomal dominant trait, with male patients more severely affected than female.

Epidermolysis Bullosa Simplex (Generalized Form).—In epidermolysis bullosa simplex, bullae may be present at birth, but usually do not begin to appear until the infant is 6 to 12 months of age. They are most numerous on the hands and feet, but may be present near elbows, knees, and other sites of friction (Fig 11–27). In contrast to Weber-Cockayne disease, they occur on the dorsa of the hands and feet. This condition is autosomal dominant and worsens in warm weather.

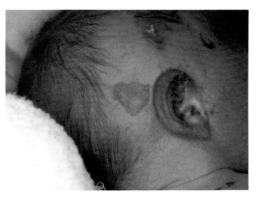

FIG 11–28.
Few blisters on scalp of newborn infant with junctional epidermolysis bullosa of Herlitz type.

Epidermolysis Bullosa Simplex Superficialis.—Onset of skin lesions in this condition occurs at birth. The lesions appear as areas of peeling skin. Pressure or heat can induce the lesions.

Epidermolysis Bullosa Letalis.—Two forms of epidermolysis bullosa letalis exist. They are very difficult to distinguish at birth in that both may start with few lesions (Fig 11–28). In the lethal form, mucous membrane lesions appear early in the disease (Fig 11–29); in the nonlethal form they do not. Failure to thrive is also a prominent symptom of the lethal form. There is considerable overlap between these two recognized forms. In epidermolysis bullosa letalis, at birth or shortly thereafter a generalized eruption of severe bullae appears on the skin and mucous membranes. The oral mucosa is severely affected, which may interfere with feeding. Tracheal and bronchiolar involvement produces respiratory distress. Infection and malnutrition often result in

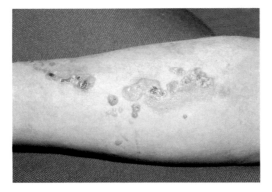

FIG 11–27.
Blisters, crusts, and healing blisters in child with generalized form of epidermolysis bullosa simplex.

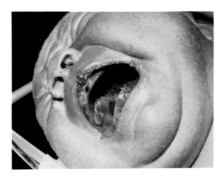

FIG 11–29.
Oral erosions in infant with Herlitz type of junctional epidermolysis bullosa.

death, but a few patients with mild blistering and occasional severe exacerbations have survived. A large bulla that has been extended at the margin by friction may be hemorrhagic and heal with scarring, but the majority of the lesions heal without scarring. The disease is inherited as an autosomal recessive trait, with a high incidence of abortion and stillbirth reported. Recurrent blisters of the nail bed result in permanent shedding of the nails.

Clinical Features: Scarring Forms

Epidermolysis Bullosa Dystrophica, Recessive Type.—In epidermolysis bullosa dystrophica of the recessive type, hemorrhagic bullae appear at birth or within a few months after birth (Fig 11–30). Removal of the blister roof leaves a raw, bleeding base that heals with a scar. Scars often entrap islands of epithelium, producing milia that appear as tiny white cysts within scars. Scarring is often sufficiently severe to result in replacement of fingernails and pseudowebbing of all digits, leading to a clublike appearance of the hands and feet (Fig 11–31). Scarring alopecia of the scalp also occurs. Blisters and erosions in the oral mucosa result in limitation of eating, immobilization of the tongue, and esophageal stricture. Laryngeal bullae will produce respiratory stridor. The teeth are malformed and carious (Fig 11–32). Anemia due to chronic blood loss and malnutrition occurs, and failure to thrive is commonly seen. Secondary bacterial infection or *Candida* infection of the skin areas is common. Squamous cell carcinoma may arise in atrophic scars on the skin or leukoplakia scars on mucous membranes. This disorder is inherited as an autosomal recessive trait.

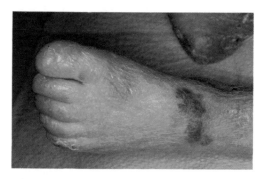

FIG 11–31.
Loss of toenails, fusion of digits, scarring, and newly formed hemorrhagic blisters in child with recessive dystrophic epidermolysis bullosa.

Epidermolysis Bullosa Dystrophica, Dominant Type.—In epidermolysis bullosa dystrophica of the dominant type, hemorrhagic bullae are seen at birth, primarily on the extremities (Fig 11–33). Atrophic scars are present, as are milia. Mucous membrane involvement, however, is unusual, and growth and development are normal in this form, in contrast to the recessive form. Ichthyosis, keratosis pilaris, thickened nails, and hyperhidrosis are often associated with the autosomal dominant form. A variant of the dominant dystrophic form occurs, in which clinical blisters are not seen, but scars and milia formation are characteristic. In this form, white atrophic lesions with numerous milia are found predominantly on the trunk.

Differential Diagnosis

The ease of blistering skin by suction or friction will differentiate epidermolysis bullosa from

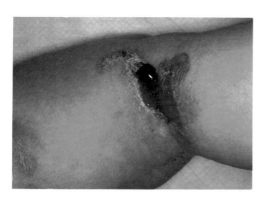

FIG 11–30.
Hemorrhagic blister in newborn infant with recessive dystrophic epidermolysis bullosa.

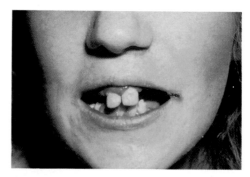

FIG 11–32.
Loss of teeth and mouth opening restricted by scarring in child with recessive dystrophic epidermolysis bullosa.

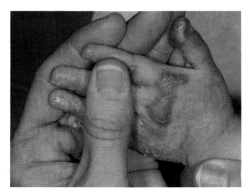

FIG 11–33.
Blister, scarring, and milia formation in dominant type of dystrophic epidermolysis bullosa.

friction blisters or spontaneous blistering disease (see Table 11–2). At birth, obstetric injuries are frequently confused because of the hemorrhagic blisters and eroded, raw areas. Urinary uroporphyrins will distinguish porphyria cutanea tarda from epidermolysis bullosa. The forms of epidermolysis bullosa may be differentiated from one another by the inheritance pattern and on the basis of a skin biopsy specimen examined by electron microscopy.

Pathogenesis

All forms of epidermolysis bullosa are inherited. The mechanism of the disease is thought to be related to deficiencies in keratinocyte-derived adhesion factors in skin. The three nonscarring forms are the result of separation of epidermal components (Fig 11–34). They are distinguished

by ultrastructural examination of the skin biopsy specimen. Recurrent bullous eruption of the hands and feet demonstrates a separation of epidermal cells just above the basal layer. Epidermolysis bullosa simplex superficialis demonstrates a separation within the granular layer of epidermis. It is the most superficial blister formation of all the forms of epidermolysis bullosa. Epidermolysis bullosa simplex separates the basal cells within the basal layer. In epidermolysis bullosa letalis, the separation occurs just below the plasma membrane of the basal cells and above the basal lamina of the dermis.

The two scarring forms show a separation below the basal lamina in the dermis. In epidermolysis bullosa dystrophica, recessive type, the anchoring fibrils, which support the basal lamina, are missing.

The biochemical abnormalities in the forms of epidermolysis bullosa are not known, but molecular biology techniques will undoubtedly identify specific defects.

Treatment

Treatment is symptomatic and supportive. One of the US centers for epidermolysis bullosa may be consulted for a comprehensive care program. For the scarring and junctional forms, skilled nursing and general health care are required. For the newborn infant, small, frequent feedings with a soft nipple are indicated. Gentle handling, soft, loose-fitting clothing, gentle sponge baths, cotton diapers, and a sheepskin pad for the crib should be instituted. Large blisters

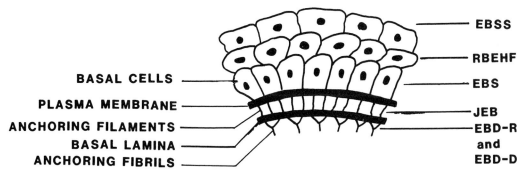

FIG 11–34.
Sites of blister formation in forms of epidermolysis bullosa: granular layer of upper epidermis in epidermolysis bullosa simplex superficialis *(EBSS)*, just above basal cells in recurrent bullosa eruption of hands and feet *(RBEHF)*, at level of basal cells in general- ized epidermolysis bullosa simplex *(EBS)*, within lamina lucida in junctional epidermolysis bullosa *(JEB)*, and beneath basal lamina in both recessive *(EBD-R)* and dominant *(EBD-D)* forms of dystrophic epidermolysis bullosa.

can be opened with sterile scissors and the roof allowed to collapse by gently compressing out the fluid. Blisters and erosions should have a topical antibiotic (mupirocin) applied gently to the surface (a wooden tongue depressor is useful).

For infants and children, a passive physical therapy program should be instituted. Water beds, egg crate padding, or sheepskin is useful for sleep. Keeping the room cool will reduce blistering and the accompanying pruritus. Wound dressings, such as Vigilon, Second Skin, and DuoDerm, may be useful for large nonhealing erosions. Keratinocyte-cultured autografts have been successful in severe nonhealing areas. If anemia is present, vitamin supplements and iron may be required. Protein and caloric requirements may be twice that recommended for size because of ongoing skin or mucosal losses. Fluids should be lukewarm, and acidic juices avoided. Ensure or other nutritional supplements may be considered. Whole grain breads and cereals may reduce constipation, which can be a major problem. A multidisciplinary approach is required in the scarring forms to deal with problems such as esophageal strictures, dental disease, pseudodactyly, laryngeal disorders, urethral meatal stenosis, conjunctival scarring, and psychosocial problems.

In recurrent bullous eruption of the hands and feet, resistance to friction may improve by painting the hands and feet one to two times a week with tincture of benzoin or spray preparations such as Tuff-Skin.

Patient Education

Much support is required for parents and patients with these disorders, which are chronic, frustrating, and, in the dystrophic form, severely debilitating. Patients should be provided with a checklist of steps to reduce friction and instructed by persons skilled in nursing techniques. The lay support group DEBRA of America, Inc. (451 Clarkson Ave., Suite 6101, Brooklyn, NY 11203) has excellent information available for parents and a North American network of local support groups to help families with children who have epidermolysis bullosa.

Follow-up Visits

A regular schedule of visits is required to monitor anemia and secondary infections. After birth, visits should be weekly or biweekly. Routine immunizations and well baby care are needed.

BIBLIOGRAPHY

Bligard C: Kawasaki disease and its diagnosis. *Pediatr Dermatol* 1987; 4:67.

Brice SL, Huff JC, Weston WL: Erythema multiforme. *Curr Probl Dermatol* 1990; 2:1–26.

Brice SL, Krzemien D, Weston WL, et al: Detection of herpes simplex virus DNA in cutaneous lesions of erythema multiforme. *J Invest Dermatol* 1989; 93:183.

Chorzelski T, Jablonska S: Evolving concept of IgA linear dermatosis. *Semin Dermatol* 1988; 7:225.

Cooper TW, Bauer EA: Epidermolysis bullosa: a review. *Pediatr Dermatol* 1984; 1:189.

Dawson TA Jr: Microscopic appearance of geographic tongue. *Br J Dermatol* 1969; 81:827.

Eady RAJ, Tidman MJ: Diagnosing epidermolysis bullosa. *Br J Dermatol* 1983; 108:621.

Fine J-D, Johnson L, Wright T, et al: Epidermolysis bullosa simplex: Identification of a kindred with autosomal recessive transmission of the Weber-Cockayne variety. *Pediatr Dermatol* 1989; 6:1.

Fry L: Fine points in the management of dermatitis herpetiformis. *Semin Dermatol* 1988; 7:206.

Hansen RC: Blindness, anonychia, and oral mucosal scarring as sequelae of the Stevens-Johnson syndrome. *Pediatr Dermatol* 1984; 1:298.

Huff JC: Therapy and prevention of erythema multiforme with acyclovir. *Semin Dermatol* 1988; 7:212.

Lechner-Gruskay D, Honig PJ, Pereira G, et al: Nutritional and metabolic profile of children with epidermolysis bullosa. *Pediatr Dermatol* 1988; 5:22.

Manzella JP et al: Toxic epidermal necrolysis in childhood: Differentiation from staphylococcal scalded skin syndrome. *Pediatrics* 1980; 66:291.

O'Brien JP: The pathogenesis of miliaria. *Arch Dermatol* 1962; 86:267.

Pessar A, Verdicchio JF, Caldwell D: Epidermolysis bullosa: The Pediatric Dermatological Management and Therapeutic Update. *Adv Dermatol* 1988; 3:99.

Rowley AH, Duffy CE, Shulman ST: Prevention of giant coronary artery aneurysms in Kawasaki disease by intravenous gamma globulin therapy. *J Pediatr* 1988; 113:290.

Schachner L, Press S: Vesicular, bullous and pustular disorders in infancy and childhood. *Pediatr Clin North Am* 1983; 30:609.

Shulman ST, Bass JL, Bierman F, et al: Management of Kawasaki syndrome: A consensus statement prepared by North American participants of the Third International Kawasaki Disease

Symposium, Tokyo, Japan, December, 1988. *Pediatr Infect Dis J* 1989; 8:663.

Sulzberger MB, et al: Studies on blisters produced by friction. *J Invest Dermatol* 1966; 47:456.

Wojnarowska F: Chronic bullous disease of childhood. *Semin Dermatol* 1988; 7:58.

Woodley DT, Briggaman RA: New immunologic techniques for the fine diagnosis of blistering disease. *Semin Dermatol* 1989; 7:178.

12 _____ Skin Cysts and Nodules

Persistent masses in the skin often result in a child's being brought in for medical examination. Frequently parents are concerned about cancer. Biopsy is usually necessary to provide an accurate diagnosis in these conditions, even though the masses are rarely symptomatic except in weight-bearing areas. A large number of skin problems can produce skin nodules. When one observes a skin-colored nodule in an infant or child, an orderly list of possibilities does not easily come to mind. One should first remember that the most common palpable superficial nodule in infants and children is the lymph node. Occipital and cervical nodes are superficial and easily palpated, and sometimes may be mistaken for skin tumors or nodules.

The most common types of superficial skin nodules in infants and children are listed in Table 12–1. An estimation of the approximate frequency of each skin nodule in infants and children is provided. Epithelial cysts and pilomatricomas together account for 70% of such superficial nodules, and one should remember particularly these two major causes of skin nodules when making a diagnosis. Overall, only 1% of such skin nodules turn out to be malignant growths. The main factors in suspecting whether one of these nodules is malignant are listed in Table 12–2. The most important factor is rapid, progressive growth. No matter what the appearance of a skin nodule is, if rapid progressive growth occurs, one should suspect malignancy and obtain a tissue sample for diagnosis.

SKIN CYSTS

Skin cysts are often solitary in children and produce skin-colored nodules that distort skin contours. They are the most common skin nodule, found predominantly on the lateral border of the eyebrow or under the scalp, both in infants and children (Fig 12–1).

Clinical Features

Epithelial Cysts, Dermoid Cysts, and Milia.—Epithelial cysts are slow-growing, firm, round nodules that reach a maximum size of 1 to 5 cm. Epithelial cysts in the newborn period are usually dermoid cysts found predominantly on the lateral border of the eyebrow or on the scalp. In adolescence, solitary cysts appear on the scalp, face, neck, and trunk in the region where acne vulgaris is seen. Multiple cysts in children or adolescents should suggest Gardner's syndrome. This is an autosomal dominant syndrome associated with possible malignant degeneration of intestinal polyposis in addition to multiple epithelial cysts, osteomas, and fibrous tissue tumors of the skin. Milia are tiny, superficial cysts seen on the face of newborn infants and within scars or sites of recent skin trauma.

Steatocystoma Multiplex.—Steatocystoma multiplex appears as firm, skin-colored or yellowish nodules 1 to 3 cm in diameter in the axillae and on the chest and arms. The condition is inherited as autosomal dominant, begins in adolescence, and is quite uncommon.

Eruptive Vellus Hair Cysts.—Eruptive vellus hair cysts begin at ages 5 to 10 years as small, 1- to 3-mm skin-colored papules appearing on the lower aspect of the chest and upper part of the abdomen, areas not usually involved with epithelial or dermoid cysts (Fig 12–2). Usually five or more lesions are present.

TABLE 12–1.

Skin Nodules and Cysts in Infants and Children

Type	Approximate Percentage of All Nodules
Epithelial cysts	60
Pilomatricomas	10
Neurofibromas	3
Lipomas	3
Lymphangiomas	3
Granuloma annulare	3
Juvenile xanthogranulomas	2
Mastocytomas	2
Fibromas	2
Malignant tumors (sarcomas)	1
Miscellaneous lesions	11

TABLE 12–2.

Factors Associated With Likelihood of Malignancy in Superficial Skin Tumors in Children*

Rapid, progressive growth
Ulceration
Fixed to deep fascia
Larger than 3 cm and firm
Occurs in first 30 days of life
*Listed in order of importance.

Differential Diagnosis

For a list of skin nodules and cysts that should be included in the differential diagnosis, see Table 12–1. Epithelial and dermoid cysts are difficult to distinguish from one another without a biopsy. Since both are usually benign, however, a biopsy is generally not necessary. Midline nasal

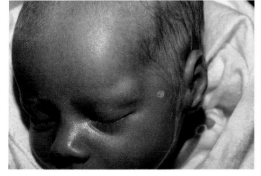

FIG 12–1.
Epithelial cyst. Cystic nodule on lateral aspect of left eyebrow of newborn infant.

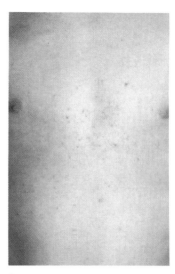

FIG 12–2.
Eruptive vellus hair cysts. Superficial cystic lesions on midportion of chest and upper aspect of abdomen.

dermoid lesions are the exception. These appear as a midline pit, fistula, or swelling anywhere from the glabella to the nasal tip. These lesions may have intracranial extensions. Steatocystoma multiplex similarly has a different distribution, with locations around the axilla, neck, and onto the arms. Gardner's syndrome should be considered when multiple epithelial cysts are seen.

Pathogenesis

Epithelial Cysts and Milia.—Although epithelial cysts are commonly called *sebaceous cysts,* they contain neither sebum nor sebaceous glands. Epithelial cysts and milia are filled with keratin in laminated layers and lined by epithelium. When they are ruptured, foreign body reactions occur around the ruptured cyst wall.

Steatocystoma Multiplex.—Steatocystoma multiplex consists of intricately folded cyst walls of epithelial cells, with flattened sebaceous gland lobules within or close to the cyst wall.

Dermoid Cysts.—Dermoid cysts represent sequestration of skin along lines of embryonic closure and contain an epithelial lining plus either mature sebaceous glands, eccrine sweat glands, or mature hair.

Eruptive Vellus Hair Cysts.—Most authorities consider eruptive vellus hair cysts a developmental anomaly of body hair follicles. Obstruction at the neck of the follicular channel results in cystic dilation of the follicle, retention of vellus hairs, and atrophy of the hair bulbs.

Treatment

Most cysts require no treatment and may be best left alone. If cosmetic improvement can be obtained, surgical excision is the treatment of choice. Midline nasal dermoid cysts require meticulous surgical excision in an effort to prevent intracranial extension and complications. No effective therapy for vellus hair cysts is available.

Patient Education

Patients should be aware of the benign nature of these growths despite their prominent size. In children with multiple epithelial cysts, bowel examination for signs of Gardner's syndrome is indicated.

Follow-up Visits

A visit 1 week after surgery to explain the pathologic findings is beneficial.

SKIN NODULES

Neurofibromas

Clinical Features

Neurofibromas may be present at birth or develop later in life. The neurofibroma is a soft skin-colored papule or nodule that may appear anywhere on the skin (Figs 12–3 and 12–4). Neurofibromas may occur as solitary lesions not associated with neurofibromatosis. When multiple neurofibromas are present, café au lait spots may accompany the neurofibroma, but few or no café au lait spots may be present at birth. The combination of six or more café au lait spots larger than 0.5 cm in greatest diameter and two or more neurofibromas is considered to be diagnostic of neurofibromatosis type 1 or Recklinghausen's disease in prepubertal children. Occasionally neurofibromas appear as soft nodules within a large café au lait spot. More commonly, however, they develop as soft nodules in adolescence in a child with multiple café au lait spots. Large plexiform neurofibromas can occur that cause hideous deformity because of the mass of hanging tissue. Solitary neurofibromas in adolescence may be observed in the absence of neurofibromatosis type 1.

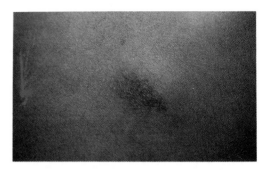

FIG 12–3.
Neurofibroma. Soft nodule with overlying hyperpigmentation.

Differential Diagnosis

The differential diagnosis of neurofibromas is listed in Table 12–3. A biopsy may be necessary to confirm the diagnosis.

Pathogenesis

Neurofibromas are benign tumors of nerve sheath cells. Some evidence suggests that the overgrowth of nerve sheath cells may be stimulated by nerve growth factor or other circulating growth factors.

Treatment

Large neurofibromas on the weight-bearing areas of the foot or on the palm of the hand are difficult, if not impossible, to treat. Surgical excision may result in severe scarring deformities, and the resulting deformity should be carefully considered before surgical intervention is undertaken.

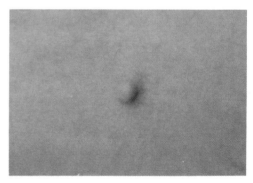

FIG 12–4.
Neurofibroma. Soft, skin-colored papule.

TABLE 12–3.

Differential Diagnosis of Neurofibromas

> Angiolipoma
> Hemangioma
> Lipoma
> Lymphangioma
> Mucous cyst
> Melanocytic nevus

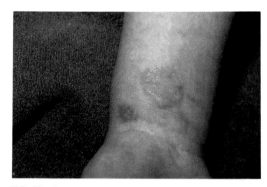

FIG 12–6.
Granuloma annulare. Large and small annular plaques on ventral surface of arm. Central resolution is seen in larger lesion.

Patient Education

The nature of neurofibromas and their association with multiple neurofibromatosis should be carefully explained to the family, and a complete family history should be obtained.

Follow-up Visits

Children with neurofibromatosis should be followed every 6 to 12 months and examined for the appearance of café au lait spots or other signs and symptoms of neurofibromatosis.

Granuloma Annulare

Clinical Features

Small, firm papules or nodules that form a circle or semicircle are characteristic of granuloma annulare. They may be skin colored, but more often a dusky, violaceous hue is seen. Stretching the skin reveals the ring of papules or nodules. The lesions occur predominantly in acral areas (Figs 12–5 and 12–6), on the digits, ankles, and wrists; 50% of the children have a single ring of lesions. Occasionally large subcutaneous nod-

ules may be seen, or multiple small papules are found (Fig 12–7). Lesions are usually asymptomatic.

Differential Diagnosis

Small, annular lesions are often mistaken for dermatophyte infections. The lack of epidermal change or scaling and the deep palpable portion help distinguish granuloma annulare from tinea corporis. Large nodules of granuloma annulare may mimic rheumatoid nodules, and subcutaneous granuloma annulare may be histologically and clinically indistinguishable from rheumatoid nodules. In granuloma annulare, no systemic symptoms are noted. Occasionally other annulare lesions (e.g., lichen planus, sarcoidosis, syphilis, necrobiosis lipoidica diabeticorum) are confused with granuloma annulare, and a biopsy will be necessary to confirm the diagnosis.

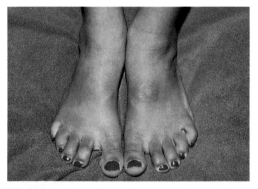

FIG 12–5.
Granuloma annulare. Unilateral oval lesion on dorsum of foot.

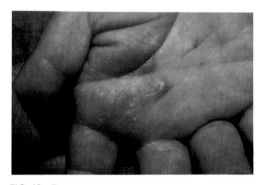

FIG 12–7.
Granuloma annulare. Grouping of firm papules on palm of hand.

Pathogenesis

Focal areas of collagen degeneration surrounded by lymphocytes and epithelioid cells are seen in the middermis and reticular dermis in granuloma annulare. The presence of immunoreactants around cutaneous blood vessels has been interpreted as indicating that a chronic vasculitis produced the granuloma. The mechanism of the disease is unknown, however. The term "pseudorheumatoid nodule" is sometimes used by pathologists to distinguish granuloma annulare from rheumatoid nodules. The term "granuloma annulare" is preferred.

Treatment

Since lesions are asymptomatic, only reassurance is necessary. Although it is tempting to treat such conditions, spontaneous remission within 2 years is the rule, and no effective therapy is available.

Patient Education

The benign nature of this disorder and its natural history should be stressed. Its distinct separation from rheumatoid disease states should be explained.

Follow-up Visits

Follow-up visits are unnecessary.

Rheumatoid Nodules

Clinical Features

True rheumatoid nodules are uncommon in children with rheumatic disease. They are seen in rheumatoid arthritis, rheumatic fever, and systemic lupus erythematosus as 1- to 4-cm subcutaneous nodules not attached to overlying skin. They develop over bony structures such as a joint and are usually associated with severe rheumatoid disease with positive rheumatoid factor. The overlying skin has a normal color, and the lesion may not be attached to the overlying epidermis (see Fig 12–7).

Differential Diagnosis

Rheumatoid nodules are most often confused with granuloma annulare. Epithelial cysts, adnexal tumors, lipomas, and other skin nodules may also be confused with rheumatoid nodules, however.

Pathogenesis

Foci of collagen degeneration surrounded by macrophages are seen in the reticular dermis and subcutaneous fat. The mechanism of production of rheumatoid nodules is unknown, but most investigators regard this condition as a form of immune complex disease.

Treatment

If the nodules are symptomatic, excision is the treatment of choice. Therapy used to control other rheumatic symptoms rarely influences rheumatoid nodules.

Patient Education

Information about the nature of the associated disease should be given.

Follow-up Visits

The timing of follow-up visits should be based on the severity of the associated systemic illness.

Fibromas

Clinical Features

Dermatofibromas.—The presenting symptom of dermatofibroma is a small, firm, well-defined, often pigmented nodule on the leg or trunk of children, adolescents, and adults (Figs 12–8). Dermatofibroma may follow minor skin trauma or may appear to occur spontaneously. Multiple lesions can also occur. Lateral pressure on the lesion will produce dimpling of its surface. The lesions may become as large as 1 to 2 cm in diameter, and they persist indefinitely.

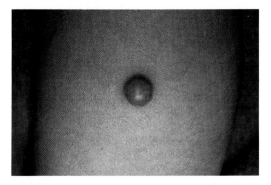

FIG 12–8.
Dermatofibroma. Firm, well-defined pigmented nodule on leg of an adolescent.

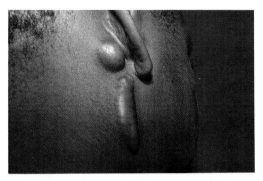

FIG 12–9.
Epithelial cyst and keloid. Superior lesion is an epithelial cyst, and lower lesion is a keloid that formed in excision scar of a previously excised epithelial cyst.

Keloids.—Keloids are firm, progressively enlarging nodules with a shiny, hairless surface. They may be painful or itch. They may occur on the extremities, but are predominantly located on the earlobes (Figs 12–9 and 12–10), presternal area, neck, and face after skin trauma. They often have stellate shapes. The tendency to form keloids may be inherited, and they are more common in blacks. They may progressively enlarge for 20 to 40 years and form lobulated or pedunculated masses.

Hypertrophic Scars.—A hypertrophic scar is an overgrowth of fibrous tissue that remains at the site of the original injury (Fig 12–11).

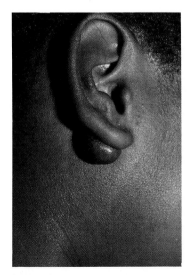

FIG 12–10.
Keloid. Nodule on ear after ear piercing.

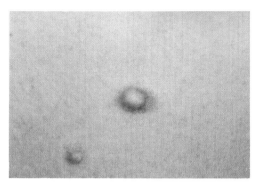

FIG 12–11.
Hypertrophic scar. Site of previous chickenpox lesion.

Digital Fibrous Tumor of Childhood.—Digital fibrous tumor of childhood is a firm nodule occurring around the fingernail or toenail. The lesion may be present at birth or will usually arise before 1 year of age. Excision often results in rapid recurrence. The lesion may initially grow rapidly and require a skin biopsy to confirm that it is not a sarcoma. It will usually spontaneously involute within several years.

Differential Diagnosis
Dermatofibromas.—Dermatofibromas may be pigmented and mimic melanoma. They are more likely to be confused with other skin nodules, however (see Table 12–1).

Keloids and Hypertrophic Scars.—Keloids are seldom misdiagnosed, but early keloids mimic ordinary scars. The keloid will extend beyond the bounds of the original injury, whereas the hypertrophic scar will remain within the area of injury.

Recurrent Digital Fibrous Tumors.—Recurrent digital fibrous tumors may mimic the fibrous thickening overlying a subungual exostosis, a callus, or a corn. An x-ray film of the digit should be obtained before biopsy.

Pathogenesis
Dermatofibromas.—Dermatofibromas contain numerous fibroblasts with excessive deposition of collagen and proliferation of the overlying epidermis. They are believed to be a reactive proliferation of fibroblasts in response to trauma.

Keloids and Hypertrophic Scars.—Keloids produce nodular patterns of collagen fibers associated with the new blood vessel formation, as expected in healing. As the vessels regress, however, collagen deposition continues and fails to thin as expected. Hypertrophic scars may be a similar process to a lesser degree.

Recurrent Digital Fibrous Tumors.—Recurrent digital fibrous tumors show proliferating fibroblasts that contain eosinophilic cytoplasmic inclusions thought to represent myofilaments.

Treatment

Dermatofibromas, if symptomatic or worrisome, may be excised. Keloids are best treated by injection of intralesional glucocorticosteroids, which results in softening and flattening. Often triamcinolone acetonide, 3 to 10 mg/mL, is injected. Surgery alone will result in rapid reappearance of the keloid, but surgery followed by frequent intralesional injections of glucocorticosteroids may be effective therapy for large keloids. Hypertrophic scars may regress with time or they can be treated as keloids. Recurring digital fibrous tumors should be allowed to involute spontaneously.

Patient Education

The benign nature of these disorders should be emphasized.

Follow-up Visits

Keloids may be injected at 4- to 6-week intervals.

Lipomas

Clinical Features

Lipomas are soft subcutaneous nodules unattached to overlying skin (Fig 12–12). They are usually solitary, begin in adolescence, and are most commonly found on the neck, upper aspect of the chest, and arms. Angiolipomas, variants of lipomas, may present as painful subcutaneous nodules.

Differential Diagnosis

Epithelial cysts, neurofibromas, and other skin nodules may mimic lipomas, but the ability to easily slide the overlying skin over the lesion helps to confirm the deep subcutaneous location of lipomas (see Table 12–3).

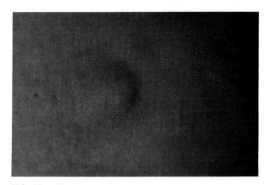

FIG 12–12.
Lipoma. Soft subcutaneous nodule unattached to overlying skin.

Pathogenesis

A lipoma is composed of nodules of normal-appearing fat cells, although unresponsiveness of fat cells to the lipolytic effects of norepinephrine occurs in multiple symmetric lipomatosis. Capillary proliferation is seen in angiolipoma in addition to an excess of normal fat cells.

Treatment

Lipomas are usually asymptomatic. Angiolipomas may be painful and may require excision for pain relief.

Patient Education

The benign nature of these nodules should be emphasized.

Follow-up Visits

Follow-up visits are unnecessary.

Juvenile Xanthogranulomas

Clinical Features

In juvenile xanthogranulomas, orange to yellow-brown firm nodules appear on the skin of infants (Figs 12–13 and 12–14). The nodules are often multiple, numbering five to ten. They may be present at birth and often involute spontaneously within a year. Lesions are seen in the iris and may be mistaken for retinoblastoma, or they may cause glaucoma. Although involvement is primarily in the skin, nodules have been described in the testes, lung, liver, spleen, and pericardium.

Differential Diagnosis

Xanthomas, spindle and epithelioid melanocytic nevi, histiocytosis, and mastocytomas all may

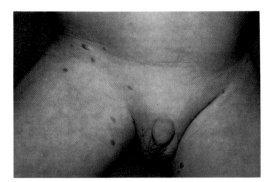

FIG 12–13.
Juvenile xanthogranuloma. Grouping of lesions on lower aspect of trunk and on thigh.

appear as orange or yellow-brown nodules at first presentation (Table 12–4). Skin biopsy is necessary to distinguish juvenile xanthogranuloma from these conditions. Stroking the skin surface covering a mastocytoma will produce urticaria within the nodule (Darier's sign).

Pathogenesis
Within the dermis, large accumulations of macrophages appear. Their cytoplasm gradually fills with lipid, creating a particular type of giant cell called the Touton giant cell. Regressing lesions show fibroblastic proliferation. There is no apparent relationship between juvenile xanthogranuloma and either abnormalities of lipid metabolism or malignant histiocytosis.

Treatment
No treatment is necessary.

TABLE 12–4.

Differential Diagnosis of Orange or Yellow-Brown Nodules
Benign cephalic histiocytosis
Histiocytosis X
Juvenile xanthogranuloma
Mastocytoma
Spindle and epithelioid cell melanocytic nevus
Xanthoma

Patient Education
The natural history of this lesion and the need for careful observation for eye involvement should be emphasized.

Follow-up Visits
Quarterly visits for examination of the eyes and observation of regression of the lesions are often beneficial.

HISTIOCYTOSIS

Clinical Features
The histiocytoses include a group of benign and fatal disorders. Lesions may be present at birth or appear during infancy or childhood (Fig 12–15). The cutaneous lesions may consist of discrete red-, orange or yellow-brown papules or nodules. The presenting symptom may be crusted, scaling dermatitis on the scalp, postauricular, perineal, and axillary areas. Presence of red-brown purpuric papules and nodules within or

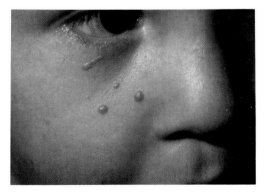

FIG 12–14.
Juvenile xanthogranuloma. Orange-brown coloration is seen on close inspection.

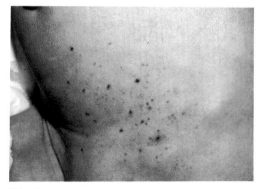

FIG 12–15.
Histiocytosis X. Crusted purpuric papules on lower aspect of abdomen, with underlying lymphadenopathy.

peripheral to areas of dermatitis should alert the physician to a diagnosis of histiocytosis.

Benign cephalic histiocytosis consists of 2 to 5 mm yellow-red to tan papules that develop on the face and upper part of the body (Fig 12–16). The lesions usually begin between 6 and 12 months of age. They consist of non–Langerhans cell histiocytes.

Congenital self-healing reticulohistiocytosis consists of papules and nodular lesions present at birth that can look like the lesions of histiocytosis X (Fig 12–17). Larger lesions can demonstrate a crateriform central erosion.

Differential Diagnosis

Histiocytosis lesions include the differential diagnosis of juvenile xanthogranulomas as well as eczema, seborrheic dermatitis, and diaper dermatitis. Presence of petechiae or purpura within or peripheral to areas of dermatitis suggests histiocytosis.

Pathogenesis

The histiocyte is a monocyte-macrophage. The Langerhans cell is a specific monocyte-macrophage within the epidermis that has characteristic cell surface markers. The associated histiocytic syndromes represent infiltrations with histiocytic cells that may or may not be Langerhans cells.

The term "histiocytosis X" refers to a group

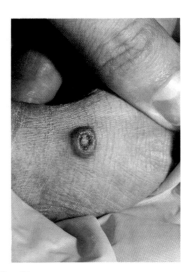

FIG 12–17.
Congenital self-healing reticulohistiocytosis. Nodule present at birth, with crateriform central erosion.

of disorders characterized by histiocytes and Langerhans cells within bone, skin, liver, spleen, lungs, and lymph nodes. The most benign form, eosinophilic granuloma, involves infiltration of Langerhans cells within bone. Chronic multifocal histiocytosis X (Hand-Schüller-Christian disease) includes patients who may have combinations of bony osteolytic defects, diabetes insipidus, or exophthalmos. The most severe form is acute disseminated histiocytosis X (Letterer-Siwe disease). At least 80% of these children have cutaneous lesions. Visceral involvement of the liver, lungs, and lymph nodes is common.

Benign cephalic histiocytosis lesions consist of non–Langerhans cell histiocytes. Congenital self-healing reticulohistiocytosis consists of Langerhans and non-Langerhans histiocytes.

Treatment

Treatment in these disorders depends on the specific diagnosis and extent of disease. A biopsy is usually necessary to confirm the diagnosis. Additional biopsies may be needed for electron microscopic examination and immunohistochemistry to confirm the specific type of histiocytosis.

Benign cephalic histiocytosis requires no therapy and should resolve during childhood. Congenital self-healing reticulohistiocytosis requires close clinical observation to confirm a benign course. Histiocytosis X survival and therapy are dependent on the number of organs involved

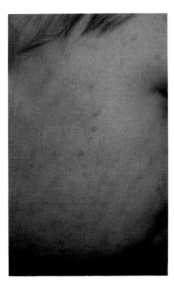

FIG 12–16.
Benign cephalic histiocytosis. Multiple tan papules on face.

and the severity of the involvement. Therapy for histiocytosis X may include surgical removal of lesions, radiotherapy, or chemotherapy. Chemotherapy usually includes prednisone and alkylating agents or vincristine. Before therapy, a systemic evaluation is required to identify the extent and severity of disease.

The dermatitis lesions of histiocytosis X often respond to topical steroid therapy in addition to systemic therapy.

Patient Education

A thorough evaluation is necessary to identify the type and extent of histiocytic syndromes. Parents should be informed of the unusual nature of histiocytosis and should be given information on the benign or malignant course that their child can expect.

Follow-up Visits

Diagnosis and treatment of these conditions require coordination with pathologist, radiologist, pediatric oncologist, and primary care physician. Follow-up visits should be arranged to inform the patient and the patient's family of the severity and extent of disease and possible therapies directed by the pediatric oncologist.

Pyogenic Granulomas

Clinical Features

Pyogenic granulomas are most common in acral areas, such as the hands and fingers, and on the face. They appear as solitary, dull-red, firm nodules that are 5 to 6 mm in diameter. The surface may be smooth and glistening (Fig 12–18), but often it is ulcerated and crusted. The lesion

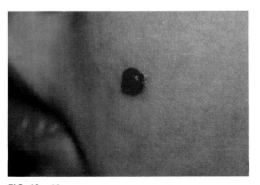

FIG 12–18.
Pyogenic granuloma. Smooth, glistening surface on an erythematous papule.

bleeds easily when traumatized. Removal has resulted in the appearance of multiple satellite lesions in a few instances. Pyogenic granuloma may occur at any age. A skin injury may precede the onset of growth.

Differential Diagnosis

Pyogenic granuloma is often misdiagnosed as a hemangioma, glomus tumor, melanocytic nevus, wart, molluscum contagiosum, or malignant melanoma. All these lesions can ulcerate and crust if traumatized. Pathologic study will distinguish pyogenic granuloma from the other lesions.

Pathogenesis

Proliferation of capillaries within a circumscribed area, with flattened or ulcerated epidermis on top and epidermal proliferation at the sides, producing a "collarette" of epidermis, is seen. Pyogenic granuloma is believed to be due to an abnormal healing response.

Treatment

Excision is the treatment of choice.

Patient Education

It should be explained that this growth is not malignant, but will not disappear without treatment and represents an abnormal healing response.

Follow-up Visits

A visit 1 week after removal of the lesion is useful to inform the patient of the pathology report on the removed tissue and to evaluate healing.

Lymphangiomas

Lymphangiomas are often present at birth and are discussed in detail in the section on Birthmarks in Chapter 19. They may, however, be overlooked until later in infancy and childhood, and their presenting symptom is solitary, soft swellings of the face, neck, trunk, or extremities, showing progressive growth.

Mastocytomas

Mastocytomas are usually present at birth and are discussed in detail in Chapters 13. They may not become apparent until 1 to 2 months of age, however, with macular red or red-brown lesions usually appearing on the trunk.

Smooth Muscle Hamartomas

Smooth muscle hamartomas are present at birth, but they may not be noted until later in infancy or childhood. The lesions may appear to have excess hair and may be hyperpigmented when compared with the normal skin. On palpation, the lesional hairs may become erect as a result of the excess smooth muscle within the lesion. Biopsy of the lesion will show abundant smooth muscle bundles within the dermis.

Calcified Nodules

Cutaneous calcinosis results from precipitation of insoluble calcium salts within cutaneous tissues. This can occur in congenital or acquired lesions. Solitary or multiple lesions can be present that are firm or rock hard. They are usually asymptomatic but can be painful and discharge chalky material through the skin. Underlying metabolic disease, connective tissue disease, or malignancy may be associated or the lesion can be idiopathic. In newborn infants, a solitary calcified nodule of the ear may form (Fig 12–19), while in children with dermatomyositis or other collagen vascular diseases, multiple nodules may form on the extensor surfaces of hands and elbows. Biopsy confirmation is necessary before a comprehensive systemic evaluation is begun.

Panniculitis

Inflammation in the subcutaneous fat may be first seen as painful lesions that feel as if they are deep beneath the skin. Biopsy will identify the in-flammation within the fat. The cause of the panniculitis may not be found, or it can be associated with infection, trauma, or metabolic or systemic disease. Biopsy confirmation may be necessary before a comprehensive systemic evaluation is begun. One type of panniculitis, subcutaneous fat necrosis of the newborn infant, is described in Chapter 19.

Sarcoidosis

Sarcoidosis is a systemic disease associated with granulomas. Skin lesions can occur with or without systemic symptoms. The skin lesions may appear as indurated papules or plaques. Skin biopsy showing the granulomas of sarcoid should prompt a systemic evaluation for sarcoidosis.

Necrobiosis Lipoidica Diabeticorum

The lesions of necrobiosis lipoidica diabeticorum are irregularly shaped yellow-red plaques on the lower leg (Fig 12–20). The lesions may show central atrophy or sclerosis. Often the lesions are bilateral and symmetric. A skin biopsy specimen of a lesion may have the histologic appearance of granuloma annulare. Children with necrobiosis lipoidica diabeticorum may have associated diabetes mellitus, and they should be evaluated with a fasting serum glucose test.

Rhabdomyosarcomas

Clinical Features

Rhabdomyosarcomas are the most common malignant soft tissue tumors occurring in child-

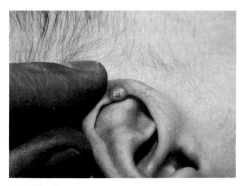

FIG 12–19.
Calcified nodule. Lesion on ear of infant.

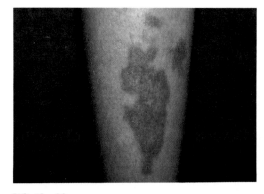

FIG 12–20.
Necrobiosis lipoidica diabeticorum. Large plaque on lower leg of female adolescent. Note elevated border and yellow-red coloration.

hood. They are far more common than melanomas in prepubertal children. The head and neck and urogenital tract are the usual sites of involvement. Two peaks of age in childhood have a higher incidence of rhabdomyosarcoma: ages 1 to 5 and adolescence. The tumor usually appears as a mass lesion of the neck, face, or extremity, or is seen as a subcutaneous or intradermal nodule covered with normal-appearing skin. Occasionally the surface of the skin covering the tumor becomes reddened. The lesion may produce local signs of destruction, depending on its location. For example, in the orbit, it may produce exophthalmos or ptosis; in the ear canal, a bloody discharge with a polypoid ear mass; and in the nasal passages, obstruction of one of the airways and bleeding. In the genitourinary tract, it may appear as urinary obstruction. Grapelike masses of tumor protruding from the vagina are another presentation of rhabdomyosarcoma.

Rhabdomyosarcoma may spread either by local extension or by hematogenous or lymphatic metastases. Seventy-five percent of the metastases will become apparent within 6 months of the appearance of the original lesion. The most frequent sites involved with metastases are the regional lymph nodes, lungs, liver, bone marrow, bone, and brain. Head and neck tumors have been reported to extend directly into the brain, and may occur as frequently as in one third of all cases.

Differential Diagnosis

The feature of rapid, progressive growth will help distinguish rhabdomyosarcoma from the other skin nodules and cysts of infants and children listed in Table 12–1. Ulceration is not an early sign of rhabdomyosarcoma, but the tumor is fixed to deep fascia, is often greater than 3 cm, and is firm in consistency.

Pathogenesis

Rhabdomyosarcoma is a malignant tumor of striated muscles. There is no hereditary pattern, and no known precipitating factors.

Treatment

Therapy has included radiation and combination chemotherapy in the initial stages of disease, following wide surgical excision. Debulking the tumor with wide surgical excision is the first treatment of choice. New therapeutic protocols are currently being evaluated.

Patient Education

Prognosis should be discussed with the family, keeping in mind that a number of factors are important in the survival rate. The location of the original lesion is an important factor, with the best prognosis found with orbital lesions, the next best with bladder lesions, and the worst with lesions beginning on the head and neck. Referral to a pediatric oncology facility as soon as the diagnosis is suspected is indicated.

Follow-up Visits

Follow-up visits should be arranged for family support, but a pediatric oncologist should be involved in determining frequency of visits.

Adnexal Tumors

A variety of benign growths arising from epithelial adnexa (sebaceous glands, hair follicles, sweat glands) produce skin nodules or tumors. Some, such as the sebaceous nevus and epidermal nevus, appear at birth and are discussed in the section on Birthmarks in Chapter 19. Most adnexal tumors do not appear until adult life, but four types, pilomatricomas, syringomas, trichoepitheliomas, and basal cell epitheliomas, may be seen in childhood or adolescence.

Clinical Features

Pilomatricomas.—Pilomatricomas (calcifying epitheliomas) appear as hard, 2 to 5 mm papules covered by normal skin on the face or extremities (Fig 12–21). They often begin in infancy or during the early school years, but are not hereditary. Pilomatricomas account for up to 10% of all skin nodules and tumors in children, and they

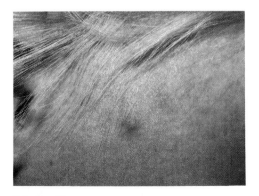

FIG 12–21.
Pilomatricoma. Firm blue papule on face of a child.

are usually solitary. They may be present in the newborn period.

Syringomas.—Syringomas appear at puberty as small (1 to 2 mm) skin-colored to yellowish soft nodules. They occur on the eyelids (Fig 12–22), cheeks, axillae, abdomen, and vulva. They are more common in girls than in boys. Most often, lesions are limited to the eyelids.

Trichoepitheliomas. — Trichoepitheliomas appear as numerous round, skin-colored nodules primarily on the midfacial area of adolescents. The nodules are 2 to 8 mm in diameter and may be seen on the upper aspect of the trunk and on the neck and scalp. A few fine telangiectases may be observed on the lesions. Multiple lesions are inherited as autosomal dominant, whereas solitary lesions may appear spontaneously without a family history.

Basal Cell Epitheliomas.—Basal cell epitheliomas are uncommon in school-age children and adolescents. They appear on the face or upper aspect of the trunk as a solitary nodule with overlying telangiectasia. They may be seen in otherwise unaffected children, but their presence should suggest three syndromes: the basal cell nevus syndrome, Bazex's syndrome, and xeroderma pigmentosum (Table 12–5). The basal cells may progress to ulceration and local invasion of the dermis and deeper tissues. They do not metastasize.

Differential Diagnosis

Pilomatricomas and basal cell epitheliomas are characteristically solitary and firm, in contrast to syringomas and trichoepitheliomas. Trichoepi-

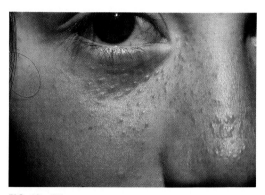

FIG 12–22.
Syringomas. Multiple skin-colored nodules on face and lower eyelid.

theliomas and syringomas may be confused with the multiple angiofibromas of tuberous sclerosis, since they occur on the face. The latter are red rather than skin colored, however. A skin biopsy will distinguish between the lesions of tuberous sclerosis, trichoepithelioma, or syringoma. Confirmatory diagnosis of all four adnexal tumors is made by skin biopsy.

Pathogenesis

Pilomatricomas.—Pilomatricoma is considered a benign hyperplasia of the cells of the hair matrix. It is an encapsulated tumor located in the reticular dermis and is composed of islands of basophilic cells and anuclear "shadow" cells. Calcium deposits appear throughout the tumor.

Syringomas.—Syringoma is a benign hyperplasia of the cells of the eccrine sweat ducts. Numerous small ducts are located in the middermis

TABLE 12–5.
Syndromes Associated With Basal Cell Epitheliomas in Children

Clinical Feature	Basal Cell Nevus Syndrome	Bazex's Syndrome	Xeroderma Pigmentosum
Inheritance	Autosomal dominant	Autosomal dominant	Autosomal recessive
Palmar pits	Present	Present	Absent
Multiple freckles	Absent	Absent	Present
Prominent dilated pores on arms and dorsa of hands	Absent	Present	Absent
Jaw cysts	Present	Absent	Absent
Defective teeth	Present	Absent	Present

to the papillary dermis, with "tennis racquet" shapes and surrounding fibrosis.

Trichoepitheliomas. — Trichoepitheliomas consist of multiple horn cysts and basophilic tumor islands in the middermis. They are believed to be derived from the cells of the hair follicle.

Basal Cell Epitheliomas.—Basal cell epitheliomas are composed of solid masses of cells that contain a large nucleus and little cytoplasm and extend down from the epidermis. Separation from the surrounding fibrous tissue by a clear space is commonly observed. The basal cell is usually oriented vertically toward the skin, seen in the basal layer of the epidermis and adnexa.

In xeroderma pigmentosum, ultraviolet light (UVL)–induced DNA damage cannot be repaired because of autosomal recessive inheritance of an enzyme deficiency. The pathogenesis of basal cell epitheliomas in the basal cell nevus syndrome and Bazex's syndrome is unknown.

Treatment

Excision is the treatment of choice for pilomatricomas and basal cell epitheliomas. Multiple syringomas and trichoepitheliomas are difficult to treat, and treatment of multiple lesions often has poor cosmetic results.

Patient Education

The benign nature and origin of pilomatricoma, syringoma, and trichoepithelioma should be discussed. Basal cell epitheliomas should be considered slowly progressing malignant tumors. In the hereditary syndromes, careful evaluation of family members is necessary.

Follow-up Visits

Children with basal cell epitheliomas should be examined every 6 months for the appearance of further skin tumors. The importance of avoidance of exposure to the sun and the use of sunscreens should be emphasized at each visit.

Corns and Calluses

Clinical Features

Corns and calluses are areas of thickened skin that appear on sites of prolonged pressure or friction. Patients who have these lesions often believe they are warts. Corns are more circumscribed (2 to 5 mm) and better demarcated than calluses (Fig 12–23). Paring the surface off the lesions will reveal a central core in a corn. They are found primarily on the feet and are the result of poorly fitting shoes. Calluses are diffuse areas of thickened skin, 5 to 20 mm in diameter, on the palmar surfaces of hands or fingers or the weight-bearing areas of the feet. Paring the surface of those lesions will reveal normal skin grooves.

Differential Diagnosis

Plantar warts are most often confused with corns and calluses. Shaving off the skin surface with a razor blade will reveal interrupted skin ridges with a central area containing black dots in a wart, interrupted skin ridges with a central core of keratin in a corn, and normal skin ridges in a callus. Patients with unexplained focal or diffuse thickening of the palms or soles may have a variety of palmoplantar keratoderma. These conditions may be associated with metabolic or structural abnormalities and may require intensive investigation.

Pathogenesis

Prolonged pressure or friction from ill-fitting shoes produces corns and calluses on the feet. Playing a musical instrument, using playground equipment, or working with tools produces corns and calluses on the hands. The thickening is due to epidermal proliferation and an increase in the number of cells in the stratum corneum.

Treatment

Reducing the lesion with a razor blade by shaving off the excess stratum corneum, followed by covering with salicylic acid 40% plaster, left on

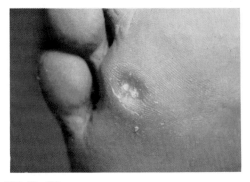

FIG 12–23.
Corn. Circumscribed epidermal thickening with central core.

for 1 to 7 days, will relieve the discomfort of corns and calluses.

Patient Education

The patient should be told that the lesion is not a wart and that prolonged pressure and friction are responsible for the genesis of the lesion.

Follow-up Visits

Follow-up visits are unnecessary.

BIBLIOGRAPHY

Altman AJ, Schwartz AD: *Malignant Diseases of Infancy, Childhood, and Adolescence.* Philadelphia: WB Saunders, 1983.

Aronson IK, Zeitz HJ, Variakojis D: Panniculitis in childhood. *Pediatr Dermatol* 1988; 5:216.

Azón-Masoliver A, Ferrando J, Navarra E, et al: Solitary congenital nodular calcification of Winer located on the ear: Report of two cases. *Pediatr Dermatol* 1989; 6:191.

Belcher RW, Czarnetzki BM, Carney JF, et al: Multiple (subcutaneous) angiolipomas. *Arch Dermatol* 1974; 110:583.

Berger TG, Lane AT, Headington JT, et al: A solitary variant of congenital self-healing reticulohistiocytosis: Solitary Hashimoto-Pritzker disease. *Pediatr Dermatol* 1986; 3:230.

Brownstein MH, Helwig EB: Subcutaneous dermoid cysts. *Arch Dermatol* 1973; 107:237.

Cohen AJ, Frank SB, Minkin W: Subungual exostoses. *Arch Dermatol* 1973; 107:431.

Coskey R, Chow C: Basal cell epithelioma in children and young adults. *Cutis* 1973; 12:224.

de Luna ML, Gilkin I, Goldberg J, et al: Benign cephalic histiocytosis: Report of four cases. *Pediatr Dermatol* 1989; 6:198.

Eldridge R, Denckla MB, Bien E, et al: Neurofibromatosis type 1 (Recklinghausen's Disease) *Am J Dis Child* 1989; 143:833.

Fitzpatrick TB, Gilchrest BD: Dimple sign to differentiate benign from malignant pigmented cutaneous lesions. *N Engl J Med* 1977; 298:1318.

Flanagan BP, Helwig EB: Cutaneous lymphangioma. *Arch Dermatol* 1977; 113:24.

Fleishmajer R, Nedwick A, Reeves JRT: Juvenile fibromatoses. *Arch Dermatol* 1973; 107:574.

Gaul LZ: Heredity of multiple cystic epithelioma. *Arch Dermatol* 1953; 68:517.

Grosfeld J, Weber TR, Weetman RM, et al: Rhabdomyosarcoma in childhood: Analysis of survival of 98 cases. *J Pediatr Surg* 1983; 18:141.

Hartsough NA, Guttman FM: Multiple pilomatricoma (calcifying epitheliomas of Malherbe). *Pediatr Dermatol* 1984; 2:23.

Howell JB: Multiple cutaneous cancers in children: The nevoid basal cell carcinoma syndrome. *J Pediatr* 1966; 69:97.

Hurwitz S: Epidermal nevi and tumors of epithelial origin. *Pediatr Clin North Am* 1983; 30:483.

James MD: The treatment of urticaria pigmentosa. *Clin Exp Dermatol* 1982; 7:311.

Juhlin L, Ijerstquist SO, Ponten J, et al: Disseminated pyogenic granuloma. *Acta Derm Venereol (Stockh)* 1970; 50:134.

Ketchum LD: Hypertrophic scars and keloids. *Clin Plast Surg* 1977; 4:2.

Kligman AM, Kirschbaum JD: Steatocystoma multiplex: A dermoid tumor. *J Invest Dermatol* 1964; 42:388.

Knight PJ, Reiner CB: Superficial lumps in children. What, when and why? *Pediatrics* 1983; 72:147.

Linares HA, Larson DL: Early differential diagnosis between hypertrophic and nonhypertrophic healing. *J Invest Dermatol* 1974; 62:514.

Lipton JM: The pathogenesis, diagnosis and treatment of histiocytosis syndromes. *Pediatr Dermatol* 1983; 1:112.

Mayron R, Grimwood RE: Familial occurrence of eruptive vellus hair cysts. *Pediatr Dermatol* 1988; 5:94.

McKenzie AW, Innes FLF, Rach JM, et al: Digital fibrous swellings in children. *Br J Dermatol* 1970; 83:446.

Mehregan AH, Nabai H, Matthews JE: Recurring digital fibrous tumor of childhood. *Arch Dermatol* 1972; 106:375.

Metzker MD, Amir J, Rotem A, et al: Congenital smooth muscle hamartoma of the skin. *Pediatr Dermatol* 1984; 2:45.

Milstone EB, Helwig EB: Basal cell carcinoma in children. *Arch Dermatol* 1973; 108:523.

Montgomery RM: Corns, calluses and warts. Differential diagnosis. *NY State J Med* 1963; 63:1532.

Muhlbauer JE: Granuloma annulare. *J Am Acad Dermatol* 1980; 3:217.

Pollard ZF, Robison ND, Calhoun J: Dermoid cysts in children. *Pediatrics* 1976; 57:379.

Ricardi VM: Pathophysiology of neurofibromatosis. *J Am Acad Dermatol* 1980; 3:157.

Rivera-Luna R, Martinez-Guerra G, Altamirano-Alvarez E, et al: Langerhans cell histiocytosis: Clinical experience with 124 patients. *Pediatr Dermatol* 1988; 5:145.

Robbins JH, Kraemer K, Lutzner M, et al: Xeroderma pigmentosum an inherited disease with sun sensitivity, multiple cutaneous neoplasms, and abnormal DNA repair. *Ann Intern Med* 1974; 80:221.

Roper SS, Spraker MK: Cutaneous histiocytosis syndromes. *Pediatr Dermatol* 1985; 3:19.

Simons FER, Schaller JG: Benign rheumatoid nodules. *Pediatrics* 1975; 56:29.

Viksins P, Berlin A: Bazex syndrome. *Arch Dermatol* 1977; 113:948.

Webster SB, Reister HC, Harmon LE: Juvenile xanthogranuloma with extracutaneous lesions. *Arch Dermatol* 1966; 93:71.

Wells RS, Smith MA: The natural history of granuloma annulare. *Br J Dermatol* 1963; 75:199.

Yasargil MG, Abernathey CD, Sarioglu AC: Microneurosurgical treatment of intracranial dermoid and epidermoid tumors. *Neurosurgery* 1989; 24:561.

Zaynoun ST, Juljulian HH, Kurban AK: Pyogenic granuloma with multiple satellites. *Arch Dermatol* 1974; 109:689.

13 _____ Vascular Reactions: Urticaria, the Erythemas, and Purpura

Urticaria, erythemas, and purpuras are considered together in a single chapter because they represent a spectrum of disease characterized by progressive signs of injury to cutaneous blood vessels. All are accompanied by vasodilation (erythema) and leakage of fluid from blood vessels (edema). Leakage of red cells also occurs in the purpuras as a further sign of vascular insult. A complex interplay of chemical mediators may be involved. Histamine is certainly involved in the urticarias, as are complement fragments with vasoactive properties, such as C3a and C5a. Eicosanoids and certain cytokines may also participate. In addition, other immunoreactants may be involved, such as IgE and circulating antigen-antibody complexes, particularly in the initial stages of vascular injury. Immune complex disease seems to be particularly important in the reactive erythemas and the purpuras.

URTICARIA

Urticarial states are common in infancy and childhood, although the exact incidence is not known. Several large studies indicate that 3% of preschool children and about 2% of older children suffer from urticaria. This high incidence undoubtedly accounts for a number with a single episode of short-lived urticaria rather than persistent urticaria. Interestingly, of all urticaria patients, only 3% to 5% have what can be documented as IgE-mediated allergic urticaria. In contrast, approximately 17% of patients have a physical urticaria, with the bulk of the patients in a large "idiopathic" group. Some children with idiopathic urticaria may have urticarial vasculitis. For purposes of presenting a clinical approach to ur-

ticaria, transient urticaria and persistent urticaria are discussed separately.

TRANSIENT URTICARIA AND ANGIOEDEMA

Clinical Features

Transient urticaria in children often follows infection, insect sting or bite, ingestion of medications (see Chapter 18) or certain foods, or inflammatory systemic disease such as collagen vascular disease or thyroiditis (Table 13–1). The eruption is sudden in onset and pruritic, with erythematous raised wheals scattered over the body. The wheals are 2 to 5 mm in diameter, flat-topped, and have tense edema (Fig 13–1). This can be appreciated by stretching the skin slightly to demonstrate whitish centers. The erythematous borders with pale centers can be mistaken for target lesions of erythema multiforme. Occasionally giant urticarial lesions up to 30 cm in diameter and with polycyclic borders will appear (Fig 13–2). Such wheals commonly last from 20 minutes to 3 hours, disappear, then reappear in other areas. The transient nature of individual lesions of urticaria distinguishes it from fixed lesions of erythema multiforme, which remain in the same skin site for at least a week. The entire episode of transient urticaria often lasts 24 to 48 hours; rarely, it lasts as long as 3 weeks. Transient urticaria, as it resolves, may leave flat, dusky areas lasting several days.

Subcutaneous extension of lesions, called angioedema, may occur. The lesions of angioedema appear as large swellings with indistinct borders around the eyelids and lips. They may also appear on the face, trunk, genitalia, and extremities (Fig

TABLE 13–1.

Causes of Transient Urticaria

Infection	Foods
Streptococcus	Nuts
Infectious mononucleosis (Epstein-Barr virus)	Eggs
Hepatitis	Shellfish
Adenovirus	Strawberries
Enterovirus	Inflammatory systemic disease
Parasites	Collagen vascular disease
Bites and stings	Lupus erythematosus
Bees	Juvenile rheumatoid arthritis
Wasps	Periarteritis nodosa
Scorpions	Dermatomyositis
Spiders	Neonatal lupus syndrome
Jellyfish	Sjögren's syndrome
Drugs	Rheumatic fever
Penicillin	Inflammatory bowel disease
Salicylates	Crohn's disease
Morphine, codeine, other opiates	Ulcerative colitis
Nonsteroidal anti-inflammatory drugs	Miscellaneous
Barbiturates	Aphthous stomatitis
Amphetamines	Behçet's disease
Atropine	Thyroiditis
Hydralazine	
Insulin	
Blood and blood products	

13–3). The face, hands, and feet are involved in 85% of patients and other areas in 15%. Up to one half of patients with transient urticaria may have angioedema, with edema of the hands and feet commonly seen.

All the persistent urticarias, when examined within the first 4 weeks of illness, may be indistinguishable from transient urticaria. Hereditary angioedema accounts for only 0.4% of cases of urticaria, but its specific diagnostic tests and high mortality rate deserve special mention. It is an au-

tosomal dominant condition with repeated attacks of swelling of the extremities, face, and throat, accompanied by abdominal pain. The onset usually follows trauma such as surgery, dental manipulation, or accidents. The presenting symptoms are diffuse, brawny swelling of the extremities in 75% of patients, abdominal pain in 52%, and swelling of the face and throat in 30%. Its onset is usually in adolescence, with the more severe symptoms

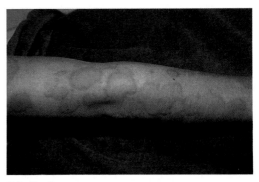

FIG 13–2.
Multiple polycyclic red wheals of different sizes in a child with urticaria. Commonly mistaken for erythema multiforme.

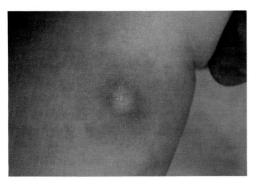

FIG 13–1.
Central wheal with red border in acute urticaria.

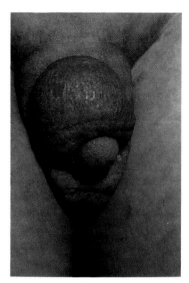

FIG 13–3.
Angioedema of scrotum in infant.

associated with the menses. Abdominal pain eventually becomes a major complaint in 93% of patients. They do not have urticarial wheals, but 26% have erythema multiforme–like lesions. Severe airway edema accounts for the mortality rate of almost 30% in untreated patients. Only 25% of patients give a positive family history. The diagnosis should be suspected if the serum C4 level is persistently low. It is confirmed by functional assay of the C1 esterase inhibitor.

Differential Diagnosis

The conditions to be considered in the differential diagnosis of urticaria are listed in Table 13–2. Urticaria, especially giant urticaria, is often confused with erythema multiforme. Urticarial lesions may blanch in the center, showing a red border and thus concentric zones of color

change, as is seen in erythema multiforme. It should be remembered, however, that individual urticarial lesions are transient, usually lasting less than 3 hours, whereas erythema multiforme lesions are fixed and stay in place at least 7 to 14 days. Also, the target lesions of erythema multiforme are dusky in the center, not lighter. Frequently, when polycyclic urticarial wheals of different sizes and shapes accompany edema of the hands and feet, an incorrect diagnosis of erythema multiforme is made.

Urticarial lesions often clear with the administration of subcutaneous epinephrine; erythema multiforme does not. A skin biopsy will distinguish the two. Urticaria can be differentiated from mastocytosis by a skin biopsy, since increased numbers of mast cells are seen in mastocytosis. Flushing states are flat rather than elevated. In juvenile rheumatoid arthritis, faint erythematous macules with a clear center are present and are associated with a spiking fever. Vasculitis lesions have purpuric centers, while psoriasis and pityriasis rosea demonstrate scaling overlying the erythematous papules.

Angioedema (Table 13–3) should be differentiated from cellulitis and erysipelas, which are seen as tender, warm red lesions. Chronic thickening of tissues occurs in lymphedema, in contrast to the acute stretching of tissue seen in angioedema. Angioedema of the hands and feet, which accompanies urticaria, may be confused with erythema multiforme. A skin biopsy will distinguish. Persistent angioedema of the face or lip should bring to mind lupus erythematosus or other collagen vascular diseases.

Considerable deep edema can develop in acute contact dermatitis, but vesiculation of the overlying epidermis and epidermal papules will help distinguish it from angioedema. Idiopathic scrotal edema of children and the Melkersson-Rosenthal syndrome are rare and can be distinguished from angioedema by the furrowed tongue and cranial nerve palsies of Melkersson-

TABLE 13–2.
Differential Diagnosis of Urticaria

Erythema multiforme
Mastocytosis
Flushing
Reactive erythemas
Juvenile rheumatoid arthritis
Vasculitis
Guttate psoriasis
Pityriasis rosea (early lesions)

TABLE 13–3.
Differential Diagnosis of Angioedema

Cellulitis and erysipelas
Lymphedema
Acute contact dermatitis
Idiopathic scrotal edema of children
Melkersson-Rosenthal syndrome

Rosenthal syndrome and the limitation of angioedema to the scrotum in idiopathic scrotal edema.

Pathogenesis

Histamine is undoubtedly the major chemical mediator of transient urticaria, and the mast cell is central in all forms of transient urticaria and angioedema. Histamine may be directly released from cutaneous mast cells in the case of certain foods or opiate drugs. Specific IgE antibodies bound to mast cell surfaces that "recognize" certain antigens, such as penicillin and other drugs, foods, and venom of certain stinging insects, result in the release of histamine after combination with antigen. Complement fragments, activated by immune complexes, may activate mast cells to release histamine or exert vasoactive effects of their own on cutaneous blood vessels. The latter mechanism is most often associated with infection, but careful documentation of the mechanism of histamine release involved with each inciting substance is not available. Eicosanoids may induce mast cell mediator release, and as more cytokines are identified and described, their role in urticaria may be important.

In hereditary angioedema, a deficiency of the C1 esterase inhibitor permits unregulated cleavage of complement proteins once the complement system is activated, with particular consumption of C4. A C2 kinin activates the clotting system via the Hageman factor in hereditary angioedema. Complement cleavage products may be responsible for the edema and erythema.

Treatment

Oral antihistamines are valuable in symptomatic control of urticaria. Hydroxyzine hydrochloride, 2 to 4 mg/kg/day in four divided doses, or diphenhydramine hydrochloride, 5 mg/kg/day in four divided doses, is the most helpful. In angioedema not controlled by antihistamines, the addition of pseudoephedrine, 4 mg/kg/day in four divided doses, is useful. The same drugs may be used to treat chronic angioedema. In acute angioedema of the airway, epinephrine 1:1,000, 0.01 mL/kg/dose to a maximum dose of 0.5 mL, may be used. There is no evidence to support the use of systemic glucocorticosteroids in urticaria or angioedema. It is unclear whether the addition of H_2 blocking drugs to H_1 antihistamines is of any additional benefit. Cromolyn sodium preparations, which may be efficacious in treatment of airway or bowel reactions, have not been particularly useful in treatment of skin diseases. Allergen avoidance is an important strategy if the allergen can be identified. Drugs such as penicillin and aspirin account for most drug-induced urticaria, and they should be specifically questioned in review of the patient's history. Similarly, foods suspected of causing the urticaria could be avoided, if nutrition is not compromised.

In hereditary angioedema, acute attacks are managed by intravenous fluid replacement and airway maintenance. Administration of danazol or stanozolol, synthetic attenuated testosterones, increases Clq esterase inhibitor levels and prevents the attacks of angioedema. Fresh frozen plasma or ϵ-aminocaproic acid may be useful before surgical procedures.

Patient Education

It should be explained that cause-and-effect relationships often cannot be found in transient urticaria and angioedema, but that lesions can be expected to resolve by 1 month in most instances. One should emphasize that control of symptoms is possible with the use of antihistamines. An extensive and expensive allergy workup is not indicated in children who have had urticaria less than 6 weeks.

Patients with angioedema should have an adrenergic agent available for airway attacks, and patients with hereditary angioedema should be advised of the high mortality rate and the need to continue taking prophylactic drugs.

Follow-up Visits

In transient urticaria and angioedema, a visit 1 week after the initial evaluation is useful for monitoring the course of the disease. Patients with hereditary angioedema should be seen after 1 month of therapy to remeasure the C1 esterase inhibitor and adjust the drug dosage.

PERSISTENT URTICARIA: THE PHYSICAL URTICARIAS

Urticaria that persists for more than 4 weeks may be simply prolonged common urticaria or due to one of the physical urticarias, urticarial vasculitis, or mastocytosis. The physical urticarias, which account for 25% of this group, consist of dermatographism, heat and exercise urticaria, delayed-pressure urticaria, cold urticaria, and familial cold urticaria.

Clinical Features

Dermatographism.—Dermatographism occurs in 1.5% to 5.0% of patients who have the physical urticarias and is characterized by wheal and erythema after minor stroking of, or pressure on, the skin (Fig 13–4). It often results in mild itching. The wheal reaches maximal size in 6 to 7 minutes and persists for 10 to 15 minutes. Wheals are commonly found around the belt area and may appear after widespread insect bites and transient episodes of urticaria. The wheal is seen in comatose children (e.g., in encephalitis, meningitis, drug overdose) and has been termed *tache cérébrale*. It is also seen in about one half of children with mastocytosis.

Dermatographism may persist for years, but most patients can expect spontaneous regression within 2 years. The natural history of dermatographism has not been thoroughly studied.

Heat and Exercise Urticaria.—Heat and exercise urticaria (cholinergic urticaria) is characterized by a large (10 to 20 mm), blotchy erythema surrounding tiny (1 to 3 mm) central wheals (Fig 13–5). It occurs in up to 15% of adolescents. Heating of the skin or exercise sufficient to raise the body temperature 0.5° C will induce attacks of multiple wheals with itching. Hot or spicy foods, febrile illnesses, and hot baths may also initiate attacks. The onset is characteristically in adolescence, but the condition tends to persist for years.

Delayed-Pressure Urticaria.—Delayed-pressure urticaria, which occurs primarily in adolescents, appears after prolonged pressure with a heavy weight. A 7 kg weight suspended

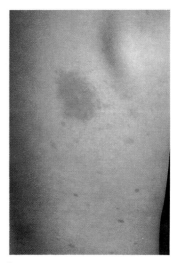

FIG 13–5.
Heat and exercise urticaria. Pinpoint central wheal surrounded by large, blotchy erythema.

from an extremity by a strap for 15 minutes will reproduce the disease. Painful, deep swellings begin 4 to 6 hours after pressure and last up to 24 hours. Spontaneous remissions have been reported, but the natural history is unknown.

Cold Urticaria.—Cold urticaria appears in three forms: It may be associated with cryoglobulins and immune complex disease; it may appear as an acquired form not associated with cryoproteins; or it may occur as autosomal dominant familial cold urticaria. In the form associated with cryoglobulins, the signs and symptoms of collagen vascular disease are often present. This disease is uncommon in children. The acquired form occurs after rewarming an area of skin exposed to cold. Wheals appear, and itching is severe. Cooling the entire body may result in widespread wheals and fainting. To test for acquired cold urticaria, an ice cube is applied to the patient's skin for 2 to 10 minutes, and the skin is allowed to rewarm. The wheal appears during the rewarming. There may be a spontaneous remission, but the natural history is not known.

Familial Cold Urticaria.—Familial cold urticaria is an autosomal dominant condition beginning shortly after birth. Erythematous macules appear in exposed areas 30 minutes after exposure to a cold wind, but not after ingestion of iced drinks or ice. Older children complain of burning

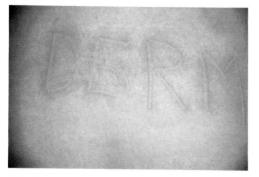

FIG 13–4.
Dermatographism. Light stroking of skin evokes intense wheal-and-flare reaction.

in the skin. Fever and chills, arthralgias, and headaches appear and last up to 48 hours. A leukocytosis occurs during the attacks. The patient tends to suffer these attacks throughout life.

Differential Diagnosis

The physical urticarias are often confused with other forms of urticaria (see Table 13–6). The role of light pressure in dermatographism and deep pressure in delayed-pressure urticaria should help distinguish these disorders from the other forms of urticaria. Heat and exercise urticaria may be distinguished from other types of urticaria by the characteristic tiny central wheal with a large rim of erythema. The cold urticarias may be distinguished by the history of cold exposure, and in the familial form, by the systemic symptoms accompanying the skin lesions. Table 13–4 represents the conditions to be considered in the differential diagnosis of cold urticaria.

Pathogenesis

The physical urticarias differ from other urticarial states in that histamine does not appear to be the chemical mediator of the disease. Histamine skin levels are normal in dermatographism, heat and exercise urticaria, cold urticaria with cryoglobulins, urticarial states, and familial cold urticaria. Histamine has been implicated in acquired cold urticaria and delayed-pressure urticaria. In dermatographism, as well as in heat and exercise urticaria, mediation through cholinergic fibers of the autonomic nervous system has been implicated. The vasoactive split products of the complement system may be involved in the cryoglobulinemic and familial cold urticarial forms.

Treatment

Many patients with physical urticaria require no therapy. If symptoms are severe enough to require therapy, hydroxyzine hydrochloride, 2 to 4

TABLE 13–4.

Differential Diagnosis of Cold Urticaria

Cryoglobulinemia and immune complex diseases
Systemic lupus erythematosus and other collagen
  vascular diseases
Macroglobulinemia
Mycoplasma infections (cold hemagglutinins)
Syphilis
Familial cold urticaria
Acquired

mg/kg/day in four divided doses, may reduce the symptoms in dermatographism as well as in heat and exercise urticaria. Delayed-pressure urticaria may respond to prednisone, 1 mg/kg/day for 4 to 5 days, but prednisone is generally not required. There is no satisfactory treatment for cold urticaria other than cold avoidance, although cyproheptadine, 2 to 4 mg three times daily, has been reported to provide relief in some patients.

Patient Education

Patients with the physical urticarias must be instructed to reduce their exposure to the precipitating factors. Patients with dermatographism and delayed-pressure urticaria should not wear backpacks or carry other heavy weights and should avoid tight-fitting clothing and excessive friction or pressure on the skin. Patients with heat and exercise urticaria need to avoid excessive heating of the skin, vigorous exercise, hot baths, and other factors resulting in increased body heat. Patients with cold urticaria should avoid ice-cold food or drinks, dress warmly in cold weather, and avoid swimming in cold water.

Follow-up Visits

A visit 2 weeks after the initial evaluation will be useful to monitor the progress of the disease and the therapeutic response.

PERSISTENT URTICARIA: URTICARIAL VASCULITIS

Clinical Features

Urticarial vasculitis is characterized by fixed wheals distributed symmetrically on the extremities. It is usually seen in adolescents and young adults. The true incidence is unknown, but it has been reported in up to 30% of patients with persistent urticaria. Lesions remain fixed in the same area for 24 to 72 hours and may be accompanied by mild arthralgias or malaise. Most patients have an elevated erythrocyte sedimentation rate and depressed serum complement levels. The natural history is not known. Although the findings are similar to those in necrotizing vasculitis with palpable purpura, most patients do not progress to palpable purpura.

Differential Diagnosis

Urticarial vasculitis may be distinguished from other conditions (see Table 13–6) by the elevated erythrocyte sedimentation rate, depressed serum complement levels, the finding of small-vessel vasculitis with skin biopsy, and the associated arthralgias.

Pathogenesis

Urticarial vasculitis has been associated with circulating immune complexes, resulting in injury to postcapillary venules in the papillary dermis. Immunofluorescence has demonstrated immunoglobulins and complement split products around inflamed venules. Skin biopsy reveals neutrophils and degenerating neutrophilic nuclei around the venules, with swelling of the venule wall and fibrin deposition. The inflammatory events are most probably mediated through the interaction of immune complexes with the complement and clotting systems.

Treatment

If a cause for immune complex disease, such as streptococcal infection, can be determined, it can be eliminated, but such associations are difficult to document. There is no known effective treatment. Both antihistamines and low-dose prednisone therapy have been utilized, with variable success.

Patient Education

Patients should be advised of the difference between urticarial vasculitis and IgE-mediated urticaria.

Follow-up Visits

Monthly visits are advisable to determine whether the disorder has progressed to involve vessels of other organs. Urinalysis, sedimentation rate, and complement levels may be used to follow the course of the disease.

PERSISTENT URTICARIA: MASTOCYTOSIS (URTICARIA PIGMENTOSA)

Clinical Features

The macular and nodular pigmented lesions of mastocytosis appear in the first 8 months of life (Fig 13–6). One or two lesions are noted initially, but numerous lesions accumulate during the next few months (Fig 13–7). The majority of lesions appear on the trunk, although some may appear on the face and extremities. Individual lesions are

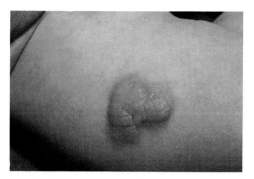

FIG 13–6.
Mastocytoma. Pink plaque on skin of infant.

often red at first and may easily become blistered (Fig 13–8). Brown pigmentation may not appear until 6 months after the onset of the lesions. Stroking the pigmented lesion will result in tense edema within the lesion and an erythematous flare surrounding the area (Darier's sign). Half the patients with mastocytosis will demonstrate dermatographism in uninvolved areas. Skin biopsy will confirm the diagnosis.

Spontaneous bulla formation within lesions may occur or may be induced by a variety of drugs (Table 13–5). These drugs or rubbing of the skin may induce enough histamine release to produce systemic symptoms, such as flushing, wheezing, tachycardia, hypotension with fainting, diarrhea, and vomiting. As the child ages, it becomes more difficult to urticate the lesions, or to induce blisters, or both. Often by age 5 they are asymptomatic, and by adolescence, only residual flat pigmentation remains.

Enlargement of the liver and spleen, systemic

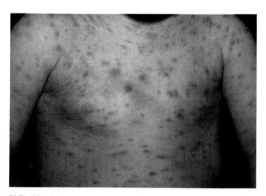

FIG 13–7.
Urticaria pigmentosa. Multiple blotchy brown macules on chest of infant.

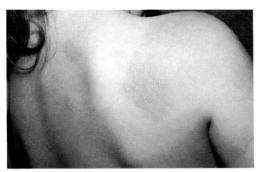

FIG 13–8.
Tense edema within tan macule of urticaria pigmentosa after stroking.

flushing episodes, and peptic ulcer symptoms should suggest systemic mastocytosis. Systemic mastocytosis occurs in up to 10% of infants with urticaria pigmentosa. Bony involvement can be documented by x-ray examination, and bone marrow examination will reveal increased numbers of mast cells. Extreme infiltration of the liver sufficient to produce cirrhosis may occur.

A solitary pigmented nodule of mast cells may be present as a birthmark.

Diffuse cutaneous mastocytosis is first seen as blisters in the neonatal period and is often accompanied by flushing episodes. The blisters are often large and peel, leaving large, eroded bases. After a severe blistering episode, 5 to 10 days may be required to regranulate mast cells, and the baby experiences recurrent episodes. When the baby is evaluated, marked dermatographism is present. A leathery thickening with yellow-tan color to the skin usually does not appear until 3 to 8 months of age. Severe syncopal episodes and death from prolonged hypotension have been reported. It is an autosomal dominant disorder.

Differential Diagnosis

Mastocytosis can be differentiated from other conditions (see Table 13–5) by skin biopsy. The bullous lesions must be differentiated from other bullous diseases of infancy. Diffuse cutaneous

TABLE 13–5.
Drugs That Produce Histamine Release in Mastocytosis

Opiates (codeine, meperidine [Demerol], morphine)
Polymyxin B
Acetylsalicylic acid

mastocytosis has been confused with the scalded skin syndrome, especially recurrent scalded skin syndrome, and with epidermolysis bullosa.

Pathogenesis

Excessive numbers of mast cells accumulate within the dermis in mastocytosis. Excessive histamine release from these mast cells results in whealing or blister formation. The blister is subepidermal and may bleed. Histamine is undoubtedly responsible for the local and systemic effects. Flushing and syncopal episodes are due to prostaglandin D_2 release, and bleeding, to heparin release by cutaneous mast cells.

Treatment

Most infants require no treatment. Flushing episodes or other systemic symptoms may be controlled by the use of hydroxyzine hydrochloride, 2 to 4 mg/kg/day divided in four doses. Solitary mastocytomas may be excised. Oral cromolyn sodium has been reported to be valuable in infants with gastrointestinal involvement. Diffuse cutaneous mastocytosis may respond to psoralens plus ultraviolet A (PUVA) therapy.

Patient Education

It is essential that the child not be given cough syrups with codeine or other medications with opiates. If surgery is contemplated, preoperative medications should be carefully selected. Substitution of other antipyretics for aspirin is also advised. The natural course should be emphasized, and parents should be provided with lists of drugs to avoid. Genetic counseling is valuable for diffuse cutaneous mastocytosis.

Follow-up Visits

A visit in 2 weeks is useful in determining the presence or absence of systemic symptoms. If treatment is given, monthly visits are advisable.

ERYTHEMAS

Erythemas of the skin without wheal production are uncommon in infants and children. Often called the reactive erythemas, they include the annular erythemas (e.g., erythema chronicum migrans), erythema multiforme, and erythema nodosum. Erythema multiforme is covered in detail in Chapter 11 and Erythema chronicum migrans, in Chapter 5.

ANNULAR ERYTHEMAS

Clinical Features

Annular, polycyclic, and partially marginated lesions are called annular erythemas. One should remember that giant urticaria can assume annular shapes.

Erythema Annulare Centrifugum.—In erythema annulare centrifugum, the lesions have erythematous borders and a dusky center (Fig 13–9). They may occur anywhere on the skin. Multiple lesions are usually present, and they slowly enlarge. Lesions last for several months and tend to recur. In infants, they may be associated with a maternal collagen vascular disorder.

Erythema Marginatum.—Erythema marginatum is a transient eruption consisting of curvilinear, migrating areas of erythema that form incomplete circles (Fig 13–10). The marginated lesions may move rapidly over the skin within several hours and disappear. Inducing cutaneous vasodilation may make the lesions more visible. Erythema marginatum is found in up to 15% of children with acute rheumatic fever and is associated with the fever and well-established carditis. A thorough evaluation for acute rheumatic fever is indicated. Erythema marginatum may also be seen after streptococcal infections without evidence of acute rheumatic fever.

Differential Diagnosis

Conditions to be considered in the differential diagnosis of annular erythemas are given in Table 13–6. Dermatophyte lesions have a scaly

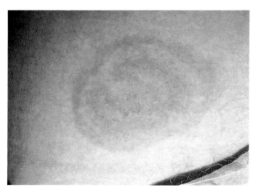

FIG 13–9.
Erythema annulare centrifugum. Concentric zones of red and dusky skin.

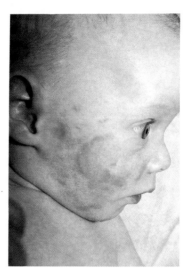

FIG 13–10.
Erythema marginatum. Fleeting, semiannular erythema on face of infant with acute rheumatic fever.

border and may be diagnosed by potassium hydroxide (KOH) examination and fungal cultures. Granuloma annulare lesions have a distinct nodular and papular border. The lesions of pityriasis rosea may be annular on occasion and have central clearing. Annular lesions may also be the presenting symptom of lupus erythematosus, sarcoidosis, and syphilis. The transient urticarial lesions of juvenile rheumatoid arthritis tend to be limited to the abdomen, and to clear slightly in the center.

Pathogenesis

Two of the erythemas demonstrate infectious agents within the skin lesions, with an attendant host response. In erythema chronicum migrans,

TABLE 13–6.
Differential Diagnosis of Annular Erythemas

Erythema annulare centrifugum
Erythema chronicum migrans
Erythema marginatum
Tinea corporis
Pityriasis rosea
Lupus erythematosus
Neonatal lupus syndrome
Sarcoidosis
Syphilis
Juvenile rheumatoid arthritis

Borrelia burgdorferi is found (Chapter 5), and in erythema multiforme, herpes simplex virus (Chapter 11). In erythema annulare centrifugum and in erythema marginatum, the mechanism of disease is unknown.

Treatment

No treatment is useful for erythema annulare centrifugum. Children with erythema marginatum are treated with penicillin.

Patient Education

It should be emphasized that such eruptions are skin reactions that do not require treatment but that serve as a clue to a systemic disorder.

Follow-up Visits

A visit 1 week after the initial evaluation is useful to discuss the results of laboratory evaluation for systemic disorders. The need for follow-up care is determined by the nature of the associated systemic disorder.

ERYTHEMA NODOSUM

Clinical Features

Erythema nodosum is characterized by the abrupt onset of symmetric, very tender, erythematous nodules on the extensor surfaces of the extremities (Fig 13–11). The nodules have indistinct borders (Fig 13–12). Occasionally erythema nodosum will be unilateral for a week. The lesions may be so painful that the patient will limp. A prodrome of cough, sore throat, and fever will occur in about 25% of children. The disease occurs most commonly in adolescents and is rare before the age of 2 years. It predominates in girls at a ratio of 1.7 to 1. Lesions last 2 to 6 weeks. Recurrences are reported in 4% of children. They resolve as a bruise, with a color change to purple, then yellow-brown. Infectious causes, such as streptococci, tuberculosis, histoplasmosis, and coccidioidomycosis, are the most common associations. A careful history should be obtained for preceding infections. Uncommonly, drugs may produce erythema nodosum, particularly oral contraceptives in female adolescents.

Differential Diagnosis

Erythema nodosum may be confused with many other processes involving the subcutaneous fat. In contrast to erythema nodosum, thrombophlebitis usually occurs on the lateral or flexor surface of the lower legs, and heals with fibrosis. The nodose lesions of periarteritis nodosa are not discolored on the surface and are associated with an exaggerated dusky, mottling pattern called livedo reticularis. Giant insect bite reactions may be confused with erythema nodosum, but a central punctum will help differentiate. Weber-Christian panniculitis and factitial panniculitis can be distinguished upon biopsy of skin to include sub-

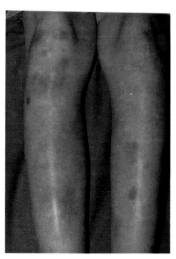

FIG 13–11.
Tender red nodules with indistinct borders in a teenage girl with erythema nodosum.

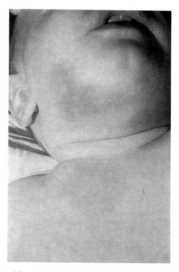

FIG 13–12.
Atypical location of erythema nodosum in infant.

cutaneous fat. The lesions of erythema nodosum are usually so characteristic that they are seldom confused with those of other disorders.

Pathogenesis

Erythema nodosum is a chronic injury of the blood vessels of the reticular dermis and subcutaneous fat. Initially, the perivascular inflammation is neutrophilic, then lymphocytic, then granulomatous as the lesions age. There is increasing evidence to implicate circulating immune complexes in the pathogenesis of erythema nodosum as a part of the host immune response to an infectious agent. Fat cell destruction usually does not occur in erythema nodosum, indicating that it is not a true panniculitis.

Treatment

Symptomatic treatment with acetylsalicylic acid or antihistamines may suffice, since in many cases the erythema nodosum resolves within 3 weeks. In patients with acutely tender lesions that interfere with walking, nonsteroidal anti-inflammatory agents, such as indomethacin, may be tried. Although some relief can be obtained with prednisone, oral steroids are not generally recommended and should not be used over an extended period of time.

Patient Education

It should be emphasized that erythema nodosum is a response to infection or to certain drugs. A search for such associations should be guided by the history and should not involve expensive laboratory tests. Parents should be reassured that most children recover within 3 weeks.

Follow-up Visits

A return visit in 1 week is useful to ascertain the need for, or response to, therapy.

PURPURAS

Purpuric lesions always prompt investigation into bleeding states. They may involve small areas (e.g., petechiae) or large areas (e.g., ecchymoses). Palpable purpura (purpuric papules), dissecting purpura, and chronic pigmented purpura are presented in this section. Neonatal purpura (Table 13–7), acral petechiae and purpura (Table 13–8), and flat generalized petechiae and purpura (Table 13–9) are not discussed, but are presented in ta-

TABLE 13–7.
Differential Diagnosis of Neonatal Purpura

Congenital infection
Toxoplasma
Enterovirus
Rubella
Cytomegalovirus
Herpes simplex
Syphilis
Coagulation defects
Autoimmune disorders
Idiopathic thrombocytopenic purpura
Systemic lupus erythematosus
Erythroblastosis fetalis
Hemangioma with platelet trapping syndrome

TABLE 13–8.
Differential Diagnosis of Flat Acral Purpura

Rocky Mountain spotted fever
Meningococcemia
Atypical measles
Coagulation disorders
Progressive pigmentary purpura

TABLE 13–9.
Differential Diagnosis of Flat Generalized Purpura

Thrombocytopenic states (idiopathic thrombocytopenic purpura, leukemia)
Coagulation disorders
Trauma (including child abuse)

ble form to allow the reader to make a differential diagnosis of these lesions.

PALPABLE PURPURA (PURPURIC PAPULES)

Clinical Features

Discrete, 1- to 3-mm papules with petechial centers characterize palpable purpura (Fig 13–13). They are usually found on the extremities and are symmetric and numerous (Fig 13–14). Palpable purpura should immediately bring to mind vasculitis or septicemia. The vasculitis that occurs is called cutaneous necrotizing venulitis (anaphylactoid purpura, Schönlein-Henoch purpura) and may be associated with vasculitis of renal, gastrointestinal, joint, or cerebral vessels. The lesions may begin as discrete urticarial wheals

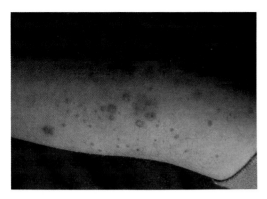

FIG 13−13.
Papules with petechial centers on leg of child with necrotizing vasculitis (Schönlein-Henoch purpura).

and then progress to papular purpura and pustular purpura. Occasionally cutaneous infarcts and gangrene with subsequent ulceration and scarring will occur. Arthralgia or arthritis of the knees and ankles is found in 80% of patients. Cramping abdominal pain, vomiting, hematemesis, and melena signal gastrointestinal involvement. Abdominal pain is common, but in most children lasts less than 24 hours. The kidney is involved in 70% of children. Most have asymptomatic microscopic hematuria, but only 25% on the first visit. In some children a nephrotic syndrome may be the presenting symptom. Up to 10% of children may progress to chronic renal failure.

Rarely, seizures, paresis, or coma occurs with involvement of the central nervous system vessels. Most episodes of necrotizing venulitis show skin changes that last from 4 to 6 weeks and then resolve. In addition to necrotizing vasculitis, at initial presentation, septicemic states are also seen

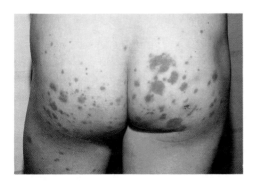

FIG 13−14.
Numerous purpuric macules and papules on buttocks of child with necrotizing vasculitis.

with palpable purpura particularly progressing to pustular purpura. Lesions are acral, symmetric, and few in number. Palpable purpura is seen in chronic meningococcemia, gonococcemia, and subacute bacterial endocarditis and is frequently associated with arthritis or arthralgias of the large joints. Blood cultures or genital cultures will confirm the diagnosis. It is difficult to culture organisms from lesions, but they may be identified by specific immunofluorescence from smears of lesions. Rarely, *Pseudomonas,* staphylococcal, deep fungal, or gram-negative septicemia is responsible.

Differential Diagnosis
Biopsy plus bacterial and fungal culture will distinguish infectious causes of palpable purpura from one another (Table 13−10).

Pathogenesis
In necrotizing venulitis and in septicemic states, circulating immune complexes have been implicated in the production of lesions through their interaction with the complement and clotting systems. The prodrome of upper respiratory infection and sometimes positive streptococcal throat cultures have implicated infectious agents as likely triggers of immune complex formation in Schönlein-Henoch purpura. Skin biopsy reveals fibrinoid necrosis of venule walls in the papillary dermis, with perivascular accumulation of neutrophils, nuclear fragments, and extravasation of red blood cells. Organisms may also be detected in the septicemic states.

Treatment
In necrotizing venulitis with skin involvement only, no treatment is required. Prednisone, 2 mg/kg/day, may be indicated with internal organ involvement. The administration of systemic antibiotics, with the choice of agent based on appropriate cultures, is indicated for septicemic states.

TABLE 13−10.
Differential Diagnosis of Palpable Purpura

Necrotizing venulitis (anaphylactoid purpura)
Meningococcemia
Gonococcemia
Staphylococcal sepsis
Pseudomonas sepsis
Subacute bacterial endocarditis

Patient Education

The serious nature of vasculitis of internal organs and septicemic states should be emphasized. Future upper respiratory illnesses should be brought to the physician's attention promptly, and appropriate cultures should be taken. Early treatment of an associated streptococcal infection may be required.

Follow-up Visits

In necrotizing venulitis, weekly follow-up visits are recommended for the first 4 weeks to monitor internal involvement, particularly of the kidney. Microscopic examination of the urinary sediment and protein determination are required. Thereafter, evaluations of renal function every 3 months are helpful to identify the children at risk of renal failure.

DISSECTING PURPURA (DISSEMINATED INTRAVASCULAR COAGULATION)

Clinical Features

Dissecting purpura, or disseminated intravascular coagulation, has an acute onset, with high fever and extensive large, dissecting purpuric areas on the extremities. It occurs in children 5 to 10 days after an infection. The purpuric "lakes" are large and are not associated with petechiae (Fig 13–15). The condition has been associated with overwhelming infections, such as meningococcemia, *Escherichia coli* septicemia, and Rocky Mountain spotted fever, or it may follow common childhood infections, such as streptococcal pharyngitis or varicella. Vascular collapse is common, and mortality is high in untreated patients.

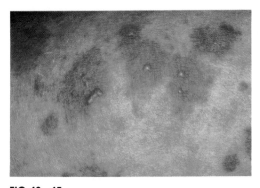

FIG 13–15.
Purpuric lakes with hemorrhagic blisters in child with disseminated intravascular coagulation.

Differential Diagnosis

The large purpuric lakes are so characteristic that they are not confused with other purpuric diseases.

Pathogenesis

The syndrome is triggered by the massive release of tissue thromboplastin with widespread fibrin deposition in the skin, lungs, and kidneys, fibrinolysis, and consumption of coagulation factors, leading to secondary bleeding. In cavernous hemangiomas, the consumption of clotting factors may be within the hemangioma.

Treatment

Replacement of consumable clotting factors with fresh plasma or platelet concentrates is the treatment of choice. Most children require hospitalization. With persistent disseminated intravascular coagulation, heparin, 100 units/kg intravenously every 4 to 6 hours, may be given. Antibiotic treatment of the triggering bacterial infection is necessary.

Patient Education

Advice is dependent on the nature of the triggering disease.

Follow-up Visits

Follow-up visits daily while the child is hospitalized to reevaluate clotting by laboratory assays is useful.

CHRONIC PIGMENTED PURPURA

Clinical Features

Chronic pigmented purpura is characterized by an insidious onset and slow progression of grouped petechiae on the extremities (Fig 13–16), developing in adolescents. Individual lesions show fresh and old petechiae intermixed and an interplay of red, brown, and yellow spots. Lesions are usually flat (Fig 13–17), but a lichenified epidermis may overlie the lesions. The grouped petechiae are oval and may begin unilaterally, but progress to become symmetric. The lower extremities are most commonly involved, with more lesions in dependent areas. Lesions may progress to involve the entire trunk and upper extremities. Itching is usually mild or absent, and no systemic symptoms are associated with chronic pigmented purpura. Spontaneous remis-

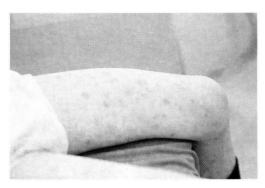

FIG 13–16.
Brown and cayenne-pepper macules on legs of child with progressive pigmentary purpura.

sion occurs within 1 to 2 years, but the natural course of the disease is not well documented.

Differential Diagnosis

The lesions of grouped petechiae of multiple ages are so characteristic that this type of purpura is seldom confused with other disorders. Occasionally, trauma (e.g., child abuse) or a mild bleeding disorder is suspected.

Pathogenesis

A mild capillaritis is seen in these disorders, with extravasation of red blood cells, hemosiderin deposits, and a mild perivascular lymphocytic infiltration of superficial dermal blood vessels. The vascular injury is mild, and its cause is unknown.

Treatment

There is no specific therapy. Reduction of venous stasis may be helpful.

Patient Education

The expected remission and the mild nature of this disorder should be emphasized.

Follow-up Visits

Follow-up visits are unnecessary.

SPIDER ANGIOMA (NEVUS ARANEUS)

Clinical Features

A spider nevus is a small, telangiectatic lesion consisting of a central arteriole from which superficial blood vessels radiate peripherally (Fig 13–18). The lesions usually appear between the ages of 2 and 6, and are located in sun-exposed areas, usually on the cheeks, nose, dorsa of the hands, and forearms. Sometimes the central arteriole is prominent and may be pulsatile on diascopy. Approximately 40% of children will have these lesions.

Differential Diagnosis

Spider angiomas must be differentiated from the telangiectatic mats of the autosomal dominant Osler-Weber-Rendu syndrome in which confluent telangiectases compose each lesion and multiple lesions are seen on the dorsa of the hands and on the lips and face. Associated epistaxis, or peptic ulcer–like symptoms, or both, may be important systemic symptoms to help differentiate the two conditions. Spider angiomas may be confused with the telangiectatic mats seen in collagen vascular diseases such as scleroderma and lupus erythematosus.

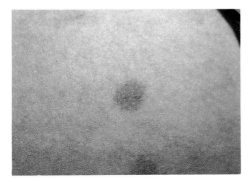

FIG 13–17.
Pigmented macules in progressive pigmentary purpura.

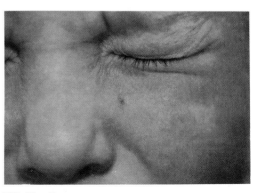

FIG 13–18.
Vascular spider on cheek of child.

Pathogenesis

The cause of these lesions is unknown.

Treatment

If the cosmetic appearance is a concern to the child, lesions may be removed with the pulsed dye laser at 585 nm.

Patient Education

The common and nonserious nature of these lesions should be emphasized.

Follow-up Visits

Follow-up visits are unnecessary.

CHERRY ANGIOMAS AND DIFFUSE ANGIOKERATOMAS

Clinical Features

True cherry angiomas are rare in childhood and usually appear as 1- to 3-mm solid-red, dome-shaped, blanching papules (Fig 13–19). The appearance of multiple cherry angiomas around the umbilicus and scrotum, which increase progressively with age, should bring to mind two diagnoses: Fabry's disease and α-fucosidosis. In Fabry's disease, attacks of pain, numbness, and tingling of the hands and feet often accompany the eruption. The usual onset of the eruption is between 4 and 12 years of age. In α-fucosidosis, severe mental retardation and neuromuscular spasticity accompany the disorder.

Differential Diagnosis

Cherry angiomas and angiokeratomas must be differentiated from small pyogenic granulomas

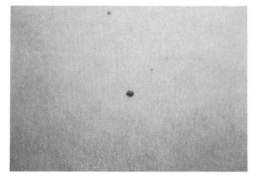

FIG 13–19.
Cherry angioma on trunk of child.

and small strawberry hemangiomas. Usually the differentiation is quite simple.

Pathogenesis

Fabry's disease is an X-linked recessive disorder in which activity of a specific lysosomal hydrolase, α-galactosidase A, is deficient. The glycosphingolipid, ceramide trihexoside, accumulates within endothelial cells and produces the cutaneous vascular lesions. On electron microscopy, the endothelial cells of the affected vessels are seen to contain multiple laminated inclusions diagnostic of the disease. In α-fucosidosis, the lysosomes of the endothelial cells are widely dilated, but the material is washed out during fixation so that the cells appear empty. Fibroblast culture and analysis of α-galactosidase A activity may be performed to confirm the diagnosis of Fabry's disease. In α-fucosidosis, an autosomal recessive trait, fibroblast cultures may also be useful in confirming the diagnosis.

Treatment

There is no effective treatment either for Fabry's disease or for α-fucosidosis. Renal transplantation has resulted in improvement in some patients with Fabry's disease. True cherry angiomas may be treated with the pulsed dye laser at 585 nm, if desired.

Patient Education

The patient should be informed about the seriousness of each of these conditions and referred for genetic counseling. The patient should be advised that prenatal diagnosis is possible for future pregnancies and that molecular probes are available to screen carrier females. Pediatric neurologic care is usually advisable. Since the condition of patients with Fabry's disease progresses to severe renal disease, and they may succumb to renal failure, evaluation of renal function with appropriate consultation should be recommended to the parents.

Follow-up Visits

Follow-up visits should be arranged with the appropriate pediatric care specialists.

BIBLIOGRAPHY

Aberg N, Engstrom I, Lindberg U: Allergic diseases in Swedish school children. *Acta Paediatr Scand* 1989; 78:246.

Alanko K, Stubb S, Kauppinen K: Cutaneous drug reactions: Clinical types and causative agents. *Acta Derm Venereol (Stockh)* 1989; 69:223.

Bisno AL, Shulman ST, Dajani AS: The rise and fall (and rise?) of rheumatic fever. *JAMA* 1988; 259:728.

Breathnach SM: Symptomatic dermographism: Natural history, clinical features, laboratory investigations, and response to therapy. *Clin Exp Dermatol* 1983; 8:463.

Cream JJ: Vasculitis. *Curr Probl Dermatol* May/June 1989; 1:67–95.

Desnick RJ, Bernstein HS, Astrin CH, et al: Fabry's disease: Molecular diagnosis of hemizygotes and heterozygotes. *Enzyme* 1987; 38:54.

Doeglas HMG, Klasen EC, Bleumink E: Alpha-1 antitrypsin deficiency and PI typing in patients with chronic urticaria. *Br J Dermatol* 1985; 112:381.

Doxiadis SA: Erythema nodosum in children. *Medicine (Baltimore)* 1951; 30:283.

Emmelin N, Feldberg W: The mechanism of the sting of the common nettle *(Urtica urens). J Physiol* 1947; 106:440.

Farley TA, Gillespie S, Rasoulpour M, et al: Epidemiology of a cluster of Henoch-Schönlein purpura. *Am J Dis Child* 1989; 143:798.

Golitz LE, Weston WL, Lane AT: Bullous mastocytosis: Diffuse cutaneous mastocytosis with extensive blisters mimicking scalded skin syndrome or erythema multiforme. *Pediatr Dermatol* 1984; 1:228–294.

Halpern SR: Chronic hives in children: An analysis of 75 cases. *Ann Allergy* 1965; 23:589.

Jacobs AH: Vascular nevi. *Pediatr Clin North Am* 1983; 30:465.

Kohen DP: Neonatal gonococcal arthritis. *Pediatrics* 1974; 53:436.

Lawlor F, Black AK, Ward AM, et al: Delayed pressure urticaria; objective evaluation of a variable disease using a dermographometer and assessment of treatment using colchicine. *Br J Dermatol* 1989; 120:403.

Leznoff A, Sussman GL: Syndrome of chronic urticaria and angioedema with thyroid autoimmunity: Analysis of 90 patients. *J Allergy Clin Immunol* 1989; 89:66.

Monroe EW: Chronic urticaria: Review of nonsedating antihistamines in treatment. *J Am Acad Dermatol* 1988; 19:842.

Ozols II, Wheat LJ: Erythema nodosum in an epidemic of histoplasmosis in Indianapolis. *Arch Dermatol* 1981; 117:709.

Quaranta J, Rohr AS, Rachelefsky GS, et al: The etiology and natural history of chronic urticaria and angioedema. *J Allergy Clin Immunol* 1987; 79:182.

Ruddy S: Hereditary angioedema. Undersuspected, underdiagnosed. *Hosp Pract* 1988; 8:91.

Schuller DE, Elvey SM: Urticaria with streptococcal infection. *Pediatrics* 1980; 65:592.

Simon M Jr, Heese A, Gotz A: Immunopathological investigations in purpura pigmentosa chronica. *Acta Derm Venereol (Stockh)* 1989; 69:101.

Stein DH: Mastocytosis: A review. *Pediatr Dermatol* 1986; 3:365.

Toews WH, Bass JW: Skin manifestations of meningococcal infection. *Am J Dis Child* 1974; 127:173.

Twarog FJ: Urticaria in childhood: Pathogenesis and management. *Pediatr Clin North Am* 1983; 30:887.

14 _____ Hair Disorders

Children may seek medical attention because of excessive hair or, more commonly, hair loss. This chapter is divided into two sections, hair loss and excessive hair.

HAIR LOSS

When evaluating hair loss in children, one should determine whether it is congenital or acquired, circumscribed or diffuse. This results in four diagnostic categories of hair loss (Table 14–1). Hair loss (alopecia) accounts for approximately 3% of children's visits to a dermatologist. It causes the parents and the child considerable anxiety and the health team considerable frustration. Three types among the numerous causes of hair loss in children account for the great majority of health visits for alopecia: alopecia areata, tinea capitis, and traumatic alopecia. All three are forms of acquired, circumscribed hair loss (Table 14–2). These three conditions should always be considered in the differential diagnosis of hair loss.

ALOPECIA AREATA

Clinical Features
Alopecia areata is characterized by complete or almost complete hair loss in circumscribed areas. Usually from one to three areas are involved (Fig 14–1). It is most commonly seen (in 90% of patients) in the frontal or parietal area of the scalp, but body hair, pubic or axillary hair, eyelashes, and eyebrows may be involved. The appearance of a circumscribed area that is completely devoid of hair without any scalp change is a constant feature. Scalp erythema or scaling may

occur in alopecia areata after sunburn. A positive family history for alopecia areata is found in 10% to 20% of the patients.

Nail pitting may accompany alopecia areata and appears as shallow, wide (1 to 2 mm) depressions in the nail plate. The pits are wider than those seen in psoriasis (Fig 14–2).

The prognosis for most children is excellent. Complete regrowth of the hair occurs within a year in 95% of children with alopecia areata. Spontaneous remission is the rule. Approximately 30% of patients will have a future episode of alopecia areata.

Ophiasis, an unusual subtype involving fewer than 5% of all patients with alopecia areata, begins in the occiput or along the frontal area of the scalp (Fig 14–3) and spreads, with many patches of alopecia along the hair margins. Ophiasis is likely to eventuate in loss of all scalp hair (alopecia totalis) (Fig 14–4) or all scalp and body hair (alopecia universalis). When this occurs, the prognosis for regrowth is extremely poor.

Differential Diagnosis
Trichotillomania or other forms of traction alopecia may mimic alopecia areata. Broken hairs, scalp petechiae, and a history of trauma are features that help distinguish these conditions. Tinea capitis, particularly the black-dot form, may be confused with alopecia areata. Careful examination of the scalp will reveal broken hairs within the follicle, and microscopic examination of these hairs in potassium hydroxide (KOH) 10% will reveal hyphae within the hair shaft. A fungal culture will help confirm the diagnosis.

The scarring alopecias may present circumscribed areas of hair loss, but the scalp thickening and color change seen in these conditions will help distinguish them from alopecia areata.

TABLE 14−1.

Diagnostic Categories of Hair Loss in Children

> Congenital circumscribed alopecia
> Acquired circumscribed alopecia
> Congenital diffuse alopecia
> Acquired diffuse alopecia

TABLE 14−2.

Major Types of Acquired Circumscribed Alopecia in Childhood

> Alopecia areata
> Tinea capitis
> Traction alopecia (including trichotillomania)

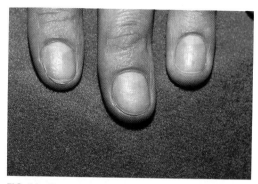

FIG 14−2.
Nail pitting in child with alopecia areata.

Circumscribed alopecia may be congenital and present from birth and is characteristic of certain birthmarks in the scalp, particularly sebaceous nevus. These alopecias may be difficult to differentiate from alopecia areata. The history of onset at birth and the yellow plaques in the scalp will differentiate congenital circumscribed alopecias from alopecia areata.

Pathogenesis

It has been presumed that alopecia areata represents an immune mechanism, since a dense perifollicular accumulation of lymphocytes precedes the hair loss. The exact mechanism of hair loss is not understood, but direct lymphocyte injury to the hair matrix has been postulated. The injury to the growing hair results in premature conversion of growing hairs to resting hairs that are shed. Thus, the margins of the circumscribed area of hair loss contain regressing hairs that are

clubbed on the end, the so-called exclamation point hairs.

Treatment

There is no reliable treatment for alopecia areata. Since spontaneous regrowth occurs in 95% of cases, the prognosis is good in most patients. The administration of systemic glucocorticosteroids and cyclosporine has been advocated for their anti-inflammatory effect. The suppression of inflammation and hair regrowth is temporary and variable, however. Withdrawal of steroids or cyclosporine results in prompt loss of the hair that has grown back. Thus the risks of side effects outweigh the benefits of temporary hair growth.

In complete hair loss, referral to a dermatologist may be useful, and prompt attention should be given to obtaining a wig for the child. Excellent children's wigs are manufactured, and a physician's prescription may allow the family to obtain a wig at reduced prices. A benefit from potent

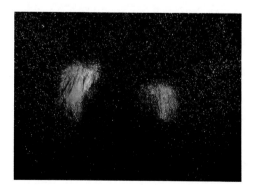

FIG 14−1.
Alopecia areata. Two circumscribed patches of completely bald scalp.

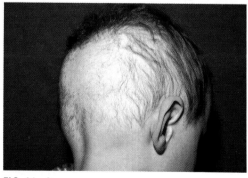

FIG 14−3.
Ophiasis pattern of alopecia areata with hair loss starting in occiput.

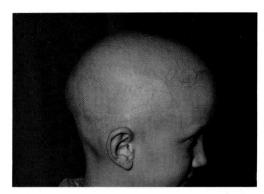

FIG 14–4.
Alopecia totalis. Ophiasis progressing to completely bald scalp.

topical or intralesional glucocorticosteroids has not been documented. A support group, the National Alopecia Areata Foundation, has a number of North American chapters that provide excellent psychologic support and the latest treatment information for persons with alopecia areata. Acceptable cosmetic improvement has been reported in some patients with the use of topical minoxidil, an antihypertensive agent.

Patient Education

In children with the usual type of alopecia areata, with one to three circumscribed patches of complete scalp hair loss, it is important to emphasize the excellent prognosis. Explaining the proposed mechanism of the disease and the excellent chances for spontaneous recovery will greatly aid understanding of the problem. Ophiasis patients should be told of the poor prognosis. The risks and benefits of all current therapy should be explained in detail, and the psychologic benefits of wearing a wig should be discussed. Patients should be informed about the National Alopecia Areata Foundation (714 C St., Suite 202, San Rafael, CA 94901). In the usual type of alopecia areata, a visit every 3 months is useful to check on progress and the chances for spontaneous regression.

Follow-up Visits

In the ophiasis type, a visit in 2 weeks to re-explain the illness and encourage the use of a wig is most helpful. Frequent visits may be necessary to establish the proper physician-patient relationship.

TINEA CAPITIS

Clinical Features

Tinea capitis involves the scalp hair in prepubertal children and is largely due to infections with two dermatophytes, *Microsporum canis* and *Trichophyton tonsurans.* Each dermatophyte produces a noninflammatory stage lasting 2 to 8 weeks, followed by an inflammatory stage. Hair loss is a regular feature of tinea capitis, although in one form of *T. tonsurans* infection, diffuse scaling without hair loss is seen. The other two clinical presentations of *T. tonsurans* infection and *M. canis* infection are characterized by circumscribed hair loss. *M. canis* will produce one or several patches of broken hairs that appear thickened and white. The hairs fluoresce yellow-green with Wood's light. In contrast, *T. tonsurans* produces hairs that break off at the follicular orifice in a circumscribed area of the scalp. This leaves small, dark hairs on the follicles, so-called black-dot ringworm. *T. tonsurans* may produce numerous circumscribed, triangle-shaped patches of hair loss throughout the scalp (see Fig 14–5). *T. tonsurans* does not fluoresce with Wood's light. Asymptomatic adults and children may carry spores of *T. tonsurans* on their scalp.

Diagnostic Procedures

The diagnosis in the noninflammatory stage should be confirmed by the following steps: (1) Wood's light examination, (2) KOH examination, and (3) fungal culture.

Wood's Light Examination.—Wood's light examination is best performed with a hand-held

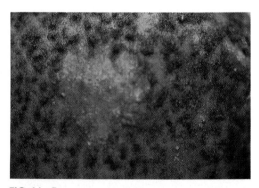

FIG 14–5.
Tinea capitis. Triangular patches of hair loss, diffuse scaling, and a circumscribed kerion with pustules in child with *T. tonsurans* infection.

ultraviolet black lamp with two fluorescent bulbs. The lamp should be held within 6 inches of the scalp, and yellow-green fluorescence of the thickened scalp hairs should be observed. Lint from clothing fluoresces white because of the addition of optical brighteners, and scale entrapped in sebum appears a dull yellow. These may be confused with true fungal fluorescence.

Potassium Hydroxide.—KOH examination should be done in every case of hair loss associated with broken hairs. If the hair fluoresces, hold the Wood's lamp in one hand and a curet in the other. Gently remove the fluorescent hairs by scraping the scalp surface for KOH examination and culture. The involved hairs are loosened in the follicle and can be extracted without pain. If the hair does not fluoresce, scrape the follicular openings in the area of the scalp hair loss with a No. 15 blade or a curet and examine the dislodged hairs under the microscope. Place the hair on a glass microscope slide, partially dissolve in KOH 20%, and place under a coverslip. Wait 20 to 40 minutes to examine the specimen (use the ×10 objective of the microscope). The outer surface of fluorescent hairs is coated with mats containing thousands of tiny spores (Fig 14–6). Hyphae may also be seen within the hair shaft. In nonfluorescent hairs, hyphae and spores are seen within the hair shaft.

Fungal Culture.—Fungal culture should be performed routinely in children with suspected tinea capitis. Sabouraud dextrose agar containing cycloheximide and chloramphenicol or modified

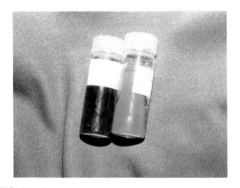

FIG 14–6.
Fungal culture on modified Sabouraud dextrose agar (dermatophyte test medium) with entire agar turned red on left (positive culture) and agar remaining yellow in negative culture on right.

Sabouraud dextrose agar with phenol red makes this procedure simple. Hair or scrapings obtained with a toothbrush or curet are inoculated so as to break the agar surface; the bottle cap is loosely applied, and the culture bottles are left at room temperature. On the modified agar, if a dermatophyte is present, the media turns from yellow to red in 4 to 5 days (see Fig 14–6). A positive culture can be subcultured on Sabouraud dextrose agar for gross and microscopic identification.

Inflammatory tinea capitis is an erythematous, boggy nodule with superficial pustules, called a kerion. These lesions are almost completely devoid of hair and, if untreated, will lead to scarring and permanent hair loss. A kerion will appear 2 to 8 weeks after infection begins and represents an exaggerated host response to the invading fungus. Approximately 40% of untreated tinea capitis due to *M. canis* or *T. tonsurans* may eventuate in kerion.

Differential Diagnosis

Alopecia areata and trichotillomania are the major considerations in the differential diagnosis of tinea capitis in children (see Table 14–2). Alopecia areata may be distinguished by the total absence of hair in a circumscribed patch, without any associated scalp change. In trichotillomania, scalp excoriations, perifollicular petechiae, and hairs broken off at differing lengths are distinguishing factors. Bacterial pyodermas are often mistaken for kerion. The pustules in kerion are sterile, however, and incision produces only serosanguineous fluid. Bacterial culture of the skin surface may yield *S. aureus* and lead to the incorrect diagnosis of pyoderma. It should be kept in mind that *S. aureus* frequently colonizes the skin surface, and such cultures do not detect bacterial invasion of deeper structures.

Less commonly, traction alopecia of other types, scleroderma, lichen planus, psoriasis, dandruff, or hair shaft defects may be confused with tinea capitis.

Pathogenesis

M. canis is harbored by cats, dogs, and certain rodents, and children handling such animals are susceptible to infection. Humans appear to be a terminal host for such infections, and human-to-human transmission does not occur. When delayed hypersensitivity to the organism occurs, a kerion may develop. Histologic study of the kerion shows a mononuclear cell infiltrate consistent with that seen in delayed hypersensitivity reactions. *M. canis* accounts for 90% of the tinea capitis seen in suburban and rural areas.

T. tonsurans is transmitted from human to human, and 4% of the general population are asymptomatic carriers. It is most prevalent in areas of crowding and accounts for 90% of tinea capitis in inner city children, with a major epidemic in North America.

Treatment

Griseofulvin, 10 to 20 mg/kg/day, in a micronized form is recommended for treatment of tinea capitis. A minimum of 8 weeks of therapy is required. Topical antifungal agents are unable to reach the hyphae within the hair shaft and are ineffective. It is not unusual to administer griseofulvin for 2 to 3 months. In *M. canis* tinea capitis, with successful treatment, the lesions become nonfluorescent 13 days after beginning griseofulvin. Although many side effects of griseofulvin are known, including agranulocytosis and aplastic anemia, side effects are rare, and it is a relatively safe drug in children. Absorption is enhanced by a fatty meal, and griseofulvin to be taken twice a day with ice cream is a popular prescription. Recently, in addition to oral griseofulvin, the topical application of selenium sulfide 2.5% shampoo to the scalp has resulted in negative cultures and a rapid return of the child to school. Shampooing twice weekly for the entire household may prevent infection of other children in the case of *T. tonsurans* infection.

Patient Education

If *M. canis* is found, the animal source should be identified and the animal, if a dog or cat, treated by a veterinarian to prevent infection of other children. In *T. tonsurans,* identification and treatment of the likely contacts is necessary. Patients should be informed that hair regrowth is slow, often taking 3 to 6 months. If a kerion is present and untreated, some scarring and permanent hair loss may result.

Follow-up Visits

A first visit in 2 weeks is helpful for ascertaining the effectiveness of griseofulvin therapy. The findings on reexamination for fluorescence and repeat culture will serve as guidelines for increasing the dosage. If at 2 weeks test results for fluorescence are negative, or the culture is negative, or both, a total of 6 weeks of therapy may be all

that will be required. Treatment 4 to 6 weeks after the culture becomes negative is a useful rule of thumb. A follow-up visit every 2 to 4 weeks until hair regrowth begins is advised.

TRAUMATIC ALOPECIA

Traumatic alopecia results from the hair injury produced by traction, friction, chemical, or other injury to hair. The common types seen in childhood include trichotillomania (hair pulling) and the traction alopecia seen with various popular hair styles.

TRICHOTILLOMANIA

Clinical Features

Circumscribed areas of hair loss with irregular borders and hairs broken off at different lengths are seen in trichotillomania (Fig 14–7). Frequently scalp excoriations and perifollicular petechiae are present (Fig 14–8). Commonly only one area of the scalp is involved, with the frontoparietal and frontotemporal scalp areas being the most usual sites. Rarely the eyebrows or eyelashes may be plucked. Children with trichotillomania exhibit obsessive-compulsive behavior. In severely emotionally disturbed children, extensive areas of the scalp may be involved.

Differential Diagnosis

The diseases considered in the differential diagnosis of trichotillomania are the same as

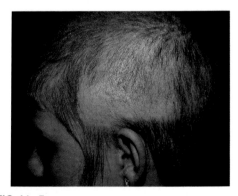

FIG 14–7.
Trichotillomania. Hair broken at many different lengths in child with hair pulling as a nervous habit.

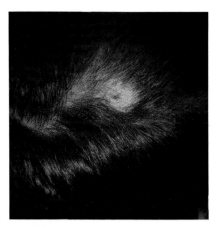

FIG 14–8.
Scalp excoriations in trichotillomania.

those for alopecia areata and tinea capitis (see Table 14–2).

Pathogenesis

Most investigators regard trichotillomania as a nervous habit. The hair pulling is most often done subconsciously at study times, while watching television, or while reading. The child may exhibit other obsessive or compulsive behavior patterns. Parents often vehemently deny such hair pulling, since they have not personally observed it. Rarely severe psychologic disturbances may be found in children who have trichotillomania.

Treatment

Explaining that hair pulling is a nervous habit relieves the child and the parents. Equating this habit with nail biting is a useful comparison to clarify the problem. Behavior modification, that is, substituting another activity, is useful, as is the daily application of oils to the scalp to make the hair so slippery that it cannot be pulled. In most children relief of stress will result in ending the nervous habit. Some children persist with trichotillomania into adult life. In severe forms that are associated with other signs of emotional stress, psychiatric referral may be indicated. Recently clomipramine was demonstrated to be useful in adult women with trichotillomania, but its efficacy in children has yet to be demonstrated.

Patient Education

A careful explanation of nervous habits and reassurance are crucial to patient and parent education. One should avoid blaming the child or one or more family members. Explain that this habit is a difficult one to break. Tell the parents that this is a compulsive behavior that may be the result of significant stress and that counseling may be useful.

Follow-up Visits

A follow-up visit in 1 to 2 months is useful in evaluating progress. Continued reassurance should be given. If the habit is persisting, referral to a child psychologist or psychiatrist is indicated.

TRACTION ALOPECIA

Clinical Features

Thinning of hair in particular areas of the scalp may result from constant traction or friction. Very few fractured hairs are found in the involved areas, although the hairs may be smaller in diameter than those found in adjacent areas (Fig 14–9). The thinning is often patchy, depending on the nature of the trauma. The history of methods of hair care and types of hair style is crucial for the diagnosis.

Differential Diagnosis

The differential diagnosis is the same as for alopecia areata and tinea capitis (see Table 14–2).

Pathogenesis

Several different sources of traction or friction have been identified as responsible for traction alopecia. The hair style or chemical or thermal treatment or friction produces incomplete and complete fractures of hair. One should always consider child abuse (e.g., pulling the child by the

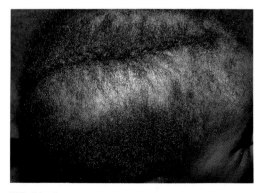

FIG 14–9.
Traction alopecia. Hair loss due to tight braiding.

hair). Neonatal occipital alopecia is physiologic hair loss exacerbated by the rubbing of the baby's head on the sheet or mattress. Massage alopecia may occur from vigorous scalp massage and frequent shampooing. Marginal alopecia is seen with hair straightening or tight hair curlers. Cornrow alopecia, ponytail alopecia, and braid alopecia are all related to tight hair styles. Hot-comb alopecia occurs on the vertex of the scalp and may involve scarring. It is the result of use of a hot comb to straighten or style hair. Marginal alopecia is sometimes seen in hot-comb alopecia.

Treatment

Discontinuation of the trauma to the hair is the obvious treatment of choice. The use of mild shampoos and wide-toothed combs with rounded ends, infrequent shampooing, and gentle brushing are all important components of therapy. Recovery may take 3 to 6 months.

Patient Education

The susceptibility of certain hair types to such trauma should be explained, and the benefits of being gentle with the hair emphasized.

Follow-up Visits

A follow-up visit in 3 to 6 months is useful to assess hair regrowth.

OTHER FORMS OF HAIR LOSS

The remaining types of hair loss are uncommon or rare. No attempt is made to consider these numerous conditions in detail, but an orderly approach to them is presented. One should first determine whether the hair loss is circumscribed or diffuse; then determine whether it has been present from birth or was acquired later in life. This results in four diagnostic categories: congenital circumscribed alopecia, acquired circumscribed alopecia, congenital diffuse alopecia, and acquired diffuse alopecia (see Table 14–1). In congenital diffuse alopecia, a further diagnostic step, the hair mount examination is necessary. Only the general clinical features of each group and the differential diagnoses are given. Two forms of diffuse hair loss, telogen effluvium and ectodermal dysplasia, are discussed in more detail later in this chapter.

The mechanisms of hair loss in most of these unusual forms of alopecia have not been uncovered. Certain associations are of therapeutic importance, however. There are an extraordinary number of clinical conditions associated with hair loss, and one should characterize hair loss into one of the four types to permit proper diagnosis and therapy.

CONGENITAL CIRCUMSCRIBED ALOPECIA

Clinical Features

Localized areas of scalp hair loss present from birth usually overlie a birthmark, such as a sebaceous or epidermal nevus. The scalp surface is smooth, particularly in newborn infants or infants with circumscribed hair loss, and it is yellow to tan in color (Fig 14–10). As the child gets older, a plaque is noted. A congenital circumscribed alopecia may also occur in aplasia cutis congenita.

Differential Diagnosis

A scalp biopsy will help in identifying and characterizing these birthmarks, which represent hyperplasia of epidermal cells or sebaceous structures. Aplasia cutis congenita demonstrates scarring of the scalp in a circumscribed area and represents failure of formation of one or more layers of the scalp. In the other rare forms, circumscribed patches of hair loss without scalp changes are present. The differential diagnosis of this type of alopecia is given in Table 14–3.

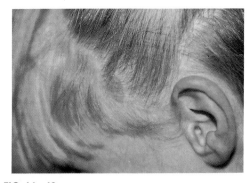

FIG 14–10.
Nevus sebaceus. Absence of hair in area of yellow-orange plaque of birthmark.

TABLE 14–3.
Differential Diagnosis of Congenital Circumscribed Hair Loss

Birthmark
Sebaceous nevus
Epidermal nevus
Hair follicle hamartoma
Aplasia cutis congenita (scarlike)
Conradi's disease
Incontinentia pigmenti
Sutural alopecia in Hallermann-Streiff syndrome
Triangular alopecia of frontal area of the scalp

ACQUIRED CIRCUMSCRIBED ALOPECIA: SCARRING FORMS

Clinical Features
Circumscribed hair loss acquired during childhood, other than alopecia areata, tinea capitis, and traction alopecia, is usually scarring in nature, that is, the hair follicles are replaced by fibrous tissue after injury to the hair follicles from infection, trauma, or inflammatory skin disease.

Differential Diagnosis
Table 14–4 presents the conditions to be considered in the differential diagnosis.

CONGENITAL DIFFUSE ALOPECIA

Clinical Features
Diffuse scalp hair loss present from birth usually results in the complaint that the child's

TABLE 14–4.
Differential Diagnosis of Congenital or Acquired Scarring Circumscribed Hair Loss

Postinfectious
Kerion due to tinea capitis
Pyoderma
Varicella
Postinflammatory
Lichen planus
Lupus erythematosus
Darier's disease
Porokeratosis of Mibelli
Postinjury
Physical trauma (abrasions, cuts)
Chemical or thermal burns
Radiation injury

hair simply will not grow. Such children never require haircuts. Included in this group are the hair shaft defects in which the failure of hair growth is the result of structural defects that result in the breaking off of hairs (Fig 14–11). The child has short, broken hairs of equal length. In many forms of ectodermal dysplasia, reduced numbers or absence of hair follicles produces the clinical picture of congenital diffuse alopecia.

Differential Diagnosis
Removing hairs and placing them on a microscope slide with mounting fluid will allow demonstration of the particular type of structural hair defect. Many rare forms of diffuse congenital hair loss are associated with syndromes, and complete examination of the child is necessary for accurate diagnosis. The differential diagnosis of this type of hair loss is given in Table 14–5.

ACQUIRED DIFFUSE ALOPECIA

Hair loss with onset in childhood after a period of normal hair growth usually results from an underlying systemic disorder. In these children, a careful search for endocrine, metabolic, and chemical abnormalities is warranted (Table 14–6). A rigorous and detailed history should be

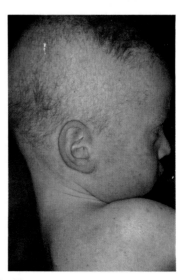

FIG 14–11.
Congenital hair shaft defect. Child who has never had a haircut at age 5 years has trichorrhexis invaginata (bamboo hairs) in Netherton's syndrome.

TABLE 14—5.

Differential Diagnosis of Congenital Diffuse Hair Loss

Hair shaft defects
  Trichorrhexis nodosa (broomstick fractures)
    Familial form
    Arginosuccinic aciduria
  Pili torti (twisted hair)
    Classic form
    Menkes' syndrome
  Monilethrix (beaded hair)
  Trichorrhexis invaginata (bamboo hair)
    (Netherton's syndrome)
Congenital hypothyroidism
Ectodermal dysplasias
  Hidrotic ectodermal dysplasia
  Anhidrotic ectodermal dysplasia
  Trichothiodystrophy
  Atrichia congenita
  Cartilage-hair hypoplasia
  Follicular atrophoderma
Progeria
Marinesco-Sjögren syndrome

TABLE 14—6.

Differential Diagnosis of Acquired Diffuse Hair Loss

Endocrine
  Hypothyroidism
  Hypopituitarism
  Hypoparathyroidism
  Diabetes mellitus
  Androgenetic alopecia (male pattern) in
    adolescents
Chemical
  Thallium poisoning (rat poison)
  Antithyroid drugs
  Heparin
  Coumarin
  Antimetabolites (e.g., cyclophosphamide)
Nutritional
  Hypervitaminosis A
  Acrodermatitis enteropathica (zinc deficiency)
  Marasmus

taken and appropriate laboratory studies ordered if the clinical data so indicate. Since most of the endocrine, metabolic, and nutritional causes are correctable, one should consider undertaking a thorough laboratory evaluation in such children.

TELOGEN EFFLUVIUM

Telogen effluvium is the name given to the acquired diffuse alopecia that results from rapid conversion of scalp hairs from the growing state to the resting state. In physiologic circumstances, an infant or child has 88% of scalp hair in a growing, or anagen, state and only 12% of hair in a resting, or telogen, state. Each individual scalp hair grows for 3 years, then regresses over a 2- to 3-week period, and rests for 3 months. This growth throughout the scalp is asynchronous in that the majority of hairs are growing at any time of observation. Acutely stressful events such as birth, auto accidents, illnesses with high fever, and acute psychiatric problems may result in a rapid conversion of growing hairs to resting hairs. Two to 4 months after the event the hairs are shed and usually continue to shed over a 3- to 4-month period. Each hair shed is a resting hair and will be replaced by a normal-growing hair. In the newborn infant, the hairs are shed in two phases from the frontal area of the scalp to the occipital area and are not asynchronous in growth phase until about 12 months of age.

Diagnosis of telogen effluvium can be made by plucking at least 50 hairs from a child's scalp and examining the roots to determine whether they are growing or resting. This is best done by cutting away the remainder of the hairs and mounting the roots in a commercial slide-mounting medium. A growing, or anagen, hair will have a pigmented core and a bulbous root that is larger in diameter than the hair shaft. Often the external root sheath is present. In a telogen, or resting, hair, the external root sheath is absent or fragmented, pigment is often absent, and the root of the hair is narrower than the caliber of the other hair and is frequently curved.

One can reassure the patient with telogen effluvium that complete regrowth is possible. Telogen effluvium has been reported after operations, crash diets, and the use of anticoagulants and antithyroid drugs. Anagen effluvium, in which growing hairs are lost, is an expected result of cancer treatment in children, in which the antimetabolites interfere with hair growth or radiation to the head injures the growing hair.

ECTODERMAL DYSPLASIA

Clinical Features

Two major forms of ectodermal dysplasia have been recognized, the anhidrotic form and the hidrotic form. In addition, in a number of uncommon and rare forms of ectodermal dysplasia, hair is thin or absent. Both common forms may be characterized by thin, sparse scalp hair. Absence of the eyebrows and eyelashes in the newborn infant may be an important clue to the diagnosis. Other clinical findings may be less obvious.

In anhidrotic ectodermal dysplasia, sweating is reduced or completely absent. Fever of unknown origin or recurrent high fever may be the presenting symptom in such infants. The facies of such children are very distinctive, with everted lips, prominent frontal ridges, saddle nose, and absence of eyebrows and eyelashes. Temporary and permanent teeth are reduced in number or may be entirely absent. If teeth erupt, they are often cone shaped, and this may be observed by dental x-ray examination even in the preeruptive stage (Fig 14–12). Atrophic rhinitis and frequent upper respiratory symptoms may lead to the mistaken diagnosis of respiratory allergy. Scalp hair is seldom totally absent, but it is very sparse and is often the first concern of the parents. Fingernails and toenails are normal in at least half of the patients, but they may be thin or brittle. A careful genetic history should be obtained.

The hidrotic form is characterized by nail dystrophy as the most prominent clinical finding. The nails are thickened, slow growing, and brittle. Thick nails may be apparent early in infancy. In one third of the families, the only feature present is nail disease. As in the anhidrotic form, the scalp hair is thin and sparse and eyebrows are thin, but sweating is normal. Teeth are often normal. The palms and soles may be diffusely thickened, and

thickening on the knuckles, knees, and elbows may be prominently observed.

Differential Diagnosis

The major conditions to be considered in the differential diagnosis are listed in Table 14–5. The findings of disorders of nails, skin, and teeth in the same patient in addition to the hair loss will suggest ectodermal dysplasia. Within a single family with ectodermal dysplasia, the features may be quite variable.

Pathogenesis

Anhidrotic ectodermal dysplasia is inherited in an X-linked recessive pattern or, rarely, an autosomal recessive pattern. The hidrotic form is inherited as autosomal dominant and has been observed in a large French-Canadian family, surnamed Clouston. In the anhidrotic form, sweat glands are absent or rudimentary, as are scalp hair follicles, sebaceous glands, and the mucous glands of the respiratory passages. Lack of sweating results in poor thermal control and high fevers. Lack of hair follicles is expressed as sparse hair, and lack of respiratory mucus produces frequent infections and watery rhinorrhea. A disorder of keratinization is thought to be important in the hidrotic form to explain the nail disease and hyperkeratosis of the palms and soles.

Treatment

Fever control with the use of cool compresses is vital in the newborn or in the infant with recurrent fevers. There is no specific therapy otherwise available. The use of wigs and dental corrective devices may be necessary.

Patient Education

Genetic counseling is very useful, as is the explanation of the cause of the febrile responses and respiratory symptoms in the infant.

Follow-up Visits

At least one follow-up visit within 4 weeks of the initial visit is most useful to reexplain the genetic factors and the symptoms of disease.

EXCESSIVE HAIR

Excessive hair may be congenital or acquired.

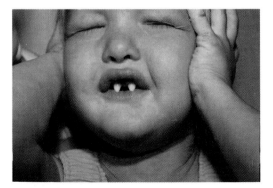

FIG 14–12.
Absence of eyebrows and cone-shaped teeth in child with hypohidrotic ectodermal dysplasia.

CONGENITAL HYPERTRICHOSIS

Clinical Features

Excessive hair may be generalized (hypertrichosis lanuginosa) or circumscribed (nevoid hypertrichosis). Excessive body hair in the newborn may be a transient problem, especially in premature infants, and resolves by 6 months of age, or may represent the rare hypertrichosis lanuginosa in which long, fine lanugo hairs cover the entire glabrous skin (Fig 14–13). Hypertrichosis lanuginosa is thought to be autosomal dominant, but most cases are sporadic. Excessive body hair may also be seen in patients with congenital hypothyroidism. Circumscribed hypertrichosis may be seen as one to six patches of excessive, long hair over various body regions. It is persistent. Circumscribed hypertrichosis when in the midline may be associated with nervous system abnormalities. Hypertrichosis on the lumbosacral spine (the "human tail") may be a clue to spina bifida; over the occiput, to meningocele or encephalocele. Facial hypertrichosis may be seen in a number of syndromes, as listed in Table 14–7.

Differential Diagnosis

Circumscribed areas of hypertrichosis must be differentiated from congenital smooth muscle and pilar nevus and congenital pigmented nevi (Table 14–8). A skin biopsy is required. Differentiating hypertrichosis lanuginosa from the tran-

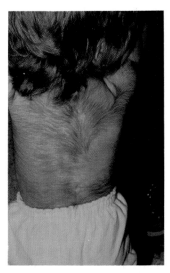

FIG 14–13.
Hypertrichosis lanuginosa.

TABLE 14–7.

Syndromes With Hypertrichosis

Cornelia de Lange syndrome
Rubinstein-Taybi syndrome
Gingival hyperplasia with hypertrichosis
Winchester syndrome
Recessive dystrophic epidermolysis bullosa
Fetal hydantoin syndrome
Erythrohepatic porphyria

sient lanugo overgrowth may be difficult the first few months of life, although the body and facial hairs in hypertrichosis lanuginosa are longer, often reaching 2 inches in length.

Pathogenesis

In nevoid hypertrichosis, excessive numbers of hair follicles are found. In hypertrichosis lanuginosa, body hairs appear as terminal hairs. Endocrine evaluations are normal.

Treatment

There is no satisfactory treatment for either diffuse or circumscribed hypertrichosis. Cutting or shaving hair may be considered. Hair removal chemicals may be too irritating to the skin of an infant or child.

Patient Education

In circumscribed hypertrichosis, an explanation of a malformation with excessive follicular structures in that segment of skin should be given. In hypertrichosis lanuginosa, genetic counseling may be useful.

Follow-up Visits

Support and counseling are very useful for parents and children, as are regularly scheduled visits.

TABLE 14–8.

Differential Diagnosis of Circumscribed Congenital Hypertrichosis

Congenital pigmented nevus
Pilar and smooth muscle hamartoma
Nevoid hypertrichosis
Midline nevoid hypertrichosis with spinal or CNS malformations

ACQUIRED EXCESSIVE HAIR (HIRSUTISM)

Clinical Features

Hirsutism is the growth of terminal hair in part or all of the male sexual pattern. It is observed predominantly in female adolescents. In Mediterranean races, females may have some male pattern hair, and it may be impossible to distinguish clinically from true hirsutism. Oriental females, in contrast, have no racial pattern of hirsutism. Excessive facial hair in the beard or moustache area may or may not be accompanied by excessively long body hairs. Other features of virilization may be seen, such as increased muscle mass, clitoral hypertrophy, and deepening of the voice. A history of abnormal menses is often obtained.

Differential Diagnosis

Racial forms that mimic hirsutism lack other signs of virilization, there are female family members with similar findings, and endocrine abnormalities are lacking (Table 14–9). Patients with porphyrias may have facial hirsutism but have a history of photosensitivity and scars from previous skin lesions.

Pathogenesis

Hirsutism is androgen dependent, and a careful gynecologic and endocrine evaluation will detect underlying disease (see Table 14–9).

Treatment

Treatment depends on the underlying endocrine abnormality and whether it is of ovarian or adrenal origin. Treatment with spironolactone is effective in some female adolescents.

Patient Education

It should be explained that hirsutism is just one feature of an endocrine disorder, and cor-

TABLE 14–9.
Conditions Resulting in Hirsutism

> Racial hirsutism
> Polycystic ovaries
> Ovarian tumors
> Congenital adrenal hyperplasia
> Cushing's syndrome
> Exogenous androgens

recting the underlying endocrine disease is required.

Follow-up Visits

Follow-up 2 weeks after gynecologic or endocrine consultation is obtained is useful.

UNMANAGEABLE HAIR

The uncombable hair syndrome and woolly hair nevus result in hair that is difficult to comb. In the uncombable hair syndrome, an autosomal dominant condition, the entire scalp hair is blond or silvery and does not lay flat when combed (Fig 14–14). In woolly hair nevus, there are one to three patches of scalp hair that are curly and coarse, different from the remaining hair. It is associated with epidermal nevi in up to half the children. Also, the cowlick of long, straight hairs over the scalp vertex is seen in 7% of children. In all cases, allowing the hair to grow long will make it more manageable, and spontaneous improvement at puberty is the rule.

SCALP WHORLS

A single whorl in the parietal scalp is found in 98% of children. In 45% it is in the midline, in 40% to the right of the midline, and to the left in

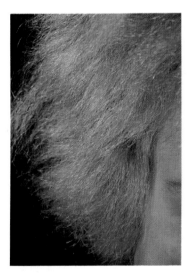

FIG 14–14.
Unmanageable hair.

the remainder. Abnormal locations of scalp whorls may be clues to CNS disease. For example, Down's syndrome, trisomy 13, Prader-Willi syndrome, and Rubinstein-Taybi syndrome show anterior scalp whorls, while malformations of cranial bones often display widely spaced biparietal whorls.

BIBLIOGRAPHY

Allen HB, Honig PJ, Leyden JJ, et al: Selenium sulfide: Adjunctive therapy for tinea capitis. *Pediatrics* 1982; 64:81.

Baden HP, Katz A: Trichothiodystrophy without retardation: One patient exhibiting transient combined immunodeficiency syndrome. *Pediatr Dermatol* 1988; 5:257.

Bailey-Pidham DD, Sanfillipo JS: Hirsutism in the adolescent female. *Pediatr Clin North Am* 1989; 36:581.

Barth JH: Normal hair growth in children. *Pediatr Dermatol* 1987; 4:173.

Barth JH, Cherry CA, Wojnarowska F, et al: Spironolactone is an effective and well tolerated antiandrogen therapy for hirsute women. *J Clin Endocrinol Metab* 1989; 68:966.

Cox NH, McClure JP, Hardie RA: Naevoid hypertrichosis—report of a patient with multiple lesions. *Clin Exp Dermatol* 1989; 14:62.

Hebert AA: Tinea capitis. Current concepts. *Arch Dermatol* 1988; 124:1554.

Matis WL, Baden H, Green R, et al: Uncombablehair syndrome. *Pediatr Dermatol* 1987; 4:215.

Price VH: Management of hair problems. *Int J Dermatol* 1979; 18:95.

Samlaska CP, James WD, Sperling LC: Scalp whorls. *J Am Acad Dermatol* 1989; 21:553.

Swedo SE, Leonard HL, Rapoport JL, et al: A double-blind comparison of clomipramine and desipramine in the treatment of trichotillomania. *N Engl J Med* 1989; 321:497.

Stroud JD: Hair loss in children. *Pediatr Clin North Am* 1983; 30:641.

Thiers BH, Bergfeld WF, Fiedler-Weiss V, et al: Alopecia areata symposium. *Pediatr Dermatol* 1987; 4:136.

Vogt BR, Traupe H, Hamm H: Congenital atrichia with nail dystrophy, abnormal facies, and retarded psychomotor development in two siblings: A new autosomal recessive syndrome? *Pediatr Dermatol* 1988; 5:236.

15 _____ Nail Disorders

Nail disorders are uncommon in children. Nail changes may be useful in the clinical identification of systemic disorders, however. Normal variations are important to recognize and distinguish from nail disease. Concave nail shapes are normal from birth to 3 years of age. Normal nails may have a few small pits in the nail plate. Scattered white spots are common in the nail plate and are caused by minor trauma. Longitudinal ridging is also common in normal nails and worsens with age.

THICK NAILS

Clinical Features

Nails thicken in proliferative epidermal disease. In psoriasis and lichen planus of children, all 20 nails may be involved. In psoriasis, thickening begins distally and is associated with distal nail separation (onycholysis), giving a yellow color to the nails (Fig 15–1). The entire nail plate may then be involved. Pitting of the nail surface also occurs (Fig 15–2). In lichen planus there is thickening of the nails, with a pinched-up central ridge and synechia formation on the nail surface (Fig 15–3).

The presenting symptom of the so-called 20-nail dystrophy of childhood is also thickened nails with exaggerated longitudinal ridges (Fig 15–4). At least in some children, this disease may be a hereditary disorder.

Psoriasis, lichen planus, and 20-nail dystrophy account for most cases of thick nails. Nails may be thickened, shiny, and contain horizontal ridges in dermatitis that involves the hands and cuticular skin. Pachyonychia congenita, an autosomal dominant disorder, presents with thickened

nails at birth that become more thickened by age 2 or 3 (Fig 15–5). Dermatophyte infections of the nail (onychomycosis) are unusual in children, with a prevalence of 0.2%, and usually involve only one or two nails (Fig 15–6).

Differential Diagnosis

Conditions to be considered in the differential diagnosis of thick nails are listed in Table 15–1. Longitudinal nail biopsy may be useful in differentiating nail disorders. Involvement of all 20 nails should suggest psoriasis, lichen planus, or 20-nail dystrophy, but not fungal infection. Finding characteristic papulosquamous skin lesions will help in the diagnosis of psoriasis and lichen planus. Thickened nails may be seen in children with scabies who cannot scratch.

Pathogenesis

The increased turnover time in the nail matrix results in a thickened, often dystrophic nail. This occurs primarily in psoriasis and lichen planus.

Treatment

There is no satisfactory treatment for hypertrophic disorders of the nail. In dermatophyte infection, griseofulvin, 20 mg/kg/day for 3 months, is effective in only about 30% of cases.

Patient Education

One must be careful to explain that nail thickening merely reflects overgrowth of nail cells and that it does not represent a specific disease.

Follow-up Visits

Visits every 6 months may be useful in following the course of these conditions.

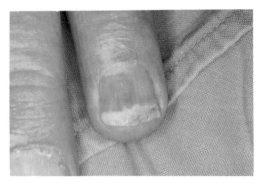

FIG 15—1.
Psoriasis of nail. Yellowing within nail represents separation of nail plate from nail bed.

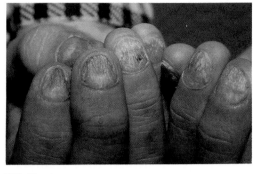

FIG 15—4.
Twenty-nail dystrophy. Exaggerated longitudinal ridging and rough surface on all 20 nails.

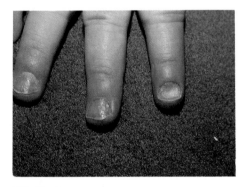

FIG 15—2.
Nail pitting in child with psoriasis.

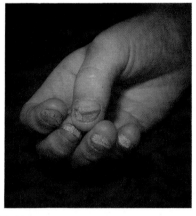

FIG 15—5.
Pachyonychia congenita type I. Distal thickening and elevation of nails.

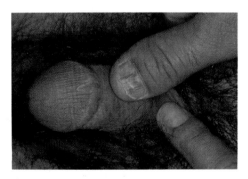

FIG 15—3.
Lichen planus of nail. "Pincer" deformity with lichen planus lesion of penis.

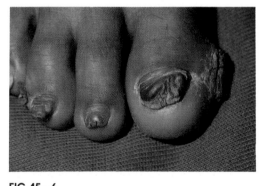

FIG 15—6.
Pachyonychia congenita type II. Distal thickening of nails associated with painful circumscribed keratoses of feet.

TABLE 15—1.

Differential Diagnosis of Thick Nails

Psoriasis
Lichen planus
Onychomycosis
Twenty-nail dystrophy
Dermatitis
Pachyonychia congenita
Ectodermal dysplasia
Palmoplantar keratodermas (Unna-Thost, mal de
    Meleda, Papillon-Lefèvre) focal dermal
    hypoplasia, dyskeratosis congenita
Norwegian scabies

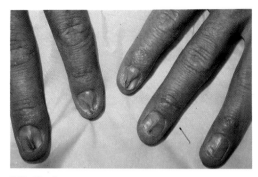

FIG 15—8.
Thin nails with pincer nail deformity in child with
hidrotic ectodermal dysplasia.

THIN OR ATROPHIC NAILS

Clinical Features

Poorly developed or absent nails are characteristic of a wide variety of congenital syndromes. These nail plate abnormalities generally reflect nail matrix disorders. Most often this is the result of ectodermal dysplasia (Figs 15—7 and 15—8), but intrauterine injury to the nail, such as that caused by epidermolysis bullosa, may be responsible. Usually most of, or all, of the nails are affected. The nails are often narrow and the nail plate thin and fragile.

Congenital anonychia, or complete absence of some or all nails, has been described as an isolated dominant or sometimes recessive condition or associated with congenital ectodermal defects. With anonychia, neither the nail plate nor the nail bed is present.

The nail-patella syndrome deserves special comment. It is thought to be an autosomal domi-

nant syndrome with both ectodermal and meso-dermal manifestations. The nail matrix of, usually, the thumb, index fingers, and great toes is hypoplastic (Fig 15—9). Occasionally it is absent. Other nails may be involved. The lunula is often characteristically triangular. In addition, there are multiple bone abnormalities: rudimentary or absent patellas, bony spurs on the posterior iliac crest, subluxation of the elbows, and thickening of the scapulas are seen. Other anomalies described include skin laxity, heterochromia iridis, and proteinuria. Periodic shedding of one or more nails is inherited as an autosomal dominant trait. This is a rare problem, and during the period of regrowth the nails may be dystrophic.

The more important causes of acquired thin or atrophic nails include trauma, infection, lichen planus, erythema multiforme, and bullous drug eruptions. Poor acral circulation, such as in Raynaud's disease, may also contribute.

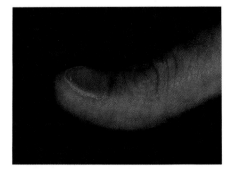

FIG 15—7.
Thin nail in ectodermal dysplasia leading to concave nail deformity.

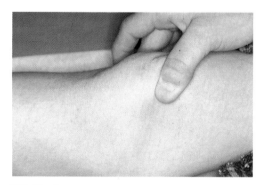

FIG 15—9.
Thin, hypoplastic thumbnail and dislocated patella in nail-patella syndrome.

Differential Diagnosis

One must first determine whether the nail disorder is congenital or acquired. Most often, the associated clinical features are very useful in distinguishing one cause of nail disease or atrophy from another. Table 15–2 lists the conditions to be considered in the differential diagnosis of thin, absent, or atrophic nails.

Treatment

There is no treatment.

Patient Education

It should be emphasized that the cells responsible for nail growth are poorly formed or injured.

Follow-up Visits

Follow-up visits are unnecessary.

PARONYCHIA

Clinical Features

Acute paronychia is most often due to *Staphylococcus aureus* or *Candida albicans;* occasionally gram-negative organisms such as *Pseudomonas* and *Proteus* are implicated. This is a common, painful infection of the nail fold in which the red, inflamed, swollen periungual tissue has a purulent exudate. Herpes simplex infection may also occur in the paronychial area and is distinguished by grouped vesicles on an erythematous base.

Chronic paronychia is a difficult but common problem, primarily in thumb suckers, nail biters, and nail pickers. It appears as dull-red swelling of the cuticle area that is usually not tender. Hobbies and habits that recurrently traumatize the nail fold are important causes. Chronic or recurrent dermatitis often occurs around the nail folds and may be the underlying cause. The nail fold is red, indurated, and raised, and the cuticle margin is lost (Fig 15–10). Often there is proximal separation of the nail plate from the nail bed. *C. albicans* is the most important causative organism.

Differential Diagnosis

Paronychia is so characteristic that it is not easily confused with other conditions.

Pathogenesis

Alterations in the integrity of the cuticle area, such as maceration and trauma, alter the epidermal barrier and allow microbial invasion.

Treatment

Treatment is complicated by the fact that avoiding the underlying cause may be extremely difficult. Systemic antibiotics are required in acute bacterial paronychia. Treatment with nystatin (Mycostatin) is useful in *Candida* infection, and good success may be achieved with the nightly application of nystatin cream followed by airtight occlu-

TABLE 15–2.
Differential Diagnosis of Thin, Absent, or Atrophic Nails

Congenital	Acquired
Ectodermal dysplasia (anhidrotic, hidrotic)*	Trauma
Epidermolysis bullosa	Infection
Incontinentia pigmenti	Lichen planus
Nail-patella syndrome*	Erythema multiforme
Acrodermatitis enteropathica	Focal dermal hypoplasia
Anonychia with/without ectrodactyly*	Ellis–van Creveld syndrome (chondroectodermal dysplasia)
Coffin-Siris syndrome*	Turner's syndrome
Hallermann-Streiff syndrome*	Dyskeratosis congenita
Progeria	Trisomy 13
	Trisomy 18
	Periodic shedding
	Severe Raynaud's phenomenon
	Vascular disease
	Bullous drug eruptions

*May be absent from birth.

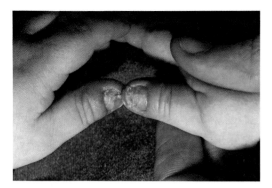

FIG 15–10.
Candida paronychia. Swelling and redness of proximal nail fold in a thumb sucker.

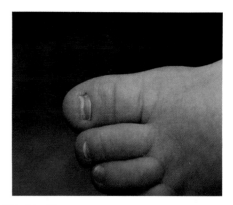

FIG 15–11.
Ingrown toenails with lateral nail fold hypertrophy.

sion. One must avoid the aspiration of occluding material in thumb suckers by covering the thumb with a cotton sock taped around the wrist. Other topical agents, such as gentamicin cream, sulfonamide solutions, and gentian violet, have limited efficacy.

Patient Education

Elimination or reduction of the causes of maceration and trauma should be emphasized.

Follow-up Visits

A visit in 1 month will be useful to determine the response to therapy.

INGROWN TOENAILS

Clinical Features

The large toes have a particular predilection for penetration of their nails into the lateral nail fold, producing a tender and sometimes erythematous swelling (Fig 15–11). Limping and discomfort on walking are frequent complaints. Purulence is sometimes seen resulting from bacterial invasion, usually due to *S. aureus*. This may proceed to cellulitis. In infants it may appear at 1 to 2 months of age with hypertrophy of the lateral nail folds.

Differential Diagnosis

Ingrown toenail is usually so characteristic that it is not confused with other processes.

Pathogenesis

Ingrown toenails are caused by the penetration of ragged edges of the nail plate into the lateral nail fold, giving rise to a foreign body inflam-

matory response with eventual formation of granulation tissue. Tight-fitting shoes and improper nail cutting promote crowding of the nail plate. In infants, asynchronous growth of the nail plate and the lateral nail folds may produce the penetration of the edge of the nail plate within the nail fold.

Treatment

The majority of cases resolve with simple local measures. The foreign body, namely, the ragged lateral spicules of the nail plate, must be removed. This can be done by excising the lateral portion of the nail plate and inserting a small cotton wad to keep the nail plate separated from the inflamed area. Frequent soaking softens the indurated area. Systemic antibiotics should be used in infected lesions. When granulation tissue is present, it can be surgically curetted and then cauterized. Occasionally surgical removal of the lateral one fourth of the nail plate is necessary to reduce its size. Avulsion of the complete nail is unnecessary.

Patient Education

Instructions in cutting the toenails are invaluable. The lateral margins must remain smooth. One should not cut the toenail until it grows beyond the distal end of the lateral nail fold. Trimming the nail straight across rather than in an arc is required. Patients should be instructed to avoid tight-fitting shoes. In infants, an explanation of a slow-growing nail plate penetrating a rapidly growing lateral nail fold may be given.

Follow-up Visits

A visit in 1 month is useful in evaluating therapy and reemphasizing toenail care.

TABLE 15–3.

Causes of Specific Color Changes in Nails

Black	Gray
Peutz-Jeghers syndrome	Silver salts
Vitamin B deficiency	Phenolphthalein
Pinta	Malignant melanoma
Ammoniated mercuric sulfide	Green
Hair dyes	*Pseudomonas*
Film developer	*Aspergillis*
Irradiation	Red
Junctional nevus	Resorcinol (nail lacquer)
Malignant melanoma	Hemorrhage
Fungus	Half-and-half nail of renal
Blue lunulae	disease
Wilson's disease	Red lunulae
Purpura	Collagen vascular diseases
Cyanosis	Systemic lupus erythematosus
Antimalarial agents	Rheumatoid arthritis
Argyria	Carbon monoxide poisoning
Yellow	Cardiac failure
Yellow nail syndrome	Cirrhosis
Onycholysis	Psoriasis
White	Twenty-nail dystrophy
Arsenic (Mees' lines)	Brown
Partial onycholysis	Resorcinol (nail lacquer)
Leukonychia (hereditary, traumatic,	Film developer
idiopathic)	Fungus infection
Hypoalbuminemia	Tobacco staining

COLOR CHANGES IN THE NAIL

It is beyond the scope of this chapter to discuss nail color changes in detail, but Table 15–3 lists the disorders to be considered when specific color changes in the nail are encountered.

BIBLIOGRAPHY

Arias AM, Yung CW, Rendler S, et al: Familial severe twenty-nail dystrophy. *J Am Acad Dermatol* 1982; 7:349.

Barth JH, Dawber RPR: Diseases of the nails in children. *Pediatr Dermatol* 1987; 4:275.

Commens CA: Twenty nail dystrophy in identical twins. *Pediatr Dermatol* 1988; 5:117.

Dawber RPR, Baran R: Nail abnormalities. *Semin Dermatol* 1988; 7:73.

Hammerton MD, Shrank AB: Congenital hypertrophy of the lateral nail folds of the hallux. *Pediatr Dermatol* 1988; 5:243.

Horn RT, Odom RB: Twenty-nail dystrophy of alopecia areata. *Arch Dermatol* 1980; 116:573.

Kleinman FK: Congenital lymphedema and yellow nails. *J Pediatr* 1973; 83:454.

Leyden J, Wood MG: The half and half nail. *Arch Dermatol* 1972; 105:591.

Lucas GL, Opitz JM: Nail-patella syndrome. *J Pediatr* 1967; 68:273.

Magid M, Esterly NB, Prendiville J, et al: The yellow nail syndrome in an 8 year old girl. *Pediatr Dermatol* 1987; 4:90.

Muehrcke RC: The finger-nails in chronic hypoalbuminemia. *Br Med J* 1956; 1:1322.

Philpott CM, Shuttleworth D: Dermatophyte onychomycosis in children. *Clin Exp Dermatol* 1989; 14:203.

Wilkerson MG, Wilkin JK: Red lunulae revisited: A clinical and histopathologic examination. *J Am Acad Dermatol* 1989; 20:453.

16 _____ Disorders of Pigmentation: White Lesions and Brown Lesions

Loss of skin color or increase in skin color may cause concern in parents. Pigmentary changes are common in infants and children. Infants' skin color is always light at birth and becomes darker with age. Hyperpigmentation of the scrotum and of the linea alba is common in dark-skinned infants. Mongolian spots are expected in dark-skinned newborn infants, and café au lait spots are common. Hypopigmented lesions, in contrast, are less common in infants, with piebaldism or ash leaf macules occurring in less than 1% of babies. Hypopigmented macules are the earliest clue to tuberous sclerosis, and café au lait spots are the earliest clue to neurofibromatosis.

Acquired pigmentary changes are also common. The prevalence of vitiligo is estimated to be 5.5 per 1,000 school-age children, while the average number of acquired benign pigmented nevi is 3 per prepubertal child. This chapter is divided into discussions of white lesions and brown lesions.

WHITE LESIONS

Circumscribed Flat Hypopigmentation: Congenital Piebaldism

Localized areas of hypopigmented skin are uncommon in infants and newborns. A hypopigmented area of the skin is found in approximately 8 per 1,000 live births, and a hypopigmented tuft of hair is found in 3 per 1,000 live births (Fig 16–1). *Piebaldism* is the name designated to circumscribed areas of absence of pigment in the newborn. Most commonly this disorder is transmitted in an autosomal dominant pattern. Although completely devoid of melanocytes, the white patches of skin may be difficult to detect at birth because of the light color of most newborn

skin. The use of a Wood's lamp to examine the infant's skin may accentuate differences in color. In several kinships, the piebald trait has been linked to cerebellar ataxia, neurosensory hearing loss, or retardation. A hypopigmented tuft of hair, usually in the frontal region, is a feature of Waardenburg's syndrome. This autosomal dominant syndrome exhibits a white forelock, white patches on the skin, heterochromia of the irises, and deafness in one or both ears. Most authorities view Waardenburg's syndrome as a variant of piebaldism.

White Patches of Tuberous Sclerosis (Ash Leaf Macules)

The white spots of tuberous sclerosis appear as hypopigmented macules, which may be leaf-shaped (ash leaf macules) (Fig 16–2). The macules may be rounded on one end, pointed on the other, and range from 5 to 50 mm at their greatest diameter. In the newborn period, they may be the only sign of tuberous sclerosis, and in families in which this condition occurs, involvement of the newborn infant may be first suspected by the presence of these lesions. A Wood's lamp examination is often necessary to detect the lesions in the newborn, and not all macules are leaf shaped. They may be found anywhere on the skin, but are most predominant on the posterior aspect of the trunk and the extremities.

The other signs and symptoms of tuberous sclerosis do not appear until later in life. The angiofibromas found on the nose and face, which may mimic acne, usually begin to appear between the ages of 5 and 10 years (Fig 16–3). Seizure disorders may appear within the first 10 years of life, but renal tumors and periungual fibromas usually appear after adolescence. A large connective tissue nevus, designated as a shagreen patch, may be

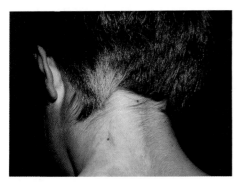

FIG 16–1.
Piebaldism. Segmental white patch on neck with tuft
of white hair present from birth.

present at birth or become more apparent as the
child becomes older. It is skin to ivory colored
and feels thickened (Fig 16–4). The red fibrous
forehead plaque (Fig 16–5) is one of the primary
criteria for tuberous sclerosis (Table 16–1). Tuberous sclerosis is an autosomal dominant condition with variable penetrance. Often a family history is difficult to obtain on a first visit. Neurorad-
iologic examination such as magnetic resonance
imaging (MRI) is indicated if suspect CNS symptoms accompany criteria listed in Table 16–1.

Hypomelanosis of Ito

Newborns with hypomelanosis of Ito have bizarre hypopigmented swirls on their skin that follow Blaschko's lines (Fig 16–6). The hypopigmentation may be zosteriform in distribution or
may be quite extensive, involving the entire half
of the body; in some circumstances it may even
be found bilaterally. No matter what the distribu-

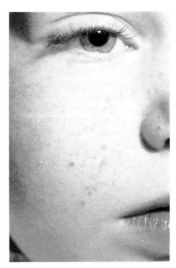

FIG 16–3.
Facial angiofibromas of tuberous sclerosis that mimic
acne.

tion, the hypopigmentation results from a decreased number of melanosomes within the pigment cells and within keratinocytes. The inheritance of hypomelanosis of Ito is not known. Hypomelanosis of Ito is often confused with
incontinentia pigmenti, linear and whorled hypermelanosis, or the linear hypermelanosis associated with the *Proteus* syndrome, all of which follow Blaschko's lines and have sharp midline demarcation of pigmentation. Hypomelanosis is
lighter than normal skin color, rather than darker.
It is thought that a mishap early in embryogenesis
is responsible, with two distinct genetically different melanocyte populations produced. Some children with hypomelanosis of Ito have been shown
to have mosaic chromosome patterns with chro-

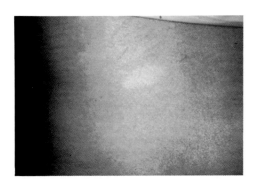

FIG 16–2.
Ash leaf white macule of tuberous sclerosis.

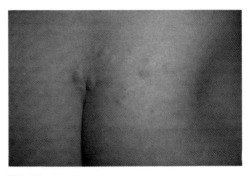

FIG 16–4.
Shagreen patch on sacral skin (tuberous sclerosis).

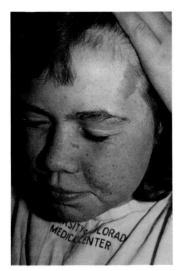

FIG 16–5.
Red forehead plaque of tuberous sclerosis.

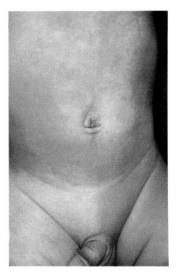

FIG 16–6.
Hypomelanosis of Ito. Whorls of hypopigmentation of trunk with demarcation at midline.

mosome 2 or 9 involved. As with other chromosomal defects, association with CNS or eye abnormalities is frequent.

Chediak-Higashi Syndrome

Infants born with Chediak-Higashi syndrome have white skin (as in albinism, but in a patchy distribution), blond hair, and blue eyes. Melanosomes in the skin and hair are dispersed in an irregular fashion and are large and abnormal. Such melanosomes cannot be transferred to keratinocytes. Patients also have abnormal lysosomes within their circulating white cells and have an inability to kill bacteria, which may result in cutane-

ous and severe respiratory infection. The respiratory infections usually do not appear until later in life.

Circumscribed Flat Hypopigmentation: Acquired Vitiligo

Clinical Features

Vitiligo is a patchy loss of skin pigment. The patches are flat, completely depigmented, and have distinct, often hyperpigmented borders (Fig 16–7). Hair within the patch of depigmentation is often depigmented as well. The distribution of patches has been used to distinguish two types of vitiligo. In type A, the distribution is roughly sym-

TABLE 16–1.
Diagnostic Criteria for Tuberous Sclerosis

Primary Criteria (only one required for diagnosis)	Secondary Criteria (two required for diagnosis)
Fibrous forehead plaque	Hypopigmented macules
Angiofibromas of face	Shagreen patch
Periungual fibromas	Single retinal hamartoma
Brain cortex tubercle	Bilateral renal cysts or
Subependymal	angiomyolipomas
hamartomas	First-degree relative with
Multiple retinal	tuberous sclerosis
hamartomas	Infantile spasms
	Cardiac rhabdomyoma

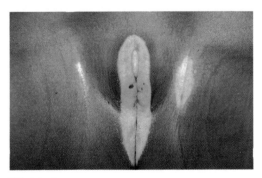

FIG 16–7.
Vitiligo type A. Involvement of perineal and inguinal skin. Note distinct borders.

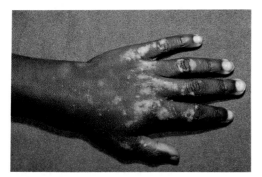

FIG 16–8.
Vitiligo type A of child's hand.

metric, whereas is type B it is in a segmental, dermatomal distribution. The extensor surfaces of the extremities and the face and neck are the areas most commonly involved in type A (Fig 16–8), which is slightly more common than type B in childhood. Type A continues to spread and develop new lesions for years, whereas type B spreads rapidly and then stops spreading after 1 year (Fig 16–9). Uncommonly, type A vitiligo may be associated with diabetes mellitus, asthma, alopecia areata, pernicious anemia, Addison's disease, hypothyroidism, or hypoparathyroidism. Vitiligo of the face, eyelashes, and scalp hair in association with uveitis, dysacousis, and alopecia areata occurs in the rare Vogt-Koyanagi syndrome. Complete spontaneous repigmentation is unusual in vitiligo. Partial repigmentation occurs in about one half of the affected children during the months when they are exposed to the sun. Pigmentation returns first around hair follicles. In

black and other dark-skinned children, the appearance produces great distress.

Differential Diagnosis

The conditions to be considered in the differential diagnosis are listed in Table 16–2. In pityriasis alba and tinea versicolor, in contrast to vitiligo, the abnormally pigmented areas are hypopigmented rather than depigmented and often have scaling, as well as indistinct borders. In postinflammatory hypopigmentation, irregular mottling of both hyperpigmented and hypopigmented areas is often seen. In piebaldism, lesions are present from birth and rarely have hyperpigmented borders. Presenting symptoms of scleroderma and lichen sclerosus et atrophicus are immobilized skin and hypopigmentation.

Pathogenesis

It has long been presumed that vitiligo is an immune disorder because of the lymphocytic infiltrate that precedes the injury to melanocytes. A few melanocytes may be present, but show reduced tyrosinase activity, or melanocytes may be completely lacking. Recently, antibodies directed against melanocytes have been detected in patients with type A vitiligo, and antibody-dependent cellular cytotoxicity may be one method of destruction of melanocytes.

Treatment

There is no entirely satisfactory treatment. Skin stains, such as dyes and walnut oil, may be used, but children generally will not comply. Psoralen, a furocoumarin derived from plants, is a potent stimulator of melanocytes. Its use has re-

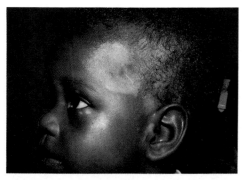

FIG 16–9.
Vitiligo type B with segmental involvement of child's forehead. Seen early during rapid color loss before complete color loss.

TABLE 16–2.
Differential Diagnosis of Patchy Pigment Loss in Children

Vitiligo
Pityriasis alba
Tinea versicolor
Postinflammatory hypopigmentation
Piebaldism
Scleroderma
Lichen sclerosus et atrophicus
Waardenburg's syndrome
Chediak-Higashi syndrome
Hypomelanosis of Ito
White spots of tuberous sclerosis
Halo nevus

sulted in successful repigmentation in more than half the patients treated. It is best used by an experienced dermatologist, since it is easy to produce severe sunburns with this photosensitizing drug. Most investigators use 10 mg of methoxsalen 2 hours before ultraviolet (UVL) exposure and treat for 3 to 6 months. Older, motivated children achieve the best results. Some repigmentation has been noted with topical steroids.

Patient Education

The natural history of vitiligo should be discussed and the need to follow a strict regimen emphasized in those motivated to undergo therapy.

Follow-up Visits

During therapy, monthly visits are advisable.

Pityriasis Alba

Clinical Features

Pityriasis alba is characterized by multiple oval, scaly, flat, hypopigmented patches on the face, extensor surfaces of arms, and upper part of trunk (Fig 16–10). The lesions range from 5 to 20 mm in diameter, and 10 to 20 patches are often seen. The borders are indistinct. It occurs predominantly between the ages of 3 and 16, and up to 30% of all children may be affected. The lesions do not itch, and medical help is sought because of the child's appearance. It is particularly distressing in dark-skinned children. It is a chronic dermatitis and often lasts several years.

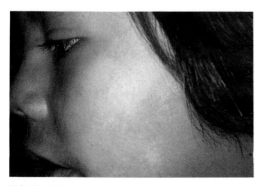

FIG 16–10.
Pityriasis alba. White, slightly scaly patches with indistinct borders on child's cheek.

Differential Diagnosis

Pityriasis alba most closely mimics tinea versicolor, which can be excluded by findings in a negative potassium hydroxide (KOH) examination (see Figs 16–5 and 16–6). (See Table 16–2 for the list of conditions to be considered in the differential diagnosis.)

Pathogenesis

On pathologic examination the lesion resembles that seen in chronic dermatitis. The stratum corneum is thickened, and edema is present within the epidermis. The cause of the hypopigmentation is not known, but the thickened stratum corneum reduces UVL penetration and thereby the tanning effect; the edema prevents or retards pigment transfer from melanocytes to keratinocytes. Some regard this as a form of atopic dermatitis, but in many children it occurs without the features of atopic dermatitis.

Treatment

There is no satisfactory treatment. Topical glucocorticosteroids have some influence on the disorder. Dyes or stains are occasionally useful.

Patient Education

The natural history of this disorder should be emphasized.

Follow-up Visits

Follow-up visits should be scheduled at monthly intervals if a treatment program is considered.

Postinflammatory Hypopigmentation

Clinical Features

After any inflammatory skin disease, particularly in dark-skinned children, irregular hypopigmented areas may appear. They are usually in a mottled pattern and associated with hyperpigmented areas (Fig 16–11). They resolve several months after the inflammatory disorder.

Differential Diagnosis

Postinflammatory changes are associated with hyperpigmentation and epidermal thickening, in contrast to the other forms of hypopigmentation (see Table 16–2).

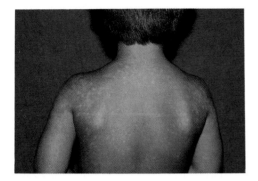

FIG 16–11.
Postinflammatory hypopigmentation with numerous hypopigmented patches on child's back.

Pathogenesis

Inflammatory injury to melanocytes as well as to epidermal cells results in decreased pigment production and transfer.

Treatment

Treatment is not necessary.

Patient Education

The patient should be informed of the nature of the pigment loss and told that recovery is expected.

Follow-up Visits

Follow-up visits are unnecessary.

Diffuse Hypopigmentation: Albinism

At least seven genetic varieties of albinism have been described in humans, most of them inherited in an autosomal recessive pattern. A newborn with albinism has fine white hair, pink skin, severe nystagmus, photophobia, and nevi, which may be pigmented. The disease is due to complete lack of functional tyrosinase in its most common form. Tyrosinase is the enzyme necessary for the final assembly of the pigment melanin. In one subtype of albinism, tyrosinase enzyme is present. These children are born with fair complexions and gray eyes, and have poor visual acuity and nystagmus.

BROWN LESIONS

In considering a hyperpigmented state, one should first determine whether the hyperpigmentation is circumscribed or diffuse.

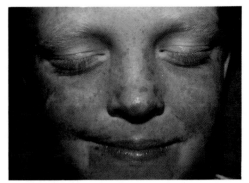

FIG 16–12.
Freckles. Note sunburn between freckled areas.

Circumscribed Flat Hyperpigmentation

Clinical Features

Freckles.—Freckles are small, 1- to 5-mm, light-brown pigmented macules that occur in UVL-exposed skin (Fig 16–12). They are autosomal dominant and first appear at ages 3 to 5 years, predominantly on the face and extensor surfaces of the extremities. They are most frequent in light-haired, blue-eyed children.

Lentigines.—Lentigines are brown or brown-black 1- to 2-mm macules found sparsely scattered over the body, including the mucous membranes (Fig 16–13). They do not change with sun exposure. They usually first appear during school age and average 30 in number per child. Lentigines on the lips are seen in the Peutz-Jeghers syndrome associated with multiple bowel polyps. Multiple lentigines are associated with cardiac abnormalities in the so-called leopard syndrome (*l*entigines, *e*lectrocardiograph abnormalities, *o*cular hypertelorism, *p*ulmonary stenosis, *a*bnormalities of the genitalia, growth *r*etardation, *d*eafness). Central facial lentigines have been de-

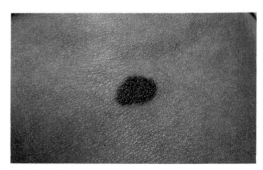

FIG 16–13.
Lentigo. Dark brown lesion.

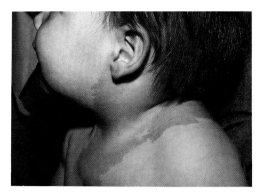

FIG 16–14.
Café au lait spot. Large lesion on child's neck.

scribed in association with cardiac defects and malignancies in NAME syndrome (*n*evi, *a*trial myxomas, *m*yxoid neurofibroma, *e*phelides).

Café au Lait Spots.—Café au lait spots are tan, flat, oval macules with distinct borders (Fig 16–14). They frequently have a diameter greater than 0.5 cm. One café au lait spot more than 0.5 cm in diameter is found in 10% of white children and in 22% of black children. Multiple café au lait spots may help with the diagnosis of type 1 neu-

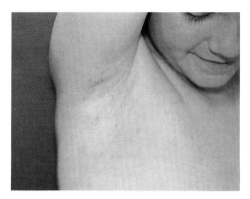

FIG 16–15.
Numerous café au lait spots in child's axilla in neurofibromatosis type 1.

rofibromatosis (Table 16–3) when there are six or more or when found in the axilla or inguinal areas (Fig. 16–15).

Café au lait spots are rarely present at birth (in 19 of 1,000 live births), but appear between the ages of 2 and 16 and tend to persist until the ages of 60 to 70. They are also seen in Albright's syndrome, tuberous sclerosis, and the *Proteus* syndrome. The *Proteus* syndrome can be mistaken for neurofibromatosis type 1 because of the skeletal overgrowth and large hamartomas that are confused with plexiform neurofibromas. In type 1 neurofibromatosis, more café au lait spots appear with age, and may be accompanied by soft cutaneous neurofibromas (Fig 16–16). Café au lait spots are not an important feature of type 2 neurofibromatosis (see Table 16–3).

TABLE 16–3.

Diagnostic Criteria for Neurofibromatosis Types 1 and 2

Neurofibromatosis type 1 (Recklinghausen's disease) (two or more must be found)
Six or more café au lait spots >5 mm in diameter in prepubertal children; >1.5 mm in postpubertal children
Two or more neurofibromas of any type
One plexiform neurofibroma
Axillary freckling
Inguinal freckling
Two or more Lisch nodules (iris hamartomas)
Distinctive osseous lesion such as sphenoid dysplasia or thinning of a long bone with or without pseudarthrosis
First-degree relative with type 1 neurofibromatosis
Neurofibromatosis type 2
Bilateral eighth nerve masses found on CT scan or MRI
First-degree relative with type 2 plus either unilateral eighth nerve mass or two of the following: neurofibroma, meningioma, glioma, schwannoma, juvenile posterior subcapsular lenticular opacity

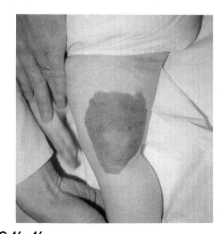

FIG 16–16.
Soft cutaneous neurofibroma beneath a large café au lait spot in neurofibromatosis type 1.

Mongolian Spots.—The mongolian spot is a blue-black macule found in the lumbosacral area in up to 90% of Oriental, black, and American Indian babies. Mongolian spots occur in 255 per 1,000 live births. They are occasionally noted on the shoulders and back, and may extend to the buttocks and extremities (Fig 16–17). Pathology of mongolian spots consists of spindle-shaped cells that contain pigment and that are located between collagen fibers deep within the dermis. Mongolian spots tend to fade with time, being darkest at 1 year of age but fading by the age of 3 years. The difference in the pigmentation from normal skin pigment becomes less obvious as a newborn infant's skin darkens in color. Some traces of mongolian spots may persist into adult life.

Junctional Melanocytic Nevi.—Junctional melanocytic nevi are flat, well-demarcated, brown to brown-black lesions (Fig 16–18). They may be present at birth, but usually appear later in childhood. They characteristically have irregular borders and may have a light brown rim and a dark brown center. They usually measure 2 to 5 mm, but may occasionally be larger. Most nevi found in infants and children are junctional nevi and average three nevi per prepubertal child. If many nevi appear before the age of 5 years, the child is likely to have a large number of moles after puberty. After puberty, the number of moles increases, with an average of 23 per adolescent. They may appear anywhere on the skin. A large, pigmented, hairy nevus, called Becker's nevus, occurs on the shoulder and is often first noticed in adolescence. Becker's nevus is considered a hamartoma of hair follicles and associated arrec-

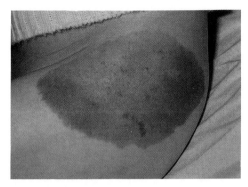

FIG 16–18.
Nevus spilus. Large, flat, tan lesion containing numerous small, dark brown areas.

tores pilorum muscles. Junctional nevi within a café au lait spot form the nevus spilus (see Fig 16–18).

Linear and Whorled Nevoid Hypermelanosis.—Hypermelanotic macules arranged in streaks corresponding to Blascko's lines, with sharp demarcation at the midline, characterize linear and whorled nevoid hypermelanosis (Fig 16–19). It may be an isolated cutaneous finding or associated with congenital malformations such as clubfoot.

Nevus of Ota, Nevus of Ito.—Flat, blue-black, speckled pigmentary discoloration may be noted in the skin surrounding the eye (nevus of

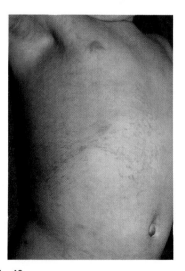

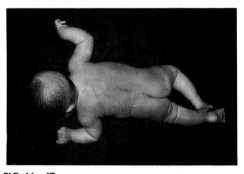

FIG 16–17.
Mongolian spots. Extensive lesions on back and buttocks.

FIG 16–19.
Linear and whorled hypermelanosis. Brown whorls on trunk of child.

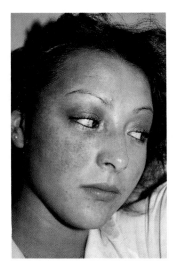

FIG 16–20.
Nevus of Ota. Speckled blue macules in periorbital skin and sclera.

Ota) (Fig 16–20) or around the chest and shoulder (nevus of Ito). Each is first noticed between 2 and 12 years of age, and the discloration becomes progressive. The sclera may be involved in nevus of Ota.

Postinflammatory Hyperpigmentation.— In children with dark skin, any inflammatory skin disorder may heal with hyperpigmentation. Often the pigmentation persists for months.

Differential Diagnosis

Skin biopsy may differentiate the acquired flat pigmented lesions from one another. The congenital lesions are often blue-black with deep pigmentation. The conditions to be included in the differential diagnosis are given in Table 16–4.

TABLE 16–4.
Differential Diagnosis of Circumscribed Flat Pigmented Lesions

Acquired
Freckles
Lentigo
Café au lait spots
Junctional melanocytic nevi
Postinflammatory hyperpigmentation
Congenital
Mongolian spot
Nevus of Ota
Linear and whorled nevoid hypermelanosis

Pathogenesis

Freckles.—Freckles are areas with increased pigment within epidermal cells but no increase in the number of melanocytes. They represent cloning of sun-responsive melanocytes that produce more pigment than do neighboring melanocytes.

Lentigines and Café au Lait Spots.—In lentigines, increased numbers of melanocytes are dispersed along the basal layer of the epidermis, and the epidermal rete ridges are elongated. In café au lait spots, melanocyte activity is increased, as is the melanin in melanocytes and in epidermal cells. The number of melanocytes is not increased.

Mongolian Spots.—Mongolian spots contain spindle-shaped pigment cells in the reticular dermis. Their exact pathogenesis is uncertain.

Junctional Melanocytic Nevi.—Clumps of increased numbers of melanocytes are located at the dermoepidermal junction in junctional nevi. In Becker's nevus, the number of melanocytes is slightly increased, and melanin is seen throughout the epidermis.

Linear and Whorled Nevoid Hypermelanosis.—Epidermal melanocytes are increased in number and keratinocytes have increased melanin in the affected area. It is thought that two genetically distinct populations of melanocytes are produced, perhaps through chromosomal mosaicism, but chromosomal analysis has not been performed to the extent done in hypomelanosis of Ito.

Nevus of Ota, Nevus of Ito.—Similar to mongolian spots, spindle-shaped melanocytes are found within the dermis.

Postinflammatory Hyperpigmentation.— The excess pigment is related to loss of pigment from damaged epidermal keratinocytes and melanocytes into the dermis, where the large polymer melanin sits free in the dermis or is engulfed by macrophages to form melanophages. Breakdown of the dermal pigment is slow.

Treatment

No treatment is necessary.

Patient Education

The common and benign nature of these pigmented areas should be emphasized.

Follow-up Visits

Follow-up visits are unnecessary.

Circumscribed Raised Hyperpigmentation

Clinical Features

Dermal Melanocytic and Compound Nevi.—Dermal melanocytic nevi and compound melanocytic nevi appear as small, raised, dome-shaped, brown to brown-black papules 10 to 15 mm in diameter (Fig 16–21). They frequently have an irregular border. Some have an irregular surface. It is common for the center to be darker than the periphery (Fig 16–22). They may appear skin colored, with little melanin production (Fig 16–23). They begin in childhood and frequently darken at puberty, with pregnancy, or with the use of oral contraceptives. Dermal nevi are usually few in number before the preadolescent growth period, averaging one or two. More appear during adolescence. Children with dozens of pigmented nevi, both junctional and dermal, are at increased risk of development of dysplastic nevi or melanoma in adult life. They typically regress after the age of 60, but may regress during childhood. A halo may appear around an intradermal nevus that is regressing in childhood (Fig 16–24), producing the "halo nevus." Blue nevi, which are uncommon, are blue to blue-black 5-mm solitary papules that begin in childhood (Fig 16–25).

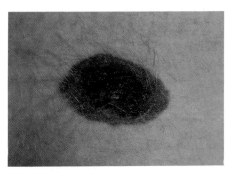

FIG 16–22.
Intradermal nevus darker in center.

Spitz Nevus.—The Spitz, or spindle and epithelioid cell, nevus begins as a solitary red or red-brown nodule, usually on the extremities or face (Fig 16–26). It appears in school-age children and tends to persist.

Congenital, Raised Nevocellular Nevi.—Skin-colored to tan, or brown, solitary papules with smooth surfaces represent congenital intradermal nevi. Most such nevi present at birth are small, measuring less than 1.5 cm at their greatest diameter (Fig 16–27). There is currently controversy over the cancer potential of large melanocytic nevi, which are defined as being larger than 10 cm at their greatest diameter. Large melanocytic nevi are very uncommon, occurring 1 in 20,000 live births. Large melanocytic nevi are often not uniform in color and contain flat tan areas, brown areas, blue-black plaques, and pigmented, long, thick hair (Fig 16–28). Numerous smaller nevi located at skin sites distant from the large nevi are found. These "satellite lesions" are more often uniform in color. The estimate of cancer potential in a large congenital nevus is ap-

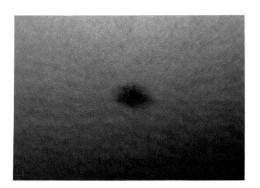

FIG 16–21.
Intradermal nevus. Irregular borders and irregular surface on raised lesion.

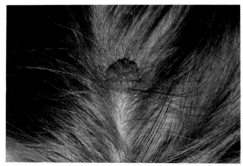

FIG 16–23.
Nonpigmented intradermal nevus of scalp.

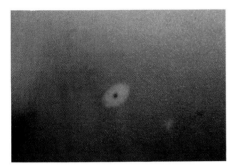

FIG 16–24.
Halo nevus. Loss of pigment around regressing central intradermal nevus.

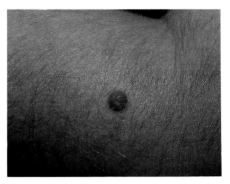

FIG 16–26.
Spitz nevus. Red-brown papule on teenager's arm.

proximately 1%, an incidence greater than in infants without these lesions. There is a slightly increased frequency of large congenital pigmented lesions in blacks and in those infants born to mothers with acute illnesses. There is no correlation of large pigmented nevi with sex, twins, parental consanguinity, parental age, birth order, radiation exposure, or drug intake. If malignant melanoma occurs, it is likely to develop within the large lesion, not any satellite lesion. About 10% of reported melanomas in children arise from large congenital nevi, 20% from acquired nevi, but the remainder from skin that did not have a previous pigmented lesion.

Malignant Melanoma.—Malignant melanomas are rare in childhood and appear as pigmented nodules of variegated colors. Within a single lesion (Fig 16–29) red, white, and blue may be seen, as well as brown and tan. The most important clinical feature is rapid, progressive growth of a pigmented lesion. Notching of the

border of a pigmented nodule and a nonuniform irregular surface should also arouse suspicion of melanoma; ulceration and bleeding are far-advanced signs. Melanomas arising in congenital pigmented birthmarks are uniformly fatal. In familial malignant melanoma, multiple primary melanomas may be found, usually first appearing in late adolescence or early adult life. There is a correlation with large numbers (greater than 50) of nevi in childhood and melanoma later in life.

Differential Diagnosis

The conditions to be considered in the differential diagnosis are listed in Table 16–5. Skin biopsy will differentiate the raised pigmented lesions from one another.

Pathogenesis
Dermal Melanocytic and Compound Nevi.—Dermal melanocytic nevi represent accumulations of groups of immature melanocytes within the middermis to the papillary dermis. When associated with clumps of melanocytes at

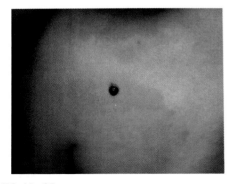

FIG 16–25.
Blue nevus. Blue-black papule on child's shoulder.

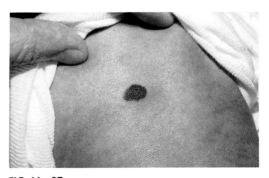

FIG 16–27.
Small congenital nevus.

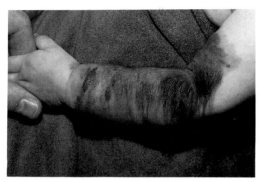

FIG 16–28.
Large congenital nevus with long, pigmented hair and a mixture of tan, brown, and blue-black within lesion.

the dermoepidermal junction, such a nevus is called a compound nevus. A blue nevus represents clumps of mature melanocytes located in the reticular dermis; often these melanocytes are present throughout the dermis.

Spitz Nevus.—Spindle and epithelioid cell nevi (Spitz nevi) are composed of collections of melanocytes with irregular cytoplasmic and nuclear shapes. They are located throughout the dermis. These nevi are associated with a proliferation of blood vessels. The bizarre nuclear shapes often result in confusion with melanoma. An experienced dermatopathologist should review all pigmented lesions in which the diagnosis of melanoma is considered.

Congenital Nevocellular Nevus.—Nests of pigment cells are found within the epidermis and dermis. Sometimes the pigment cells are large and of unusual shape. In giant congenital

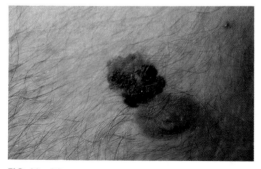

FIG 16–29.
Malignant melanoma on chest of male adolescent.

TABLE 16–5.

Differential Diagnosis of Circumscribed, Raised Pigmented Lesions

Dermal melanocytic nevus
Compound melanocytic nevus
Blue nevus
Spindle and epithelioid cell nevus
Malignant melanoma
Dermatofibroma
Hemangioma
Pyogenic granuloma
Mastocytoma
Juvenile xanthogranuloma

nevocellular nevi, pigment cells may populate the entire dermis and extend around hair and eccrine sweat structures. Most authorities consider congenital nevocellular nevi to be developmental.

Malignant Melanoma.—In malignant melanomas, the tumor originates at the dermoepidermal junction and has a radial growth phase before it demonstrates a vertical growth phase. Melanomas arising in congenital pigmented birthmarks may begin in the reticular dermis with a vertical growth phase. The tumor cells within a melanoma show great variation in size and shape and invade epidermal structures. The depth of invasion is an important prognostic factor and is the basis for histologic classification of melanomas. There are compelling data to support a role of sunlight in melanomas arising from acquired nevi or nonpigmented skin.

Treatment

In any raised pigmented lesion in which melanoma is suspected, surgical excision is the treatment of choice. Although malignant melanoma is rare in childhood, a high index of suspicion of malignant melanoma should be maintained for any rapidly growing pigmented skin lesion. Any excised skin lesion, particularly pigmented skin lesions, should be sent to the pathologist. It is unnecessary to remove the common dermal melanocytic nevus that is uniform in color, however. Many authorities recommend prophylactic removal of large congenital nevocellular pigmented nevi within the first year of life. This recommendation is controversial, based on the very small likelihood of occurrence of malignant melanoma. Currently it is advisable to take into consideration the potential for cosmetic improvement and surgical risk before recommending removal of such lesions. There is no compelling reason to remove these in the child's first year. For best cosmetic results, the use of tissue expanders is preferred for large lesions. Small lesions can be removed during adolescence. There is no urgency to remove small congenital nevi before puberty. There is a small risk of melanoma arising in a small congenital nevus in late adolescence or in young adults.

Patient Education

After confirmation by the pathologist, the nature of the lesion can be explained to the patient. Since there is no uniform agreement among authorities as to the best management for large congenital nevi, this should be explained to the parents, with the positive and negative reasons detailed.

Follow-up Visits

A visit 1 week after surgical removal is necessary to inform the patient of the diagnosis and suggested further treatment, if any.

Acanthosis Nigricans

Clinical Features

Acanthosis nigricans is characterized by hyperpigmentation and a velvety thickening of irregular folds of skin of the posterior aspect of the neck and the axilla (Figs 16–30 and 16–31). It is common in dark-skinned children, found in as many as 7% of pubertal children. Often parents complain that their child's skin is dirty and cannot be cleaned. Small papillomatous growths (skin tags) may be found within the irregular folds. Acanthosis nigricans can be found in other skin

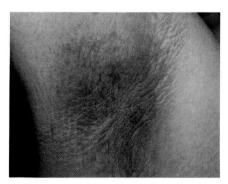

FIG 16–30.
Acanthosis nigricans of child's axilla. Velvety, brown rows of hyperpigmentation.

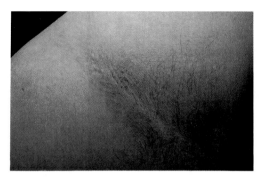

FIG 16–31.
Acanthosis nigricans of child's neck.

areas as well, such as elbows, inguinal creases, areolae, and knuckles. It is associated with obesity, and correlates well with hyperinsulinemia and insulin resistance. With obesity, the age of onset correlates with the onset of obesity. Less commonly it is associated with various lipodystrophies, hirsutism, hypogonadism syndromes such as Prader-Willi, Cushing's syndrome, estrogen therapy, acromegaly, Addison's disease, and hypothyroidism.

Differential Diagnosis

Acanthosis nigricans is so distinctive that it is seldom misdiagnosed. A lichenified chronic dermatitis may mimic.

Pathogenesis

The epidermis is papillomatous, with no abnormality of pigmentation. The association with insulin resistance is so striking that a role for insulin or insulin-like receptors in the papillomatous overgrowth is suspected.

Treatment

Weight loss has resulted in reversal of the acanthosis nigricans, as has stopping hormone therapy or treating the hypothyroidism.

Patient Education

Parents should be told that this is not dirt and that it is unrelated to hygiene. If the child is obese, its relationship to obesity should be emphasized, and the institution of a weight control program should be considered.

Follow-up Visits

Follow-up visits should be determined by therapy.

TABLE 16–6.

Differential Diagnosis of Diffuse Hyperpigmentation

Addison's disease
Acromegaly
Cushing's syndrome of pituitary origin
Thyrotoxicosis
ACTH administration
Subacute bacterial endocarditis
Lymphomas and leukemia
Scleroderma, dermatomyositis
Renal failure
Hemochromatosis
Familial progressive hyperpigmentation
Chronic arsenism
Argyria

Diffuse Hyperpigmentation

Diffuse hyperpigmentation is rare in infancy and childhood, but may occur as a result of endocrine disturbances. Adrenal insufficiency, with overproduction of adrenocorticotropic hormone (ACTH) and its melanocyte-stimulating fragments, or hyperfunction of the pituitary gland may result in diffuse hyperpigmentation. Pigmentation of the scrotum, linea alba, and palmar creases may occur. Table 16–6 lists the conditions to be included in the differential diagnosis of diffuse hyperpigmentation.

BIBLIOGRAPHY

Alper JC, Holmes LB: The incidence and significance of birthmarks in a cohort of 4,641 newborns. *Pediatr Dermatol* 1983; 1:58.

Bauer BS, Vicari F: An approach to excision of congenital giant pigmented nevi in infancy and early childhood. *J Pediatr Surg* 1988; 23:509.

Bolognia JL, Pawelek JM: Biology of hypopigmentation. *J Am Acad Dermatol* 1988; 19:217.

Braffman BH, Bilaniuk LT, Zimmerman RA: The central nervous system manifestations of the phakomatoses on MR. *Radiol Clin North Am* 1988; 26:773.

Castilla EE, Da Graca Dutra M, Orioli-Parreiras IM: Epidemiology of congenital pigmented naevi: II. Risk factors. *Br J Dermatol* 1981; 104:307.

Cramer SF: The melanocytic differentiation pathway in congenital melanocytic nevi: Theoretical considerations. *Pediatr Pathol* 1988; 8:253.

Eldridge R, Denckla MB, Bien E, et al: Neurofibromatosis type I (Recklinghausen's disease). *Am J Dis Child* 1989; 143:833.

Gari LM, Rivers JK, Kopf, AW: Melanomas arising in large congenital nevocytic nevi: A prospective study. *Pediatr Dermatol* 1988; 5:151.

Glover MT, Brett EM, Atherton DJ: Hypomelanosis of Ito: Spectrum of disease. *J Pediatr* 1989; 115:75.

Guzzo C, Johnson B, Honig PJ: Cockarde nevus: A case report and review of the literature. *Pediatr Dermatol* 1988; 5:250.

Hogan DJ, Murphy F, Bremner RM: Spontaneous resolution of a giant melanocytic nevus. *Pediatr Dermatol* 1988; 5:170.

Hurwitz S: Pigmented nevi. *Semin Dermatol* 1988; 7:17.

Huson SM: Recent developments in the diagnosis and management of neurofibromatosis. *Arch Dis Child* 1989; 64:745.

Huson SM, Compston DAS, Clark P, et al: A genetic study of von Recklinghausen neurofibromatosis in south east Wales. I: Prevalence, fitness, mutation rate, and effect of parental transmission on severity. *J Med Genet* 1989; 26:704.

Huson SM, Compston DAS, Harper PS: A genetic study of von Recklinghausen neurofibromatosis in south east Wales. II: Guidelines for genetic counseling. *J Med Genet* 1989; 26:712.

Jacobs AH, Walton RG: The incidence of birthmarks in the neonate. *Pediatrics* 1976; 58:218.

Kalter DC, Griffiths WAD, Atherton DJ: Linear and whorled nevoid hypermelanosis. *J Am Acad Dermatol* 1988; 19:1037.

Kikuchi I: The biological significance of the mongolian spot. *Int J Dermatol* 1989; 28:513.

Koga M, Tango T: Clinical features and course of type A and type B vitiligo. *Br J Dermatol* 1988; 118:223.

Mackie RM, English J, Aitchison TC, et al: The number and distribution of benign pigmented moles (melanocytic naevi) in a healthy British population. *Br J Dermatol* 1985; 113:167.

National Institutes of Health Consensus Development Conference. Neurofibromatosis Conference Statement. *Arch Neurol* 1988; 45:575.

Norris DA, Kissinger MR, Naughton GM, et al: Evidence for immunologic mechanisms in human vitiligo: Patient's sera induce damage to human melanocytes in vitro by complement-mediated damage and antibody-dependent cellular cytotoxicity. *J Invest Dermatol* 1988; 90:783.

Piepkorn M, Meyer LJ, Goldgar D, et al: The dysplastic melanocytic nevus: A prevalent lesion that correlates poorly with clinical phenotype. *J Am Acad Dermatol* 1989; 20:407.

Rampen FHJ, de Wit PEJ: Racial differences in mole proneness. *Arch Derm Venereol (Stockh)* 1989; 69:234.

Renfro L, Grant-Kels J, Brown SA: Multiple agminate Spitz nevi. *Pediatr Dermatol* 1989; 6:114.

Rhodes AR: Pigmented birthmarks and precursor melanocytic lesions of cutaneous melanoma identifiable in childhood. *Pediatr Clin North Am* 1983; 30:435.

Sampson JR, Scahill SJ, Stephenson JBP, et al: Genetic aspects of tuberous sclerosis in the west of Scotland. *J Med Genet* 1989; 26:28.

Stuart CA, Pate CJ, Peters EJ: Prevalence of acanthosis nigricans in an unselected population. *Am J Med* 1989; 87:269.

Trozak DJ, Rowland WD, Hu F: Metastatic malignant melanoma in prepubertal children. *Pediatrics* 1975; 55:191.

Viljoen DL, Saxe N, Temple-Camp C: Cutaneous manifestations of the *Proteus* syndrome. *Pediatr Dermatol* 1988; 5:14.

Weinstock MA, Colditz GA, Willett WC, et al: Nonfamilial cutaneous melanoma incidence in women associated with sun exposure before twenty years of age. *Pediatrics* 1989; 84:199.

17 ————————

Immobile and Hypermobile Skin

Certain skin changes are distinguished by palpation rather than by visual assessment of morphology. Skin mobility and elasticity are two qualities that are distinguished by this method.

Skin that is immobile is fixed to the underlying fascia, sometimes to muscle or bone, or to both. A growth or nodule that is fixed to the underlying fascia might indicate a malignant tumor in childhood. Far more common, however, are fibrous thickenings that attach dermis to the fascia, as in the localized forms of scleroderma. Testing for this feature is performed by grasping the skin with the thumb and forefinger and determining its movement. Hypermobile skin is often associated with hypermobile joints and brings to mind the various forms of the Ehlers-Danlos syndrome.

SKIN THICKENINGS

Skin may become thickened and immobile in certain areas. Nodules are not formed, but the thickened, slightly raised, or slightly depressed area can be appreciated on palpation.

LOCALIZED SCLERODERMA (MORPHEA)

Clinical Features

Circumscribed areas of scleroderma may occur as solitary or multiple oval lesions, or as a linear lesion. Solitary linear lesions on the extremities (Fig 17–1), forehead, or chest are present in 60% of the children. About 25% of patients have an associated vertebral abnormality, such as scoliosis, kyphosis, or spina bifida occulta. Atrophy of an extremity, digital contracture, or facial hemiatrophy may occur. Linear lesions of the forehead

often extend into the frontal area of the scalp, producing a scarring hair loss (Fig 17–2). The immobile area will be exaggerated by having the child wrinkle the forehead. The surface of the immobile, bound-down skin of morphea is often shiny and hypopigmented, and it may be surrounded by a violaceous hue (lilac border) (Fig 17–3). About one third of children with morphea have arthralgias. In guttate morphea, depressed, dusky appearing, slightly thickened lesions that are not completely bound down may be present (Fig 17–4). Often this is confused with atrophoderma, but the lesions will evolve to more typical bound-down circumscribed morphea. Some children have lesions of guttate morphea and linear morphea simultaneously or have guttate morphea lesions accompanied by fine wrinkling and thinning of the skin of the hands, the so-called acrodermatitis chronica atrophicans. Concurrent lesions of morphea and lichen sclerosus et atrophicus have also been noted in childhood. Dysesthesias of lesions or spinal radiculopathies have also been recognized in children with morphea.

If Raynaud's phenomenon is present, the erythrocyte sedimentation rate is elevated, or the antinuclear antibody (ANA) test results are positive, the probability of progression to systemic sclerosis is high.

Differential Diagnosis

Lichen sclerosus et atrophicus shows many features that overlap those of morphea, but its characteristic epidermal thinning and lichenoid papules will help differentiate it from morphea.

Pathogenesis

The mechanism of the disease is unknown, but recent evidence implicating a *Borrelia* infection by positive serology, presence of a spirochete

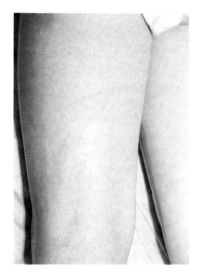

FIG 17–1.
Linear morphea (scleroderma). White, bound-down plaque extending down back of thigh of female adolescent.

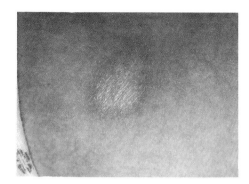

FIG 17–3.
Lilac borders with white center of "active" lesion of guttate morphea.

by immunoperoxidase staining of affected skin biopsy tissue, and recovery of a spirochete by culture of morphea lesions is intriguing. The associated neurologic symptoms and coexistence with known *Borrelia* infections such as acrodermatitis chronica atrophicans strengthen the possible role of spirochetal infection producing the condition. An inflammatory stage precedes the sclerotic stage and is characterized by a predominantly lymphocytic infiltrate around dermal blood vessels and collagen bundles. In the sclerotic stage, thickened dermal collagen replaces the subcutaneous fat. Injury to the underlying muscle fibers, with separation and inflammation of muscle, occurs in linear forms.

Treatment

There is no specific treatment. Symptomatic relief may be achieved with the use of topical lubricants three times daily or topical glucocorticosteroids twice daily. Whether penicillin or other antispirochetal therapy is indicated is yet to be determined.

Patient Education

The duration of lesion activity is 3 to 5 years, and residual pigmentation may last several years longer. Atrophy of the limbs or facial hemiatrophy will persist.

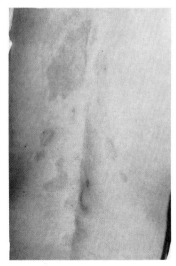

FIG 17–4.
Slightly depressed, tan, slightly bound-down lesions of early morphea.

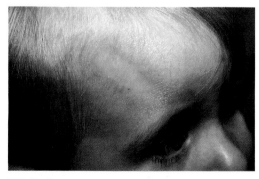

FIG 17–2.
Linear scleroderma of forehead in child.

Follow-up Visits

Examination at 3-month intervals is useful to determine whether systemic symptoms or signs have appeared. A repeat antinuclear antibody test for laboratory evidence of systemic collagen vascular disease is useful.

LICHEN SCLEROSUS ET ATROPHICUS

Clinical Features

White papules and immobile plaques occur primarily in the anogenital area in grade school or adolescent girls (Fig 17–5). Purpura, vesicles, and telangiectasia may be seen within the plaques in the genital area. As the lesions age, the skin surface becomes thinned and finely wrinkled (Fig 17–6). Ulcerations and excoriations may be superimposed on these primary lesions. The anogenital lesions in girls tend to surround both the vulva and the anus in a figure eight pattern. Itching and burning of the skin are frequent complaints.

Extragenital lesions appear as asymptomatic white papules on the upper part of the back or chest (see Fig 17–6) and occasionally on the neck, face, or extremities. About one half of the patients with anogenital lesions will also have distal lesions. Koebner's phenomenon occurs in lichen sclerosus et atrophicus, and lesions may develop in surgical scars or other sites of skin trauma. Coexistence of lichen sclerosus et atrophicus with morphea is observed in children.

Differential Diagnosis

The skin immobility will suggest localized scleroderma, but the atrophic skin, white color, and papular lesions will help distinguish lichen

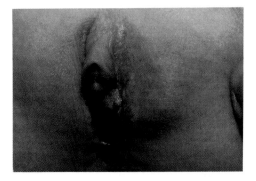

FIG 17–5.
Lichen sclerosus et atrophicus of child's vulva.

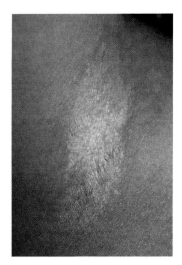

FIG 17–6.
Extragenital lichen sclerosus et atrophicus of neck. Telangiectasia and fine wrinkling within white area.

sclerosus et atrophicus from scleroderma. Anogenital lesions may be confused with candidiasis, intertrigo, or irritant dermatitis. Atrophic areas of lichen planus may mimic lichen sclerosus et atrophicus, but the purple papular border of lichen planus is a useful differentiating feature.

Pathogenesis

The area that is sclerotic or thick is the dermis, and the thinned portion is the epidermis. A bandlike accumulation of lymphocytes is present in the middermis, and features of epidermal injury are also seen. Atrophy of the epidermis and hydropic degeneration of the basal epidermal cells are present. Hyperkeratosis occurs, so that the stratum corneum layer is much thicker than the remainder of the epidermis. Edema and homogenization of collagen in the papillary dermis are also seen. As the lesions progress, the collagen of the reticular dermis thickens, mimicking circumscribed scleroderma. The mechanism of this inflammatory disease is unknown, although, like morphea, some investigators have linked lichen sclerosus et atrophicus to *Borrelia* infections.

Treatment

There is no specific treatment. Itching often responds to topical glucocorticosteroids applied three times daily. Topical lubricants and cleanliness of the anogenital area are useful in preventing superimposed infection. Whether penicillin or other antispirochetal drugs will help is yet to be determined. Androgen creams offer no benefit and may virilize the child.

Patient Education

It is helpful to explain to patients that the course is irregularly progressive, although lesions may remain stable for long periods. Patients should be informed that areas of whitish thickening (leukoplakia) may appear on the mucosa or adjacent mucosal surfaces, and that these may rarely progress to carcinoma. Carcinomas have been reported in childhood, but are exceedingly rare.

Follow-up Visits

Yearly examinations are useful to monitor the progress of the disease and examine lesions for possible malignant changes, which require biopsy.

EHLERS-DANLOS SYNDROME

Clinical Features

Ehlers-Danlos syndrome is a phenotype in which there is excessive stretching of skin and joints. Ten different subtypes of Ehlers-Danlos syndrome have been described, but most patients

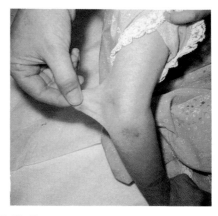

FIG 17–7.
Hyperextensible skin in child with Ehlers-Danlos syndrome.

have autosomal dominant inheritance (Table 17–1). The increase in skin stretchability is often spectacular; however, the skin returns to its normal position (Fig 17–7). Injury often results in large hematomas that heal with a large fibrotic nodule covered by thin, wrinkled epidermis. These are usually prominent on the lower part of the legs (Fig 17–8). The nodules may calcify.

Hematemesis and bleeding in the lower intestine may occur. Aortic aneurysms, arteriovenous fistula, retinal detachment, and lens abnormalities have been described. Premature births are common.

Hyperextensible joints may result in sublux-

TABLE 17–1.
Subtypes of Ehlers-Danlos Syndrome and Their Clinical Features

Subtype	Inheritance	Skin/Joints	Other
I	Dominant	Hyperextensible, lax skin and joints	Premature birth, hernias, scars, varicosities
II	Dominant	Soft, bruisable/lax hands and feet	
III	Dominant	Normal skin/lax joints	
IV	Recessive or dominant	Thin, prominent veins, pale skin, ecchymoses	Bowel and arterial rupture
V	X-linked	Hypermobile skin, scarring, bruising	Floppy mitral valves
VI	Recessive (lysyl hydoxylase deficiency)	Hyperextensible skin/lax joints	Blue sclerae
VII	Recessive or dominant	Soft/hyperextensible hip dislocation, lax joints	Retinal detachment
VIII	Dominant	Fragile/lax joints	Short stature
IX	X-linked	Lax skin/lax joints	Periodontitis
X	Recessive (fibronectin defect)	Soft, lax skin/lax joints, bruising	Pectus excavatum

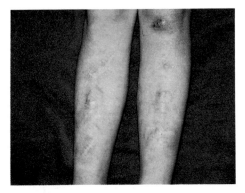

FIG 17–8.
Large scars and pseudotumors of anterior aspect of lower legs of child with Ehlers-Danlos syndrome.

ation of the joints, particularly of the knees, and flat feet, kyphosis, and scoliosis may occur (Fig 17–9).

Differential Diagnosis

The hyperextensible skin is characteristic and usually is not confused with other disorders.

Pathogenesis

The common problem in all ten subtypes is faulty formation of collagen. Since collagen limits the stretchability of skin, joints, and blood vessels, defective collagen results in hyperextensible skin and joints and fragile blood vessels. In two subtypes, deficiencies of enzymes necessary for crosslinking collagen molecules have been identified. In type IV, four separate defects in synthesis of type III collagen have been identified, two at the messenger RNA (mRNA) level and two at the structural protein level. Molecular biology tech-

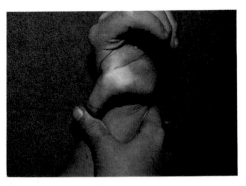

FIG 17–9.
Hyperextensible, lax joints of child with Ehlers-Danlos syndrome.

niques are likely to clarify the mechanisms of types currently unknown.

Treatment

Protective measures to prevent skin trauma, particularly during the toddler stage, are most useful. Otherwise no satisfactory treatment is available.

Patient Education

Informed genetic counseling should be given if a parent is affected. The expectation of premature birth should be emphasized. The skeletal and eye difficulties that may occur as the child grows should also be stressed.

Follow-up Visits

Yearly ophthalmologic and orthopedic examinations are recommended.

BIBLIOGRAPHY

Aberer E, Kollegger H, Kristoferitsch W, et al: Neuroborreliosis in morphea and lichen sclerosus et atrophicus. *J Am Acad Dermatol* 1988; 19:820.

Aberer E, Stanek G: Histological evidence for spirochetal origin of morphea and lichen sclerosus et atrophicus. *Am J Dermatopathol* 1987; 9:374.

Aberer E, Stanek G, Ertl M, et al: Evidence for spirochetal origin of circumscribed scleroderma (morphea). *Acta Derm Venereol (Stockh)* 1987; 67:225.

Berth-Jones J, Graham-Brown RAC, Burns DA: Lichen sclerosis. *Arch Dis Child* 1989; 64:1204.

Byers PH, Wenstrup RJ, Bonadio JF, et al: Molecular basis of inherited disorders of collagen biosynthesis: Implications for prenatal diagnosis. *Curr Probl Dermatol* 1987; 16:158.

Claman HN: On scleroderma. Mast cells, endothelial cells, and fibroblasts. *JAMA* 1989; 262:1206.

Hammerschmidt DE, Arneson MA, Larson SL: Maternal Ehlers-Danlos syndrome type X. *JAMA* 1982; 248:2487.

Pope FM, Narcisi P, Nicholl HC, et al: Clinical presentations of Ehlers-Danlos type IV. *Arch Dis Child* 1988; 63:1016.

Rizzo R, Contri MB, Micali G, et al: Familial Ehlers-Danlos syndrome type II: Abnormal fibrillogenesis of dermal collagen. *Pediatr Dermatol* 1987; 4:197.

18 _____ Drug Eruptions

DRUG ERUPTIONS

The diagnosis of a drug eruption is usually only suspected and not confirmed with absolute certainty. Evaluation of the possibility of a drug eruption is dependent on the patient's previous experience with specific drugs and the experience of the general population with drugs to which the patient has been exposed. The morphology of the patient's lesions and the relative frequency of the similar-type reactions in the general population are of assistance. Specific medications have a higher frequency of causing drug eruptions and specific types of a drug eruption than other medications. These are listed in Tables 18–1 through 18–7. The timing of the eruption in relationship to the commencement of drug therapy may assist in establishing the association of the drug with the drug eruption. The clinician will look for alternate explanations for the eruption, which include infection or the primary illness. Depending on the type of eruption and the drug involved, rechallenge to that drug in the future may be indicated to confirm the diagnosis, but rechallenge is usually not done because of concern of a more severe reaction. Removal of the suspected drug from the patient may or may not assist in more rapid resolution of the drug eruption. Fortunately the incidence of adverse drug reactions in infants and children appears to be less than in adults.

Clinical Features

Morbilliform Drug Eruptions.—Cutaneous drug reactions often have specific patterns. The morbilliform or so-called maculopapular eruption is probably the most common of all drug-induced eruptions in children. The term *morbilliform* means measles-like because of the development of a maculopapular erythematous rash that becomes confluent (Figs 18–1 and 18–2). This rash often starts on the trunk and extends onto the extremities. It is frequently symmetric and often has areas of totally normal skin that is surrounded by the eruption (Fig 18–3). The initial macules may become papular and then large plaques may form from the confluence of the individual lesions. The patient may have associated fever as well as malaise and arthralgias. In Table 18–1 drugs associated with morbilliform drug eruptions are listed.

Urticarial Drug Eruptions.—Drug eruptions associated with hives are called urticarial drug eruptions. Their presenting symptom is edematous, flat, erythematous papules that usually last less than 24 hours (Fig 18–4). New lesions appear almost continuously. The lesions may begin as small discrete papules that become confluent large figurate plaques (Fig 18–5). Occasionally the edema can be so intense in the center of the erythematous papules and plaques that the center appears less erythematous than the periphery, giving a target appearance. Lesions may resolve, leaving a macular blue-brown appearance that looks like a bruise. The absence of epidermal injury and more typical urticarial papules and plaques on the rest of the body confirms that this is an urticarial drug eruption and not erythema multiforme. Drugs associated with urticarial drug eruptions are listed in Table 18–2.

If the lesions show a deep dermal component with induration and swelling of the subcutaneous tissue, the reaction is called angioedema. If angioedema involves the mucous membranes, it can become life threatening, with airway obstructions associated with anaphylaxis reactions.

Fixed Drug Eruptions.—Fixed drug eruptions may be first seen as solitary to multiple,

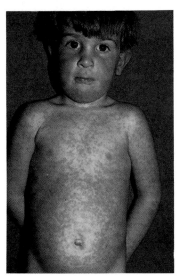

FIG 18–1.
Morbilliform drug eruption. Trimethroprim sulfameth-oxazole–induced eruption with discrete macules and papules on the trunk and confluent erythema on the face.

sharply demarcated, erythematous lesions that go on to give an intense macular hyperpigmentation (Fig 18–6). The initial lesions may appear edema-tous like urticaria or become bullous (Fig 18–7). In several days the edema and erythema will fre-

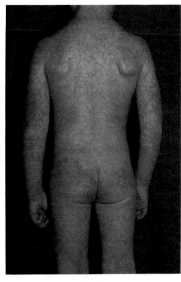

FIG 18–2.
Morbilliform drug eruption. Trimethroprim sulfameth-oxazole–induced eruption with confluence of lesions on upper arms and buttocks.

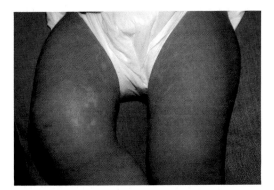

FIG 18–3.
Morbilliform drug eruption. Confluent intense eryth-ema with islands of normal skin in a patient treated with both phenobarbital and trimethroprim sul-famethoxazole.

quently decrease within the lesion, leaving a mac-ular hyperpigmentation with sharply demarcated outlines in a figurate pattern. Rechallenges with the same medication may cause lesions to de-velop in precisely the same spot as well as in new locations. In Table 18–3 the drugs commonly causing fixed drug eruptions are listed.

Vasculitis.—Palpable purpuric lesions asso-ciated with cutaneous necrotizing vasculitis can be associated with drugs. The vasculitis is usually on the lower extremities in dependent areas, but can occur anywhere on the body (Fig 18–8). The lesions may begin as soft, small erythematous papules or urticarial papules, which blanch when pressure is applied to the skin. Within several

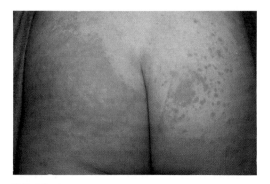

FIG 18–4.
Mixed urticarial and morbilliform drug eruption. Tri-methroprim sulfamethoxazole–induced urticarial plaques on left buttock with maculopapular lesions on right buttock.

TABLE 18–1.

Drugs Associated With Morbilliform Drug Eruptions

Analgesics, antipyretics, antirheumatics
    Gold
    Nonsteroidal anti-inflammatory drugs
        Meclofenamate sodium
        Piroxicam
        Sulindac
        Zomepirac sodium
Antibiotics
    Amoxicillin
    Ampicillin
    Cephalosporins
    Chloramphenicol
    Erythromycin
    Gentamicin sulfate
    Isoniazid
    Penicillins
    Sulfonamides
    Trimethroprim
    Trimethroprim and sulfamethoxazole
Drugs acting on the CNS
    Barbiturates
    Carbamazepine
    Phenytoin
Other
    Allopurinol

TABLE 18–2.

Drugs Commonly Associated With Urticarial Drug Eruptions

Analgesics, antipyretics, antirheumatics
    Acetylsalicylic acid
Antibiotics
    Amoxicillin
    Ampicillin
    Cephalosporins
    Penicillins
    Sulfonamides
    Trimethroprim and sulfamethoxazole
Other
    Horse serum

TABLE 18–3.

Drugs Associated With Fixed Drug Eruptions

Barbiturates
Carbamazepine
Phenazone derivatives (phenylbutazone)
Phenolphthalein
Sulfonamides
Tetracycline
Trimethroprim
Trimethroprim and sulfamethoxazole

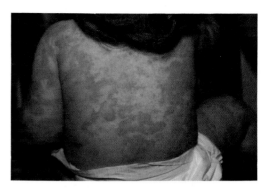

FIG 18–5.
Urticarial drug eruption. Large urticarial plaques in child given cefaclor.

hours to days the lesions become firm in texture and dark red-blue or purple in color. Drugs associated with vasculitis are listed in Table 18–4.

Exfoliative Dermatitis.—Diffuse erythema followed by bullae and loss of large sheets of epidermis can be associated with drugs. This is called Lyell's syndrome, toxic epidermal necrolysis, or erythema multiforme major. Drugs commonly associated with this condition are listed in Table 18–5. The presenting symptom is usually morbilliform or urticarial eruptions that show desquamation or become bullous within several hours or several days (Fig 18–9). The condition is considered in depth in Chapter 11.

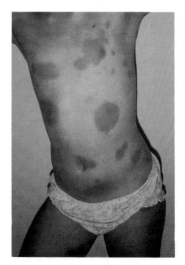

FIG 18–6.
Fixed drug eruption. Trimethroprim sulfamethoxazole induces oval erythematous macules with diffuse hyperpigmentation within several lesions.

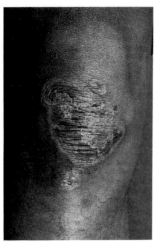

FIG 18–7.
Fixed drug eruption. Bullous reaction to tetracycline. Lesions have a necrotic hyperpigmented epidermis with sharp demarcation of normal and involved skin.

Differential Diagnosis

Morbilliform Drug Eruptions.—Morbilliform drug eruptions usually appear within a week after beginning therapy, but with the penicillins it may be 2 weeks or more before the eruption is seen. The onset of the eruption may occur after the drug is stopped. Morbilliform eruptions may fade over time even with continuation of the responsible medication. The eruption typically lasts 7 to 14 days and may be associated with pruritus during that time. The incidence of morbilliform eruptions is higher in those patients taking ampicillin or amoxicillin associated with an infectious mononucleosis condition.

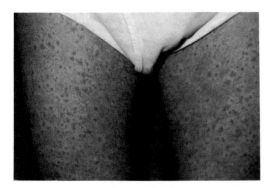

FIG 18–8.
Vasculitis. Amoxicillin induces lesions on legs.

TABLE 18–4.
Drugs Associated With Vasculitis

Allopurinol
Barbiturates
Gold
Horse serum
Penicillins
Sulfonamides
Thiazide derivatives

TABLE 18–5.
Drugs Associated With Exfoliative Dermatitis

Allopurinol
Barbiturates
Hydantoin derivatives
Penicillins
Phenazone derivatives (phenylbutazone)
Sulfonamides
Sulindac

Urticarial Drug Eruptions.—Urticarial lesions are usually pruritic and at times it is difficult to separate an urticarial eruption from a morbilliform eruption early in the course of the condition (see Fig 18–4). Urticarial lesions may occur immediately after exposure to the drug or within several days. The individual urticarial lesions usu-

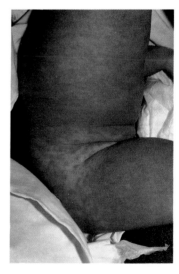

FIG 18–9.
Exfoliative dermatitis due to phenobarbital therapy. Dusky blue-red edematous lesions with epidermal necrosis and areas of noninvolvement. Epidermal necrosis is not sufficient to give a bullous reaction.

ally resolve within 24 hours, with new lesions arising. In the morbilliform drug eruption, individual lesions expand in several days, giving more of a confluent macular type eruption, whereas urticarial plaques are raised and indurated. Urticarial lesions occur commonly in children and are not associated with drugs (see Chapter 13).

Fixed Drug Eruptions.—The fixed drug eruption will usually occur within several days of the drug exposure. Biopsy of the fixed drug lesion will often help to confirm the diagnosis. Rechallenge with the suspected medication may cause recurrences of similar lesions in the same spot. The area of hyperpigmentation may take several months to resolve.

Vasculitis.—Drug-induced vasculitis can occur quickly after drug exposure or after prolonged drug exposure. Since drugs are one of many causes for cutaneous vasculitis, other conditions inducing these lesions must be considered. Sepsis with bacterial emboli and many viruses can cause palpable purpura with very similar cutaneous appearances. Biopsy of an individual lesion can confirm the small vessel vasculitis but cannot confirm the cause of the vasculitis.

Exfoliative Dermatitis.—Toxic epidermal necrolysis can be confirmed by a biopsy that demonstrates full-thickness epidermal necrosis and separation of the epidermis from the dermis. As with vasculitis, the biopsy can confirm the condition but not the cause.

Other Conditions.—Another condition that must be included in the differential diagnosis of drug eruptions is graft-versus-host disease. Also, viral or bacterial exanthems need to be recognized in order to characterize the cutaneous eruption as a response to the illness and not an adverse response to the therapy.

Pathogenesis

Drug reactions can occur as a result of immunologic reactions or nonimmunologic reactions. Immunologic reactions require host immunologic pathways and are called drug allergies. The ability of a drug to elicit an immune reaction is dependent on many characteristics. Most drugs are small organic molecules of less than 1,000 daltons. Because of their size they are unable to elicit

immune responses unless they bind to a larger molecule, which is usually a protein macromolecule. In this situation the drug functions as a hapten. Most drugs have little ability to form covalent bonds with macromolecules and are unable to form this type of immunologic antigen.

The host reacts to drugs in different manners. The body may respond differently to a drug given intravenously than to one applied topically. Patients may have variation in their ability to absorb or metabolize a given drug. The patient infected with infectious mononucleosis may be more likely to develop a morbilliform eruption as a reaction to ampicillin.

The body's immunologic response to drugs may be IgE dependent, which can be associated with pruritus, urticaria, bronchial spasm, and laryngeal edema. Drug eruptions may be associated with serum sickness caused by circulating immune complexes. Cytotoxic drug reactions can occur where the drug combines with the tissue, and that combination then becomes the target for antibodies or cellular-mediated cytotoxicity.

Nonimmunologic drug reactions can result through various modalities. Aspirin, opiates, and radiocontrast medications may directly release mast cell mediators, resulting in urticaria. Overdosage of a medicine may cause adverse cutaneous side effects by direct injury to cutaneous cells. Genetic inability to detoxify certain chemical compounds results in toxic metabolites, which can also damage cutaneous cells.

Secondary side effects of chemotherapy can include alopecia or particular types of rashes resulting from thrombocytopenia. Antibiotics can destroy the normal bacterial flora, allowing overgrowth of other organisms. Drugs may interact to compete for binding sites or cause metabolic changes. In addition, certain drugs (such as lithium, which exacerbates acne and psoriasis) can exacerbate preexisting dermatologic diseases.

Drug-induced urticaria can also be caused either by IgE mechanisms or by circulating immune complexes. The IgE-dependent urticaria reactions usually occur within 36 hours of drug exposure, but they can occur within minutes. The eruption associated with circulating immune complexes is a type of serum sickness reaction. It usually begins 4 to 12 days after exposure to the drug, at which time an equilibrium has been achieved between antibody and drug antigen, allowing for the formation of immune complexes. The serum sickness type reaction is often accompanied by fever, hematuria, and arthralgia. Liver and neurologic injury may occur.

The pathophysiology of drug-associated cutaneous vasculitis is not clear, but immune complexes may be responsible. The lesions usually begin to resolve several days or weeks after the offending drug is removed.

Treatment

Removal of the offending drug is the usual first method. Drug eruption is easily diagnosed when one can identify a specific pattern of drug eruption with a known timely exposure to only a single medication, and that medication has frequently been associated with that specific type of eruption. The infant or child exposed to multiple medications during a short period of time offers a more difficult diagnostic and therapeutic dilemma. Depending on the severity of the drug reaction, none, the most likely, or all of the drugs may need to be removed. Tables 18–1 through 18–5 are useful in identifying which drugs are most likely to be the cause of the eruption.

Morbilliform eruptions may fade with time without drug removal, especially when associated with amoxicillin or ampicillin. Urticarial eruptions may respond to antihistamine therapy. Because of fear that continued offending drug therapy can be associated with anaphylaxis or toxic epidermal necrolysis, attempts at drug removal are usually made.

Anaphylaxis associated with urticarial eruptions and angioedema is a medical emergency. Immediate therapy should be started with 1:1,000 aqueous epinephrine (0.2 to 0.5 mL given subcutaneously) and intravenous fluids. Antihistamines and systemic steroids may also be required in order to maintain an adequate airway while the symptoms subside.

Patient Education

The parents should be informed of the possible association of the cutaneous eruption with the specific drugs involved. The risk for the child from subsequent exposure to the specific or similar medications needs to be explained. For severe reactions, the child may be instructed to wear a bracelet or necklace that would alert examining health care workers to the suspected allergy. The parents should be informed of alternative forms of therapy that would omit the offending agent.

Follow-up Visits

Follow-up visits are necessary to confirm the resolution of the eruption and to recognize the response of the original illness that required drug therapy. The frequency and timing of the visits will depend on the severity of the original illness and the drug eruption.

The patient's medical records should document the possible drug-associated eruption in order to attempt avoidance of future exposures to the drug or related compounds. For penicillin-associated reaction, skin testing may be indicated to attempt to predict the future possibility of hypersensitivity reactions to the penicillins.

PHOTOSENSITIVE DRUG ERUPTIONS

Drug photosensitivity reactions can be either phototoxic or photoallergic. In either situation a combination of topical or systemic medication and exposure to light is necessary.

Photoallergic reactions are less common than phototoxic reactions. The photoallergic reaction involves an immunologic response to a chemical (drug) that is altered by ultraviolet light. The body recognizes the altered form as a foreign antigen and develops an immunologic delayed hypersensitivity response. This process requires sufficient drug and light to produce adequate antigen for immunization.

Phototoxic reactions involve direct cutaneous injury by a drug after the drug is changed by light energy. Increased light energy or increased amount of drug increases the risk of a phototoxic reaction.

Clinical Features

Photosensitive eruptions are characterized by more intense dermatitis in the areas of more intense sun exposure. Often the face, upper part of the trunk, and extensor surfaces of the arms are most involved. The lesions are usually erythematous and edematous, with associated papules, vesicles, or oozing, weeping lesions. Phototoxic reactions often are painful, similar to a severe sunburn. Photoallergic reactions may be painful or cause severe pruritus in the areas of the most intense sun exposure. Phototoxic reactions are dose dependent for both the amount of drug and the amount of light exposure. In addition to sunlight, fluorescent lamps or sunlight that comes through window glass may produce photosensitive drug reactions.

Pathogenesis

Common drugs associated with phototoxic and photoallergic reactions are listed in Tables 18–6 and 18–7. The histologic picture for photoallergic contact dermatitis and phototoxic reactions is similar, with associated epidermal spongiosis, dermal edema, and inflammatory response.

The photosensitivity may be confirmed by a photopatch test where the drug is readministered and multiple intensities of ultraviolet light exposure are given. Photosensitive reactions are usually in the ultraviolet A range. They often resolve with marked hyperpigmentation, which may take several months for resolution.

Treatment

The specific diagnosis is suggested by involvement of the light-exposed areas of the skin. A history of a combination of drug and light exposure will strongly support the diagnosis.

Treatment involves removal of the offending drug. The acute dermatitis can be treated as listed for treatment of sunburn in Chapter 10. If a true photoallergic reaction exists with severe pruritus, systemic steroids may be necessary for more rapid relief.

Patient Education

The cause of the photosensitivity should be fully described to the family and the child. If the drug that caused a phototoxic reaction is required, it may be continued if the ultraviolet light intensity can be decreased to a level that is not adequate to cause significant dermatitis. Children who develop a phototoxic reaction to psoralen-containing plants, such as celery or limes, should avoid the combination of plant exposure and sun exposure. If possible, the photosensitizing drug should be totally withdrawn.

Follow-up Visits

A follow-up visit in 1 week may be necessary to confirm the resolution of significant dermatitis. Additional follow-up visits for photo patch testing to confirm the diagnosis are dependent on the severity of the reaction and the medical necessity to confirm the diagnosis.

BIBLIOGRAPHY

Alanko K, Stubb S, Kauppinen K: Cutaneous drug reactions: Clinical types and causative agents. *Acta Derm Venereol (Stockh)* 1989; 69:223–226.

Arndt KA, Jick H: Rates of cutaneous reactions to drugs. *J Am Acad Dermatol* 1976; 235:918–922.

Bigby M, Jick S, Jick H, et al: Drug-induced cutaneous reactions. *J Am Acad Dermatol* 1986; 256:3358–3363.

Bork K: *Cutaneous Side Effects of Drugs.* Philadelphia, WB Saunders, 1988.

Bruinsma W: *The Guide to Drug Eruptions,* ed 4. Norwood, N.J., American Overseas Book Co., 1987.

Cirko-Begovic A, Vrhovac B, Bakran I: Intensive monitoring of adverse drug reactions in infants and preschool children. *Eur J Clin Pharmacol* 1989; 36:63–65.

Croydon EAP, Wheeler AW, Grimshaw JJ, et al: Prospective study of ampicillin rash: Report of a Collaborative Study Group. *Br M J* 1973; 1:7–9.

Gutman LT: The use of trimethoprim-sulfamethoxazole in children: A review of adverse reactions and indications. *Pediatr Infect Dis* 1984; 3:349–357.

TABLE 18–6.

Drugs Associated With Phototoxic Reactions

Coal tar derivatives
Furocoumarins in plants
Furosemide
Griseofulvin
Methotrexate
Nalidixic acid
PABA esters
Phenothiazines
Psoralens
Sulfonamides
Tetracycline
Thiazides
Tretinoin

TABLE 18–7.

Drugs Associated With Photoallergic Reactions

Fragrances
PABA esters
Perfume
Phenothiazines
Sulfonamides

Kauppinen K, Stubb S: Drug eruptions: Causative agents and clinical types. *Acta Derm Venereol (Stockh)* 1984; 64:320–324.

Kauppinen K, Stubb S: Fixed eruptions: Causative drugs and challenge tests. *Br J Dermatol* 1985; 112:575–578.

Knutsen AP, Anderson J, Satayaviboon S, et al: Immunologic aspects of phenobarbital hypersensitivity. *J Pediatr* 1984; 105:558.

Knutsen AP, Shah M, Schwarz KB, et al: Graft versus host-like illness in a child with phenobarbital hypersensitivity. *Pediatrics* 1986; 78:581–584.

Kramer MS, Hutchinson TA, Flegel KM, et al: Adverse drug reactions in general pediatric outpatients. *J Pediatr* 1985; 106:305.

Shear NH, Spielberg SP: Pharmacogenetics and adverse drug reactions in the skin. *Pediatr Dermatol* 1983; 1:165–173.

Shear NH, Spielberg SP, Grant DM, et al: Differences in metabolism of sulfonamides predisposing to idiosyncratic toxicity. *Ann Intern Med* 1986; 105:179–184.

Stern RS, Bigby M: An expanded profile of cutaneous reactions to nonsteroidal anti-inflammatory drugs. *J Am Acad Dermatol* 1984; 252:1433–1437.

Stern RS, Wintroub BU, Arndt KA: Drug reactions. *J Am Acad Dermatol* 1986; 15:1282–1288.

VanArsdel PP: Allergy and adverse drug reactions. *J Am Acad Dermatol* 1982; 6:833–845.

Wintroub BU, Stern R: Cutaneous drug reactions: Pathogenesis and clinical classification. *J Am Acad Dermatol* 1985; 13:167–179.

19 _____ Neonatal Dermatology

Skin lesions appearing in the first month of life usually prompt parents to seek medical advice. A thorough knowledge of the fetal skin biology (see Chapter 1) and of the cutaneous lesions of newborns is expected of those providing neonatal care.

This chapter is divided into five sections: neonatal skin care, transient skin disease in the newborn, birthmarks, common congenital malformations that involve skin, and chronic skin conditions that begin in the newborn period. Many of the transient disorders of the newborn will be considered by their clinical features, differential diagnosis, and pathogenesis only, since no treatment is required of these self-limited problems. Acne neonatorum is also discussed in Chapter 3, miliaria in Chapter 11, and pigmentary changes in Chapter 16.

NEONATAL SKIN CARE

The full-term newborn infant's skin feels very soft and smooth. The smooth texture and softness are related to the hydration of the epidermis and the condition of the collagen and dermal matrix substances. At birth the full-term infant's skin is functionally mature. The barrier portion of the epidermis, the stratum corneum, is intact and effectively protects the infant.

Even though the infant's barrier function may be normal at birth, the infant is at increased risk for systemic toxicity of topically applied compounds (Table 19–1). The infant's surface area is great when compared with body mass. The infant's metabolism, excretion, distribution, and protein binding may be different from that of an adult. The premature infant is at much greater risk. The premature infant has markedly decreased epidermal barrier function and an even greater body surface area to body volume ratio. In addition, the immature organs of the premature infant may greatly change the metabolism, excretion, distribution, and protein binding of chemical agents. Local or systemic toxicity can occur in the premature infant from soaps, lotions, or other cleansing solutions.

The skin of the mature infant often appears dry and cracked soon after birth (Figs 19–1 and 19–2). The stratum corneum that has accumulated in utero has not yet shed. On the ankles and wrist fissures and bleeding may occur. During this time topical care should include moisturizing lotions or creams. The goal of therapy is to retain the soft flexible texture of the infant's skin by hydrating and lubricating the epidermis. For infants in a dry environment, the moisturizers may need to be used indefinitely. Infants from a more humid environment may need only intermittent use of moisturizers.

The skin care of the premature infant is much more difficult and complex (Table 19–2). Not only is the barrier portion of the epidermis absent or defective, but the skin has markedly increased fragility. Because of epidermal and dermal injury, the infant may have significant cutaneous pain, which is accentuated by routine handling. The infant is at risk of developing sepsis from skin-associated organisms. Maintaining a humid environment will decrease the infant's transepidermal water loss and assist in skin hydration. This can be done by using a humidity-controlled isolette or with thin plastic tents over infants under infrared warmers.

Dry, flaking, fissured skin of premature infants should be treated with moisturizing creams or ointments. Petrolatum-based ointments with little or no preservatives appear to offer the greatest

TABLE 19−1.

Reasons for Increased Risk of Systemic Toxicity From Topically Applied Agents in Infants

> Increased surface area/body weight ratio
> Differences in drug excretion
> Differences in drug metabolism
> Differences in drug protein binding
> Differences in drug distribution

TABLE 19−2.

Care of the Premature Infant's Skin

Gentle handling
  Adhesive tape used sparingly, in smallest possible area
  Infrequent cardiac monitor changes
  Sparing use of antibacterial cleansing solutions
  Avoid frictional trauma to skin
Intervention
  Humidify infant environment
  Skin lubrication with awareness of possible absorption of preservatives and emulsifiers within product used
  Localized use of semipermeable wound dressings

benefit and lowest risk. Ointments placed on the infant's skin under an infrared warmer will not cause cutaneous burns. Semipermeable wound dressings may offer additional cutaneous pain relief and protection, but additional studies must be done to analyze the potential for associated risk with bacterial growth under the dressings.

TRANSIENT SKIN DISEASE IN THE NEWBORN

Milia

Clinical Features

Milia are multiple, white 1 to 2 mm papules seen on the forehead, cheeks, and nose of infants (Fig 19–3). They may be present in the oral cavity as well, where they are called *Epstein's pearls*. Up to 40% of newborns have milia on the skin and 64% have them on the palate. The cystic spheres rupture onto the skin surface and exfoliate their contents within a few weeks after birth.

Differential Diagnosis

Molluscum contagiosum, an acquired viral infection, may mimic milia, but does not appear in the immediate neonatal period. Sebaceous gland hyperplasia also occurs on the nose and cheeks of infants, but is yellow, rather than whitish.

Pathogenesis

On histologic examination, milia appear as superficial epithelial cysts in the papillary dermis, just beneath the epidermis. The cyst cavity is filled with keratin.

Sebaceous Gland Hyperplasia

Clinical Features

Tiny (1-mm) yellow macules or yellow papules are seen at the opening of each pilosebaceous follicle on the nose and cheeks of newborns. They recede completely by 4 to 6 months of age.

FIG 19−1.
Dry, flaking skin on term infant 36 hours old.

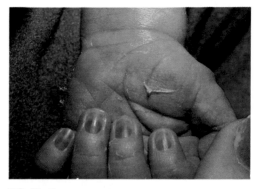

FIG 19−2.
Postmature infant. Long fingernails and peeling of palms can be seen in this 2-day-old infant.

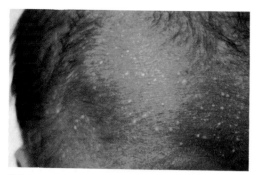

FIG 19–3.
Milia. Multiple white papules seen on forehead of infant.

Differential Diagnosis

Milia may mimic sebaceous hyperplasia, but are white and cystic in appearance.

Pathogenesis

Maternal androgenic stimulation is responsible for the increase in sebaceous gland volume, sebaceous cell size, and total number of sebaceous cells.

Erythema Toxicum

Clinical Features

Blotchy, erythematous macules 2 to 3 cm in diameter, with a tiny 1- to 4-mm central vesicle or

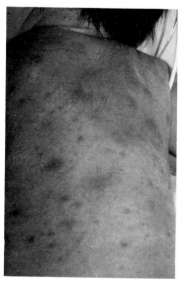

FIG 19–4.
Erythema toxicum. Blotchy erythematous macules and plaques with multiple papules and pustules.

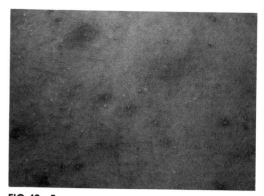

FIG 19–5.
Erythema toxicum. Closer view demonstrates vesicles and pustules with or without an erythematous base.

pustule, are seen in erythema toxicum (Figs 19–4 and 19–5). They usually begin at 24 to 48 hours of age, and occur in about 50% of term infants and less commonly in premature infants. Lesions are seen on the chest, back, face, and proximal extremities, sparing the palms and soles. The individual lesions clear in 4 to 5 days, and new lesions may occur from birth to the tenth day of life. Smear of the central vesicle or pustule contents will reveal numerous eosinophils on Wright-stained preparations. A peripheral blood eosinophilia up to 20% may accompany the tissue eosinophil accumulation, particularly in infants with numerous lesions.

Transient Neonatal Pustular Melanosis

Clinical Features

These lesions are seen at birth as vesicles, pustules, or ruptured vesicles or pustules with a collarette of surrounding scale (Fig 19–6). Pigmented macules are also often present at birth, or they develop at the sites of resolving pustules or vesicles (Fig 19–7). The vesicles and pustules usually disappear by 5 days of age, while the pigmented macules resolve during a period of 3 weeks to 3 months. These lesions are more common on black infants, and they can occur on the palms and soles. Smear of the vesicle or pustule contents will reveal numerous neutrophils and an occasional eosinophil on Wright-stained preparations.

Differential Diagnosis

Miliaria rubra is frequently confused with erythema toxicum. The erythema around miliaria

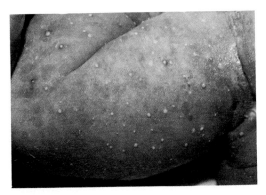

FIG 19–6.
Transient neonatal pustular melanosis. Multiple papules present at birth on arm of infant.

rubra is small in area (1 to 2 mm vs 20 to 30 mm in erythema toxicum). The central vesicle or pustule may mimic herpes simplex or bacterial folliculitis lesions. A Gram's stain of the pustules of erythema toxicum or transient neonatal pustular melanosis will be negative. The Wright-stained slide from a pustule of erythema toxicum will show a predominance of eosinophils, while the slide of a pustule of transient neonatal pustular melanosis will usually show a predominance of neutrophils.

Pathogenesis
Erythema toxicum is believed to be associated with obstruction of the pilosebaceous orifice. The cause of transient neonatal pustular melanosis is not known.

Mottling
Clinical Features
A lacelike pattern of dusky erythema appears on the extremities and trunk of neonates when exposed to a temperature decrease. This phenomenon may be sensitive to small increments of temperature change. The mottling disappears on rewarming. Mottling that persists beyond 6 months of life may be a sign of hypothyroidism or cutis marmorata telangiectatica congenita, which can be associated with musculoskeletal or vascular abnormalities.

Differential Diagnosis
Certain birthmarks, such as cutis marmorata telangiectatica congenita, may mimic mottling, but the color change will not disappear with rewarm-

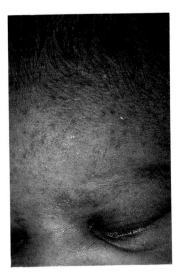

FIG 19–7.
Transient neonatal pustular melanosis. Multiple macules at sites of previous pustules in 10-day-old infant.

ing. Similarly, the livedo reticularis seen with collagen vascular disease such as neonatal lupus erythematosus will persist when the skin is warmed.

Pathogenesis
Immaturity of the autonomic control of the skin vascular plexus is believed to be responsible for mottling, with constriction of the deeper plexus and opening of the superficial plexus.

Harlequin Color Change
Clinical Features
When a low-birth-weight infant is placed on one side, an erythematous flush with a sharp demarcation at the midline develops on the dependent side. The upper half of the body becomes pale. The color change subsides within a few seconds of placing the baby in the supine position, but may persist for as long as 20 minutes.

Differential Diagnosis
The color change is seldom confused with other vascular problems.

Pathogenesis
The exact mechanism of this unusual phenomenon is not known, but the immaturity of autonomic vasomotor control is believed to be responsible.

Sucking Blisters

Clinical Features

Sucking blisters are usually solitary intact oval blisters or erosions on noninflamed skin in the newborn. They occur on the forearms, wrists, fingers, or upper lip (Fig 19–8) and resolve within a few days.

Differential Diagnosis

Herpesvirus infection or bullous impetigo is often considered when sucking blisters are encountered, but these lesions appear on an erythematous base. In incontinentia pigmenti, multiple linear blisters are present, in contrast to the solitary sucking blister. Epidermolysis bullosa usually is first seen as multiple new blisters developing after birth.

Pathogenesis

Vigorous sucking in utero has been postulated as the cause of these blisters.

Subcutaneous Fat Necrosis

Clinical Features

In subcutaneous fat necrosis of the newborn, firm, sharply circumscribed, reddish or purple nodules appear on the cheeks, buttocks, arms, and thighs (Fig 19–9). The lesions usually begin within the first 2 weeks of life and resolve spontaneously in several weeks. Occasionally the lesions can heal with atrophy leaving a skin depression. Infrequently, hypercalcemia can occur with or without associated irritability, vomiting, weight loss, and failure to thrive. Serum calcium evaluations should be repeated biweekly until the le-

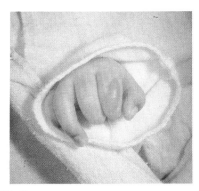

FIG 19–8.
Sucking blister. Oval, noninflammatory blister on finger of newborn.

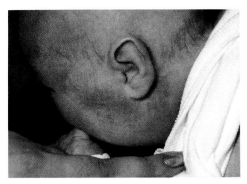

FIG 19–9.
Subcutaneous fat necrosis. Firm, indurated nodules on face of infant.

sions have totally resolved for a month or more in infants who have large plaques of involved skin or who have renal disease.

Differential Diagnosis

Bacterial cellulitis or septicemic lesions may be confused with subcutaneous fat necrosis at the onset. The infant with fat necrosis appears healthy and nurses vigorously, in contrast to infants with bacterial infections. Several separate lesion sites are often seen with subcutaneous fat necrosis and would be extremely unusual with cellulitis.

Pathogenesis

Cold injury is believed to be responsible for subcutaneous fat necrosis. The fat of the neonate contains more saturated fatty acids that have a higher melting point. Once the temperature of the skin drops below the melting point of the fat, crystallization occurs within the fat of the dermal fat cells, followed by a granulomatous reaction.

Sclerema

Clinical Features

Premature newborns who suffer hypothermia are susceptible to the development of sclerema, a diffuse hardening of the skin. The skin becomes tight, immobile, yellow, and shiny. Sclerema appears in severely ill newborns who have suffered sepsis, hypoglycemia, metabolic acidosis, or other severe metabolic abnormalities. Temperature control, nutritional replacement, correction of metabolic acidosis, and possibly repeated exchange transfusions will arrest the process. Infant mortality in sclerema is high.

Differential Diagnosis

The thickening and hardening of the skin are so characteristic of sclerema that it is not confused with other disorders.

Pathogenesis

The susceptibility of the subcutaneous fat to cold injury is believed to be the cause. Edema of fibrous septa surrounding fat lobules, without fat necrosis, is found.

Pustules in the Newborn

Clinical Features

Pustules are discrete, yellow, 1- to 9-mm raised lesions that frequently display a red base. The appearance of pustules in the newborn should immediately bring to mind the possibility of bacterial sepsis. Pustules on the newborn skin in association with other signs or symptoms of sepsis, or when prolonged rupture of maternal membranes has occurred, should make one suspect bacterial sepsis. Bacterial culture of pustules of other body fluids, such as blood, urine, and cerebrospinal fluid, should be performed. There is no rapid, completely reliable method of determining whether a baby has bacterial sepsis, and one should always maintain a high index of suspicion. The incidence of bacterial sepsis is higher in the preterm infant than in the full-term infant, and overall sepsis is an uncommon cause of pustules in the newborn. The high mortality rate of unrecognized bacterial sepsis makes it imperative for the clinician to consider this possibility, however.

Differential Diagnosis

Other causes of pustules in the newborn may be considered after bacterial sepsis is eliminated as a possibility. Erythema toxicum may occasionally be pustular, particularly if skin involvement is extensive. Transient neonatal pustular melanosis mimics erythema toxicum and is characterized by pustules present at birth. Herpes simplex skin infections may be pustular but are usually vesicular. Acne neonatorum is usually not present in the first 14 days of life, and evolution to the pustular stage may require several more weeks. Candidiasis, particularly of the diaper area or of other intertriginous areas, may be pustular, and satellite pustules are characteristically found at a distance from the margins of confluent areas of candidiasis. Congenital candidiasis, acquired in utero, may also be pustular, with discrete pustules at birth

and subsequent development of diffusely eczematous skin. Infantile acropustulosis may begin at birth or within the newborn period. Its presenting symptom may be discrete pustules limited to the distal extremities, with prominent involvement of the palms and soles. Nevus comedonicus is a birthmark consisting of patulous follicular openings in which pustule formation, or even deeper abscesses, may occur. Psoriasis rarely occurs in the newborn period, but it also may be extensive and pustular.

Pathogenesis

In bacterial infections, pustules arise as the result of accumulation of neutrophils within the skin, following dissemination of bacteria from the blood to the skin or direct bacterial invasion of the skin.

Acne Neonatorum (See also Chapter 3)

Clinical Features

Neonatal acne is rarely present at birth but may appear as multiple, discrete papules at 2 to 4 weeks of age. The face, chest, back, and groin are the usual areas for cutaneous lesions (Fig 19–10). Papules evolve into pustules after a few weeks. Neonatal acne may persist up to 8 months of age. There is some suggestion that infants with extensive neonatal acne may experience severe acne as adolescents.

Differential Diagnosis

The differential diagnosis of acne neonatorum is the same as for pustules in the newborn.

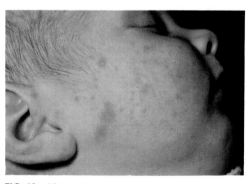

FIG 19–10.
Acne neonatorum. Multiple small inflammatory papules on face of 1-month-old infant.

Pathogenesis

Neonatal acne may be a part of the so-called miniature puberty of the newborn. Neonatal sebaceous glands are hyperplastic, and hydroxysteroid dehydrogenase activity in these structures is high in the 2 months just before birth and at birth. There is evidence that newborns with acne experience transient increases in circulating androgens.

Treatment

Neonatal acne usually resolves spontaneously without treatment. If the involvement is severe, topical therapy with 2.5% benzoyl peroxide gel can be prescribed.

Herpes Simplex Virus Infection

Clinical Features

Grouped vesicles on an erythematous base should bring to mind neonatal herpes simplex virus infection (Fig 19–11). Any area of skin may be involved, but vesicles on the scalp or buttock are particularly common. Monitoring electrodes may produce sufficient skin trauma on involved skin sites to allow invasion by the virus and to induce herpes simplex virus skin lesions. Vesicles may be present immediately at birth, but the onset after birth is more likely, with 6 days as the mean age of onset. Some infants with neonatal herpes simplex virus will not have skin lesions, but 70% of all infants infected with herpes simplex virus display lesions. Mucous membrane involvement is common. Eighty percent of neonatal infections are herpes simplex virus type 2, and 20% are herpes simplex virus type 1.

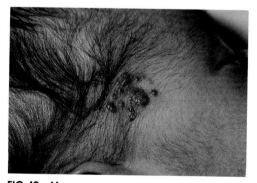

FIG 19–11.
Neonatal herpes simplex. Grouped vesicles on an erythematous base in 9-day-old infant.

Differential Diagnosis

Other blistering diseases of the newborn, such as congenital varicella, bullous impetigo, and incontinentia pigmenti, may be considered in the differential diagnosis. A Wright-stained smear of cells scraped from a vesicle base will demonstrate multinucleated giant cells and balloon cells in herpes simplex virus infection. Fluorescein-tagged antiherpes simplex virus–specific antibody may be used to examine vesicle smears or snap-frozen biopsy sections of skin to make a rapid diagnosis. Viral culture of herpes simplex virus requires 12 to 120 hours to grow, and in all infected or suspected neonates cultures of skin lesions, urine, nasopharynx, eyes, and cerebrospinal fluid are indicated. Serum antibodies for herpes simplex virus are of little assistance in making the diagnosis accurately. Rapid diagnosis of herpes simplex virus is essential, and a high index of suspicion should be maintained.

Pathogenesis

Herpes simplex virus is usually related to maternal infection in the birth canal. Infected infants are likely to have had a premature birth, may have signs that mimic bacterial sepsis, and may develop psychomotor retardation even if obvious signs of dissemination of herpes simplex virus are not evident in the newborn period. Infants born to mothers with a primary herpes genital infection at the time of delivery are more likely to develop neonatal herpes simplex than infants born to mothers with recurrent genital lesions.

Treatment

Either adenosine arabinoside or acyclovir, administered intravenously, has been demonstrated to be efficacious. Early recognition and early therapeutic intervention appear to lead to an improved outcome in the infected infant.

Varicella (see also Chapter 8)

Clinical Features

Congenital varicella is quite rare but may mimic herpes simplex virus in the newborn. This infection is associated with maternal chickenpox 2 to 3 weeks before delivery. Lesions appear as crops of macules and papules that evolve into vesicles and then crust. Age of onset is within the first 10 days after birth, and a mortality of up to 20% has been reported in infants who develop skin lesions between 5 and 10 days of age. A

Wright-stained smear of cells from a blister base or a skin biopsy demonstrates the same changes as are seen in herpes simplex virus. Maternal history of varicella and cutaneous lesions in the infant compatible with varicella are most useful in making the diagnosis.

Varicella can also develop in neonates infected postnatally. This could result in a severe infection, especially in premature infants.

Differential Diagnosis

Herpes simplex virus infection and bullous impetigo are the two most important considerations in the differential diagnosis of congenital varicella. Fluorescein-tagged antiherpes zoster virus–specific antibody may be used to examine vesicle smears or snap-frozen biopsy sections of skin to make a rapid diagnosis. Culture identification of the virus from the vesicles may require 7 to 14 days.

Pathogenesis

Maternal infection with varicella-zoster virus results in dissemination of the virus to the newborn. Maternal infection may be unrecognized.

Treatment

Immediate administration of zoster-immune globulin to the infant is recommended if maternal infection is present from 5 days before to 2 days after delivery. Infected infants may require therapy with intravenous acyclovir. Passive immunization with varicella-zoster immunoglobulin should be considered for postnatal exposure of premature and term infants exposed to varicella.

Impetigo (see also Chapter 5)

Clinical Features

Bacterial impetigo may be observed in the newborn period. Flaccid, well-demarcated bullae may be seen that evolve into erosions. Any area of skin may be involved, but the scalp, face, and diaper areas are the most common sites of infection. A collarette of scale around the erosion is characteristic of *Staphylococcus aureus* (Fig 19–12).

Differential Diagnosis

Bacterial culture of skin lesions and culture of the nasopharynx will yield the organism within 24 hours. Smear of vesicle contents and Gram's stain will demonstrate the bacteria.

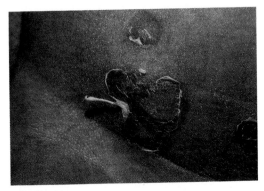

FIG 19–12.
Impetigo in suprapubic area of neonate. A collarette of scale around erythematous erosions is characteristic of *S. aureus* impetigo.

Pathogenesis

S. aureus is a predominant organism producing impetigo, including those strains capable of producing the staphylococcal scalded skin syndrome; therefore, prompt recognition and treatment are necessary. Occasionally group A streptococci or gram-negative bacteria can cause impetigo in the newborn period.

Treatment

The appropriate systemic antibiotic should be administered promptly to prevent sepsis and diminish spread of bacteria to other patients and hospital personnel.

Staphylococcal Scalded Skin Syndrome (Ritter's Disease)

Clinical Features

Infants 2 to 30 days of age may develop an abrupt onset of generalized erythema, followed in 24 hours by bullae with subsequent exfoliation of large sheets of skin within 48 hours. The lesions are commonly around the head, neck, buttocks, groin, axilla, and periumbilical area of the abdomen.

Differential Diagnosis

Toxic shock syndrome and toxic epidermal necrolysis should be considered in the differential diagnosis of the staphylococcal scalded skin syndrome. They are rarely observed in the newborn period, however.

Pathogenesis

Skin injury is the result of an intraepidermal cleavage through the granular layer of epidermis due to circulating exotoxin produced by *S. aureus.* Small amounts of staphylococci, less than 10^8 organisms, may produce enough toxin to exfoliate a human. Culture of the nasopharynx, rectum, and blisters are likely to yield the organism.

Treatment

Isolation of the affected newborn to prevent nursery epidemics is essential. Antistaphylococcal antibiotics should be administered systemically, and fluid and electrolyte replacement should be provided, much like that provided for burn therapy.

Breast Abscess

Clinical Features

Swelling, erythema, and fluctuance in one breast of a newborn infant signifies the possibility of breast abscess. Onset usually begins 5 to 20 days after birth. The infant may have fever, but usually is asymptomatic otherwise.

Differential Diagnosis

Breast hyperplasia due to miniature puberty of the newborn may produce asymmetric enlargement of one breast. The breast is not red or fluctuant to the feel in breast hyperplasia, in contrast to abscess.

Pathogenesis

S. aureus and gram-negative organisms are the most likely pathogens. A needle aspiration of the infection may be necessary to obtain a positive bacterial culture.

Treatment

Systemic antibiotic therapy with the appropriate antistaphylococcal agent is usually necessary.

Omphalitis

Clinical Features

Redness and induration of the umbilical region is characteristic of omphalitis. Often the redness is not well localized and diffusely spreads beyond the umbilicus.

Differential Diagnosis

An irritant dermatitis produced by the treatment of the umbilicus with various bacteriostatic agents may sometimes mimic omphalitis.

Pathogenesis

Bacterial infection through the cut surface of the umbilical cord is the usual cause. It is predominantly caused by *S. aureus,* and, if untreated, may progress to bacterial sepsis.

Treatment

Prophylactic bacteriostatic agents applied to the cord in the newborn period have reduced the likelihood of this infection in many nurseries. Administration of systemic antistaphylococcal antibiotic is the treatment of choice.

Caput Succedaneum and Cephalohematoma

Clinical Features

Caput succedaneum is subcutaneous edema of the presenting part of the head. Cephalohematoma is a subperiosteal collection of blood. Edema or hemorrhage of the scalp appears as deep swelling, with or without purpura. The swelling occurs primarily in vertex deliveries, particularly those with prolonged labor, and resolves spontaneously in 7 to 10 days. If the purpura is extensive, it can serve as a source of hyperbilirubinemia. Secondary bacterial infection of cephalohematoma, resulting in cellulitis, may occur rarely.

Differential Diagnosis

The caput succedaneum tends to feel soft and lacks a well-defined outline. The cephalohematoma is bounded by the suture lines of the skull and often feels fluctuant. Both lesions can mimic cellulitis or bacterial abscess. Appropriate cultures may assist in the differential diagnosis.

Pathogenesis

Both lesions are due to shearing forces on the scalp skin and skull during labor.

Petechiae and Purpura

Clinical Features

Petechiae and purpura may be presenting features of congenital infection, particularly when the newborn is small for gestational age and has hepatosplenomegaly. An acronym used for these infections is TORCH syndrome. Petechiae and purpura are the most common cutaneous symptoms for this group of congenital infections, and may be important clues to the diagnosis. Newborns with congenital infection may also demonstrate other features, such as microophthalmia, congenital heart defects, cataracts, and psychomotor retardation.

Differential Diagnosis

Toxoplasmosis, syphilis (see also Chapter 5), rubella, cytomegalovirus, and congenital herpes simplex virus infections are the usual congenital infections responsible for the production of petechiae and purpura. Serologic tests and viral cultures for these infections should be performed. Other causes of petechiae and purpura in the newborn include trauma, with face and scalp petechiae common in difficult vertex deliveries or in section-assisted deliveries (Fig 19–13). Neonatal thrombocytopenia due to maternal autoantibodies, as in idiopathic thrombocytopenic purpura, or systemic lupus erythematosus may also produce neonatal petechiae a few hours after birth. Hypoprothrombinemia may result in purpura in the newborn older than 2 or 3 days as a result of vitamin K deficiency. Protein C deficiency can also cause severe purpura in the neonate. Neonatal petechiae and purpura are unusual in the hemophilias, but bleeding from circumcision sites may be the first manifestation of hemophilia in the newborn period. Neonatal purpura resulting from platelet dysfunction may be observed in von Willebrand's disease or Wiskott-Aldrich syndrome.

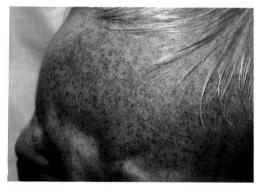

FIG 19–13.
Multiple petechiae on forehead of neonate after difficult vertex delivery.

BIRTHMARKS

Birthmarks represent an excess of one or more of the normal components of skin per unit area: blood vessels, lymph vessels, pigment cells, hair follicles, sebaceous glands, epidermis, collagen, or elastin. Birthmarks are collections of highly differentiated cells in tissue. The vascular birthmarks are the most common.

Congenital malformations are most frequently observed in skin. The two most commonly seen are flat hemangiomas of a faint-red color, the so-called salmon patch, and mongolian spots. Salmon patches are observed with high frequency in infants, both in white infants (703/1,000 live births) and black infants (592/1,000 live births). Mongolian spots are more frequently observed in Orientals (910/1,000 live births) and black infants (880/1,000 live births), but are less common in white infants (48/1,000 live births). Mongolian spots and salmon patches are observed at least 100 times more frequently than any other skin birthmark.

Vascular Birthmarks: Flat Hemangiomas (Nevus Flammeus, Port-Wine Stain)

Flat vascular birthmarks tend to persist, while raised vascular birthmarks usually regress with time.

Clinical Features

Flat hemangiomas can be divided into those that are light red or pink in color (salmon patch [nevus flammeus]) and those that are deep red or purple-red (port-wine stain). The salmon patch appears as a light-red macule on the nape of the neck, the upper eyelids, and the glabella (Figs 19–14 and 19–15). A salmon patch is present on the back of the neck in more than 40% of infants. Salmon patches fade with time, but remnants may persist well into adult life. Generally, the eyelid lesions fade by 6 to 12 months of age, and the glabellar lesions, by 5 or 6 years of age. Lesions on the nape of the neck are more likely to persist.

Port-wine stains appear as deep-red or purple-red macules on the face or extremities (Fig 19–16). They are usually unilateral (Fig 19–17). Occasionally they are extensive and cover large areas of skin. Port-wine stains on the face or an extremity may be associated with soft tissue and bony hypertrophy. A port-wine stain on the face may be a clue to the Sturge-Weber syndrome.

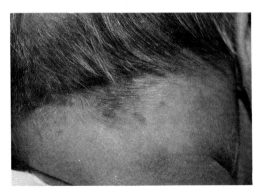

FIG 19—14.
Salmon patch. Lesion on nape of neck. Also called "stork bite," because this is where the stork carries the baby before it is delivered.

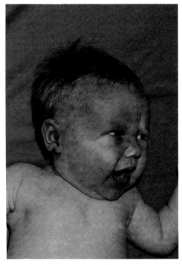

FIG 19—16.
Port-wine stain. Infant subsequently developed seizures associated with Sturge-Weber syndrome.

Overall, 8% of infants with facial port-wine stains will develop Sturge-Weber syndrome, but the incidence is higher if the lesion covers the upper and lower eyelids or if the lesion is bilateral. The Sturge-Weber syndrome is characterized by seizures, mental retardation, glaucoma, and hemiplegia. Calcification of the hemangioma in the brain in Sturge-Weber syndrome may be detected in childhood by x-ray examination of the skull. Identification of cerebral vascular abnormalities and early calcification can be detected in infancy by CT or MRI.

When port-wine stains are found on an extremity and are associated with soft tissue or bony hypertrophy of that extremity, the condition is called the Klippel-Trenaunay-Weber syndrome. Elongation of an extremity can cause orthopedic deformity. Arteriovenous fistulas are present in 25% of such patients. Absence of the deep venous channels in the affected limb may be detected by venography.

Differential Diagnosis

In an older infant, flat hemangiomas are so characteristic that they are seldom confused with other skin conditions, but in the first weeks of life the raised hemangioma may be flat and look like a port-wine stain. After several weeks of life, the raised hemangioma will begin to elevate the skin and be distinguished from a port-wine stain. Port-wine stain lesions usually cover a larger surface area and are unilateral.

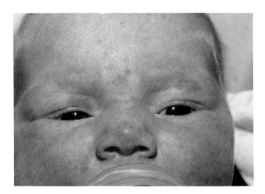

FIG 19—15.
Salmon patch. Lesion on glabella and upper eyelids.

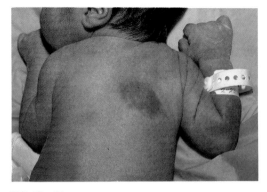

FIG 19—17.
Port-wine stain. Lesion on back of neonate.

Pathogenesis

Numerous dilated capillaries without endo-thelial change are seen on a skin biopsy specimen from lesions in an adolescent or adult. The capillaries are mature and represent a developmental malformation. In infants and children, the skin biopsy specimen may be indistinguishable from normal skin.

Treatment

Recent data support use of a pulsed dye laser that selectively causes thermal damage to cutaneous vasculature while sparing surrounding epidermal and dermal structures. This therapy can commence during infancy. Therapy for the cutaneous lesion may reverse underlying soft tissue overgrowth, but bony hypertrophy or the neurologic progressions in Sturge-Weber syndrome are not affected. In addition, flat hemangiomas may be covered with makeup.

Patient Education

The natural course of flat hemangiomas should be explained. Infants and children with port-wine stains can be referred to the nearest center with expertise in pulsed dye laser therapy for port-wine stains.

Follow-up Visits

If features of Sturge-Weber syndrome are present, ophthalmologic evaluation and follow-up should be obtained immediately. Measurements of the length and girth of the extremities should be carefully recorded every 3 to 6 months if a port-wine stain is found on an extremity. Since leg length differences can induce scoliosis, orthopedic evaluations and assistance may be required if one leg is longer than the other.

Vascular Birthmarks: Raised Hemangiomas (Strawberry Hemangioma, Cavernous Hemangioma)

Clinical Features

Raised hemangiomas may not be observed at birth, but a circumscribed area of blanched skin with a few fine telangiectases may be present, representing a developing raised hemangioma (Fig 19–18). By 2 to 4 weeks of age the skin becomes raised, with red nodules (Figs 19–19 and 19–20). The lesions grow out of proportion to the baby for the first 8 to 12 months of life. Raised hemangiomas begin to show signs of involution around

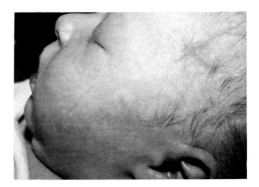

FIG 19–18.
Precursor to raised hemangioma. Blanched skin with fine telangiectasia is present at birth. Later the lesion will become raised.

15 months of age, when pale gray areas appear within the red nodule. Soon the first sign of flattening appears. The raised lesion regresses to skin level by 5 years of age in 50% of the patients, and by puberty in almost all patients. Most often, only redundant loose skin that was stretched during the rapid growth phase remains. In large, raised hemangiomas, ulceration of the epithelial surface often occurs when secondary bacterial superinfection results (Fig 19–21).

There are several major complications of raised hemangiomas: (1) platelet trapping, (2) airway obstruction, (3) visual obstruction, and (4)

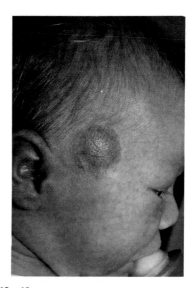

FIG 19–19.
Hemangioma on 2-week-old neonate. This lesion is raised, with blue-red coloration.

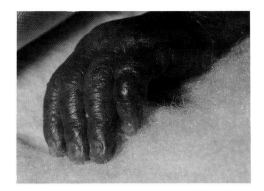

FIG 19–20.
Hemangioma developing on finger of premature infant.

cardiac decompensation. Platelet trapping (Kasabach-Merritt syndrome) occurs within the sluggish circulation of the raised hemangioma. It usually occurs in patients with a single large hemangioma, primarily within the first 6 months of life. Platelet trapping produces easy bruising and petechiae on areas of the body not involved with hemangioma and may progress to frank hemorrhage. Often the involved hemangioma will suddenly enlarge and become very firm at the onset of the platelet trapping.

Obstruction of the airway results in respiratory stridor and is usually due to subglottic hemangiomas. Infants with such hemangiomas usually have multiple hemangiomas of the skin of the head and neck. Visual acuity disturbances may occur either by growth of the hemangioma within the orbit, causing compression of the eyeball, or by swelling around the eyelid, forcing the lid to close and obstructing vision. Large, raised heman-

giomas may pool sufficient blood to produce high-output cardiac failure. Internal hemangioma may occur with or without cutaneous lesions.

Differential Diagnosis

Raised hemangiomas may be confused with pyogenic granulomas, malignant vascular tumors, and giant melanocytic birthmarks; the latter may be vascular at birth with little pigment production. Usually little confusion occurs, but occasionally a biopsy is needed to help distinguish such lesions.

Pathogenesis

Most raised hemangiomas are mixtures of dilated, proliferating capillaries and dilated venous channels. The biologic behavior of the cavernous and mixed types is similar in children, however. Blood flow through such lesions is sluggish and platelet aggregation can occur, followed by consumption of clotting factors in the Kasabach-Merritt syndrome.

Treatment

The indications for treatment are: obstruction of a vital orifice (airway, excretory channel), visual obstruction, platelet trapping syndrome, and cardiac decompensation. The treatment of choice is prednisone, 1 to 6 mg/kg/day. Alternate-day therapy may be sufficient. Treatment for 4 to 8 weeks is often necessary. Treatment initiated during the growing phase of the hemangioma (1 to 8 months of age) produces the best results. The mechanism of action of prednisone is unknown, but reduction of the capillary cell division by steroids has been postulated. X-ray therapy produces poor cosmetic results, and squamous cell and basal cell carcinomas subsequently develop within the areas of radiodermatitis. Surgical therapy results in significant blood loss and scarring. Newer methods of hemangioma control, such as the pulsed dye laser and the use of growth factors, are currently being tested.

There is often great pressure to treat for cosmetic reasons, but strict adherence to the indications for therapy are advised. Topical antibiotic or antiseptic agents will reduce secondary infection in ulcerated hemangiomas, but often oral anti-staphylococcal therapy may be necessary.

Patient Education

The rapid growth of the tumor often convinces parents that such lesions will not disap-

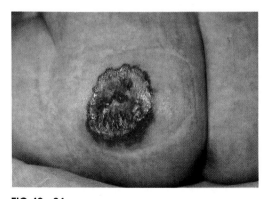

FIG 19–21.
Ulcerated hemangioma on buttock of infant.

pear. Careful explanation of the natural history of these lesions is necessary.

Follow-up Visits

Photographs and measurements are useful for following the progress of a raised hemangioma. In infants treated with prednisone, patients should be seen every 2 weeks during therapy to monitor progress and then monthly thereafter until the age of 1 year. In other infants, a single follow-up visit in 2 weeks will allow reinforcement of the concept that treatment is not required. Monthly or bimonthly follow-up visits are advised thereafter.

Cutis Marmorata Telangiectatica Congenita

Clinical Features

In cutis marmorata telangiectatica congenita, a mottled pattern of blue or dusky-red erythema is seen from birth (Fig 19–22). Often a single extremity is involved, but the lesions may occur bilaterally on the extremities or on the trunk. The skin surface overlying such areas may be depressed. A gradual increase in the size of lesions is expected during the first few years of life, but most lesions fade by adult life. Rigorous natural history studies of cutis marmorata telangiectatica congenita are not available. Associations with musculoskeletal or vascular abnormalities occur.

Differential Diagnosis

In contrast to cutis marmorata telangiectatica congenita, mottling of newborn skin is a transient vasodilation and is relieved by rewarming the

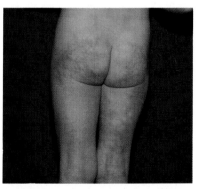

FIG 19–22.
Cutis marmorata telangiectatica congenita. Mottled areas of venous ectasia are still present on legs of this 4-year-old child.

skin. The livedo reticularis pattern of collagen vascular disease is flat, is not depressed over the discolored areas, is always bilateral, and is associated with systemic signs and symptoms.

Pathogenesis

The disorder is considered to be a vascular ectasia of veins and, possibly, of capillaries. Tortuous, dilated veins are found in the dermis and subcutaneous tissue on biopsy.

Treatment

There is no treatment. Routine evaluations should include close inspection of extremities for possible orthopedic deformity.

Patient Education

It should be explained that cutis marmorata telangiectatica congenita is a birthmark, and that some increase is expected in the area of skin involved. It should be emphasized that it is an unusual disorder and that few data are available for predicting its course. Associated deformities should be treated as necessary.

Follow-up Visits

Progress can be monitored during the usual neonatal follow-up visits.

Diffuse Neonatal Hemangiomatosis and Blue Rubber Bleb Nevus Syndrome

Clinical Features

This rare syndrome consists of multiple small, raised cutaneous hemangiomas that may or may not be associated with hemangiomas in the liver, lungs, gastrointestinal tract, and central nervous system (Figs 19–23 and 19–24). The raised hemangiomas may be present at birth, and more develop with time. The hemangiomas vary from 2 to 15 mm in diameter. Spontaneous involution of the lesions has been reported. Bleeding into the gastrointestinal tract may occur. The blue rubber bleb nevus syndrome is a rare disorder consisting of multiple cavernous hemangiomas of the skin and bowel. The lesions are blue and 3 to 4 cm in diameter.

Differential Diagnosis

The presence of skin hemangiomas is so characteristic that little difficulty in differential diagnosis is experienced. The lesions of blue rubber bleb nevus syndrome are compressible and

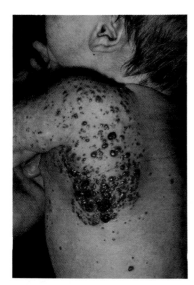

FIG 19-23.
Diffuse neonatal hemangiomatosis in 18-day-old infant.

may be painful or associated with excessive sweating. Monitoring stool samples for occult blood is helpful in identifying the presence of intestinal lesions.

Pathogenesis

Within the middermis, proliferating endothelial cells and numerous capillary lumina are observed. This syndrome has been reported in twins, but insufficient data are available to determine whether it is hereditary. The blue rubber bleb nevus syndrome lesions are more similar to cavernous hemangiomas.

Treatment

Infants with diffuse neonatal hemangiomatosis who develop complications may respond to prednisone at a dose of 2 to 6 mg/kg/day with appropriate attention to side effects. The duration of treatment may exceed 8 to 12 weeks. The blue rubber bleb nevus lesions are not responsive to systemic therapy and may require surgical resection. Frequent stool guaiac examinations will identify intestinal bleeding.

Lymph Vessel Birthmarks: Lymphangiomas

Clinical Features

Lymphangiomas may be circumscribed, superficial skin papules (Figs 19-25 and 19-26) or deep, cavernous nodules. Circumscribed lymphangiomas appear as a solitary group of 2- to 4-mm gelatinous skin-colored papules limited to a skin area less than 10 cm in diameter. They are often connected to underlying venous channels, and hemorrhage into one or more papules may occur, producing sudden darkening. They may be present at birth, but are often not noticed until late infancy or childhood.

Cavernous lymphangiomas are rubbery, skin-colored nodules that may result in grotesque enlargement of soft tissues. They are usually solitary and involve the face, trunk, and extremities. They are particularly common in the parotid area, where they are called *cystic hygromas*. They may have a rapid growth phase similar to that of raised hemangiomas.

Differential Diagnosis

Circumscribed lymphangioma may be mistaken for a disorder with grouped vesicles, such

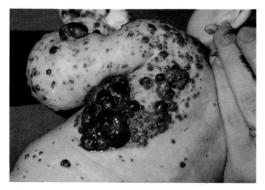

FIG 19-24.
Infant in Fig 19-20 at 30 days of age. Note rapid enlargement of size of lesions and multiple lesions on back and arm.

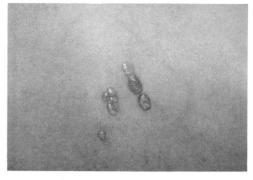

FIG 19-25.
Lymphangioma circumscriptum. Grouping of gelatinous skin-colored papules on abdomen.

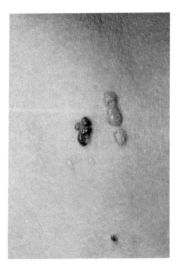

FIG 19–26.
Lymphangioma circumscriptum. After minor trauma lesions may darken, resulting from bleeding into lesion.

as herpes simplex, herpes zoster, or dermatitis herpetiformis. There is no erythematous base in circumscribed lymphangioma, however, and the lesions appear gelatinous, not fluid filled. As noted, hemorrhage into such lesions results in darkening, which may be confused with malignant melanoma.

Cavernous lymphangiomas may be confused with lipomas, neurofibromas, and other soft subcutaneous masses.

Pathogenesis
Dilated, tortuous lymph vessels appear within the dermis and subcutaneous fat. Most often, many channels are found spreading from the original lesion, so that the skin surface change reflects only the tip of a triangular lesion. Cavernous lymphangiomas may involve the muscle as well.

Treatment
There is no satisfactory treatment. Surgical excision can result in defects two or three times larger than the observed skin lesion, and the recurrence rate is high. Often the lymph channels are found to surround vital subcutaneous structures, such as major arteries or nerves. The lesions are not responsive to radiotherapy or systemic steroids.

Patient Education
The nature of these lymph vessel birthmarks should be explained.

Follow-up Visits
Monthly or bimonthly visits in which photographs of the lesions are taken and careful measurements made are indicated initially. Eventually semiannual or annual visits are sufficient to evaluate and commence therapy for complications.

Pigment Cell Birthmarks: Mongolian Spots (See chapter 16)

Infants' skin is always light at birth and becomes progressively darker with increasing age. Hyperpigmentation of the scrotum and of the linea alba is common in dark-skinned infants at birth. The most commonly observed pigmentary abnormality of infants is the mongolian spot.

Clinical Features
Mongolian spots are blue-black macules found in the lumbosacral area in up to 90% of Oriental, black, and American Indian babies (Fig 19–27). They are occasionally noted on the shoulders and back and may extend to the buttocks and extremities. Mongolian spots fade somewhat with time, and the difference in pigmentation from normal skin pigment becomes less obvious as the newborn's pigment darkens. Some traces of mongolian spots may persist into adult life.

Pathogenesis
Mongolian spots consist of spindle-shaped pigment cells located deep within the dermis. The precise mechanism of this condition is not known.

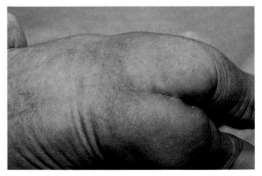

FIG 19–27.
Mongolian spot on buttock of neonate.

Pigment Cell Birthmarks: Café Au Lait Spots

Light-brown, oval macules that may appear more dark brown on black skin are found anywhere on the body and are designated *café au lait spots*. Black infants are far more likely (120/1,000 live births) than white infants (3/1,000 live births) to have a solitary café au lait spot. Café au lait spots persist through childhood and may increase in number with age. The presence of six or more larger than 0.5 cm at their greatest diameter is considered by most authorities as a major clue to neurofibromatosis type 1 in prepubertal children (see Chapter 16).

Pigment Cell Birthmarks: Junctional Nevocellular Nevi

Dark-brown or black macules with distinct borders represent clones of melanocytes found at the junction of the epidermis and dermis, and are designated *junctional nevocellular nevi*. As an infant ages, these nevi may become slightly raised and papular and develop intradermal melanocytes, creating a compound nevus. Often the surface of the lesion at birth is slightly irregular.

Pigment Cell Birthmarks: Raised Nevocellular Nevi

Clinical Features

Skin-colored to tan or brown solitary papules with smooth surfaces represent intradermal nevi. Most nevi are small, measuring less than 1.5 cm at their greatest diameter. When these localized, raised pigment cell lesions are more than 10 or 20 cm at their greatest diameter, there is a concern about their cancer potential (Figs 19–28 and 19–29). Malignant melanoma may occur in such large nevi. The precise estimate of cancer potential is unknown, but most authorities accept 1% or less.

Pathogenesis

The cause of large, pigmented nevi is not known. There is no correlation with twinning, infant sex, parental consanguinity, parental age, birth order, radiation exposure, or drug intake. They are more common in black infants.

Treatment

Prophylactic removal of large congenital nevi within the first year of life has been recom-

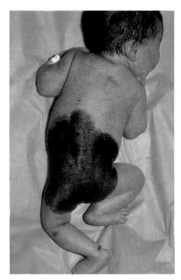

FIG 19–28.
Giant congenital nevus in bathing trunk distribution.

mended by many authorities, although the best age for removal is unknown. Equal weight should be placed on the potential for cosmetic improvement and the cosmetic deformity produced by such surgical removal. Optimal surgical results may be best when the child is older. Whether smaller lesions have any malignant potential and require removal is not known.

Hypopigmentation

Localized areas of hypopigmented skin are uncommon in infants. A hypopigmented area of skin is found in approximately 8/1,000 live births, and a hypopigmented tuft of hair is found in 3/

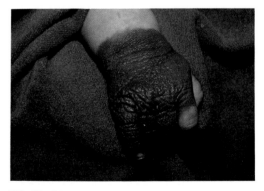

FIG 19–29.
Congenital nevus on hand of infant.

1,000 live births (see also Chapter 16 for piebaldism and hypomelanosis of Ito).

Hypopigmentation: Albinism

Clinical Features

Seven types of oculocutaneous albinism occur. Typically the newborns with albinism have fine, white hair and pink skin at birth. They may also have nevi present at birth that are raised but not pigmented. Severe nystagmus and photophobia may also be present at birth.

Differential Diagnosis

An erroneous diagnosis of albinism may be made in fair-skinned infants and infants with phenylketonuria as well as Chediak-Higashi syndrome. The presence of nystagmus often helps distinguish albinism.

Pathogenesis

The most common form of albinism involves a lack of tyrosinase, the enzyme necessary for the production of melanin. Other subtypes of albinism have tyrosinase present, but melanin formation is nevertheless impaired or slow.

Hypopigmentation: Phenylketonuria

Clinical Features

Newborns with phenylketonuria have blond hair, blue eyes, and light-colored skin. Routine screening tests for the presence of excessive amounts of phenylalanine in the blood will help detect this syndrome.

Differential Diagnosis

Phenylketonuria should be distinguished from albinism and Chediak-Higashi syndrome. Analysis of blood for phenylalanine is the most useful differentiating test.

Pathogenesis

Patients with phenylketonuria lack the enzymes needed to utilize phenylalanine. Their hypopigmentation is thought to be related to the tight binding of phenylalanine to the receptor sites of tyrosinase to the extent that the enzyme cannot oxidize phenylalanine to melanin.

Epidermal Birthmarks: Epidermal Nevi

Increases in mature epidermal cells, hair follicles, or sebaceous glands may appear as birthmarks. The majority of lesions are present at birth, but new lesions can develop up to the time of adolescence.

Clinical Features

These lesions have a warty surface and appear anywhere on the body (Fig 19–30). They are often linear or oval with the long axis of the lesion parallel to the long axis of the dermatome (Fig 19–31). The majority of lesions are present at birth, and up to 95% of the lesions are present by 7 years of age. Initially the lesion is barely palpable and may be a confluence of smooth-topped papules. In time the lesion becomes more wartlike and scaly (Fig 19–32). Most are 2 to 5 cm in length, but occasionally they may appear as long unilateral streaks involving an entire extremity or one side of the trunk (nevus unius lateris). The lesions may be so extensive as to involve most of the body. The terms *ichthyosis hystrix* or *benign congenital acanthosis nigricans* have been applied to such extensive epidermal nevi. Epidermal nevi may become erythematous and itchy with episodes of redness and inflammation, and may be designated *inflammatory linear verrucous epidermal nevi (ILVEN).*

Patients with epidermal nevi may have associated abnormalities. They have an increased number of cutaneous lesions, including café au lait spots, congenital hypopigmented macules, and congenital nevocellular nevi. They may have associated skeletal defects, seizure disorders, mental retardation, and ocular abnormalities. Patients

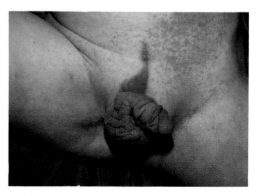

FIG 19–30.
Epidermal nevus. Unilateral lesion on right side of penis, scrotum, and pubic skin.

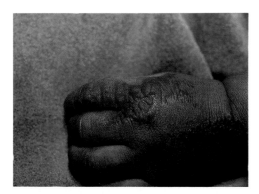

FIG 19–31.
Epidermal nevus. Linear hyperpigmented lesion on dorsum of hand. Some areas of lesion are smooth with a waxlike appearance.

with more extensive skin involvement have a higher association of other abnormalities than those with limited skin involvement.

Differential Diagnosis

Warts are commonly confused with epidermal nevi. The presence from birth and the linear arrangement will help distinguish epidermal nevi from warts. Extensive lesions may be confused with ichthyosis, and certain features of congenital bullous ichthyosiform erythroderma may exactly mimic epidermal nevi. Some investigators believe that congenital bullous ichthyosiform erythroderma is a variant of epidermal nevi. Inflammatory linear epidermal nevi may be confused with the warty stage of incontinentia pigmenti, with lichen striatus, or with a dermatitis.

Pathogenesis

Epidermal nevi show thickening of the epidermis and hyperkeratosis. In some lesions a pe-

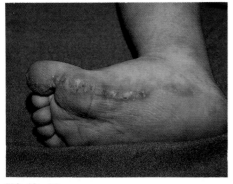

FIG 19–32.
Epidermal nevus on plantar aspect of foot.

culiar vacuolization of the granular layer appears, with separation of the cells in that layer, resulting in a microscopic blister cavity. This process is called epidermolytic hyperkeratosis. In inflammatory lesions, dermal accumulation of inflammatory cells and alternating bands of parakeratosis are described. Overgrowth of sebaceous glands and apocrine glands may be found underlying the epidermal proliferation.

Treatment

For small lesions, surgical excision is the best treatment. Extensive lesions may be improved with the use of mild keratolytics, such as retinoic acid cream 0.05% once daily, 12% ammonium lactate lotion several times a day, or with bland lubricant therapy. The lesions revert to their hyperkeratotic state when treatments are discontinued.

Patient Education

It should be emphasized to parents that this birthmark may be a clue to internal problems. Infants with extensive lesions should have careful neurologic examinations and x-ray examination of bone to detect skeletal lesions. A birth defect clinic may be a good referral source for a multidisciplinary approach to such infants.

Follow-up Visits

The frequency of follow-up visits is determined by the severity of the associated problems.

Epidermal Birthmarks: Sebaceous Nevi

Clinical Features

Jadassohn's sebaceous nevus appears at birth as a slightly raised oval or linear area with a yellow or orange color (Figs 19–33 to 19–35). These nevi are common on the scalp and are devoid of hair, producing a congenital circumscribed hair loss. They may be seen on the face as well. Sebaceous nevus may be contiguous with an epidermal nevus and constitute part of the epidermal nevus syndrome. At puberty, or with androgenic stimulation, sebaceous nevi enlarge and become warty on the surface and raised (Fig 19–36). Basal cell carcinomas will develop within the lesions after puberty in approximately 15% of children with sebaceous nevi.

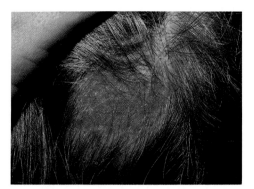

FIG 19–33.
Nevus sebaceus. Orange lesion on scalp of infant.

Differential Diagnosis

Juvenile xanthogranulomas and xanthomas are yellow or orange lesions that may mimic sebaceous nevus. Skin biopsy will distinguish them.

Pathogenesis

Sebaceous nevus is a birthmark with an increased number of sebaceous glands without hair follicles. Such lesions often have an increased number of apocrine glands as well.

Treatment

Surgical excision during puberty is the treatment of choice because of the risk of basal cell carcinoma after puberty and for improved cosmetic appearance. Lesions excised before puberty

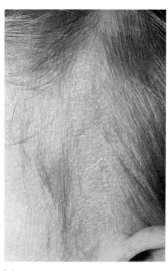

FIG 19–34.
Nevus sebaceus. Linear, yellow lesion on scalp of infant.

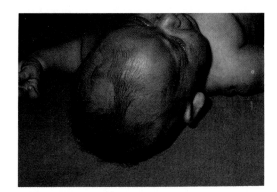

FIG 19–35.
Nevus sebaceus. Large orange lesions on scalp of newborn.

may be incompletely excised and demonstrate warty growth along the surgical scar.

Patient Education

The nature of this birthmark should be explained. The possibility that skin cancer may develop should be emphasized.

Follow-up Visits

Follow-up visits should be as usual for newborn care.

Epidermal Birthmarks: Nevus Comedonicus

Clinical Features

In nevus comedonicus, linear or oval groups of widely dilated follicular openings plugged with keratin are present at birth on the face and scalp (Fig 19–37). They may become inflamed and pus-

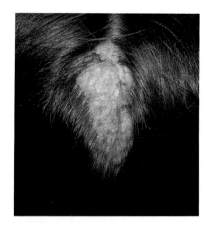

FIG 19–36.
Nevus sebaceus after puberty. Warty, raised growth on scalp.

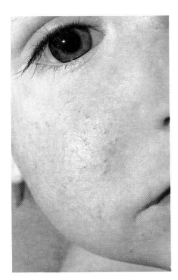

FIG 19–37.
Nevus comedonicus on cheek of child.

tular as the child ages and may mimic acne. Bilateral and widespread lesions occur rarely.

Differential Diagnosis

In contrast to nevus comedonicus, neonatal acne begins at 1 month of age and involves discrete, single lesions rather than grouped arrangements of lesions.

Pathogenesis

Nevus comedonicus is a birthmark consisting of pilosebaceous follicles with patulous openings.

Treatment

In small lesions, simple surgical excision is the treatment of choice. Large or extensive lesions may be controlled with the application of topical retinoic acid cream once or twice daily.

Patient Education

It should be explained that this is a birthmark containing pilosebaceous follicles and is not necessarily related to acne.

Follow-up Visits

Follow-up can be made on routine neonatal care visits.

Aplasia Cutis Congenita

Clinical Features

In aplasia cutis congenita, oval, sharply marginated, 1- to 2-cm depressed areas are seen pri-

marily in the midline of the posterior aspect of the scalp (Fig 19–38). They are hairless, may appear as an ulcer, or are covered by a smooth, finely wrinkled epithelial membrane. Ulcerated defects heal with scar formation. Aplasia cutis congenita is a developmental defect rather than a true birthmark. It occurs in 1 per 3,000 live births. Other developmental defects, such as cleft palate or lip, syndactyly, absence of digits, and congenital heart disease, may be associated. It may be seen as an autosomal dominant trait in some families or may be associated with dystrophic forms of epidermolysis bullosa. Although the majority of lesions appear on the scalp, lesions may be found on the trunk, face, or proximal extremities.

Differential Diagnosis

Scalp ulcers at birth may be mistaken for obstetric trauma, although a careful history will distinguish between the two. Other forms of congenital circumscribed hair loss should be considered.

Pathogenesis

Aplasia cutis congenita represents a developmental failure of skin fusion. Dermis, epidermis, and fat all may be missing, or single layers may be absent.

Treatment

If the lesion is small, surgical excision, with mobilization of the scalp and simple closure, will correct the hairless defect. Hair transplantation has been successful in large defects.

Patient Education

Explanation of the failure to form certain layers of skin will help parents understand that this

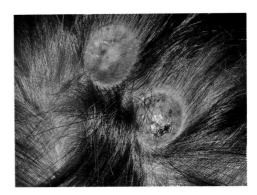

FIG 19–38.
Aplasia cutis congenita. Two oval lesions on scalp of child.

lesion does not represent mishandling of the child during the birth process.

Follow-up Visits

Follow-up visits as necessary for routine newborn care are advised.

Connective Tissue Birthmarks

Connective tissue nevi are skin lesions consisting predominantly of the elements of extracellular collagen tissue and products of fibroblasts, such as collagen, elastin, and proteoglycans. All connective tissue nevi are quite rare, although the precise incidence is not known.

Clinical Features

Connective tissue nevi are localized areas of thickened skin appearing as multiple skin-colored papules and plaques (Fig 19–39). Stretching the overlying skin will give a yellowish discoloration to the areas. They may occasionally have increased vascularity and appear red. Collagenomas are localized areas of thickened skin with multiple skin-colored papules or plaques. They may be solitary or appear in a zosteriform segmental pattern. Elastomas are solitary plaques that are present at birth and contain increases in both elastic tissue and proteoglycans. Elastomas may be solitary or they may be multiple in the Buschke-Ollendorff syndrome. This autosomal dominant syndrome appears as symmetrically distributed skin-colored papules or nodules with a predilection for the lower part of the trunk or for the extremities. Lesions may assume a thickened appearance of skin and develop a lacy pattern on the trunk. X-ray films may show sclerotic densities of the ends of long bones, pelvis, and hands, although such lesions are often asymptomatic. The shagreen patch of tuberous sclerosis is a connective tissue nevus. The nevi are subtle at birth and may go unnoticed. They tend to persist throughout life.

Differential Diagnosis

Connective tissue nevi are so characteristic that they are seldom misdiagnosed. Examinations for possible associated systemic disease may be necessary.

Pathogenesis

Connective tissue nevi show thickened, abundant collagen bundles with or without associated increases in elastic tissue. Such histologic changes are difficult to appreciate unless the skin biopsy specimen includes adjacent normal skin for comparison.

Treatment

Treatment is unnecessary.

Patient Education

Connective tissue nevus is a birthmark consisting of collagen or elastin, or both, and it should be emphasized that such lesions can occur related or unrelated to systemic or genetic disease. In the absence of associated disease, the connective tissue nevus does not represent a serious problem.

Follow-up Visits

Follow-up visits are unnecessary except for routine neonatal visits.

COMMON CONGENITAL MALFORMATIONS THAT INVOLVE SKIN

Congenital malformations involving the skin are frequently observed in newborns. They are observed in 7 per 100 live births.

Ear Anomalies

Minor abnormalities in the formation of the ear constitute the most common congenital malformations. Loss of the fold of the skin in the superior part of the helix is the most common. Low-set ears that angle away from the eye, periauricular skin tags (Fig 19–40), auricular or preauricu-

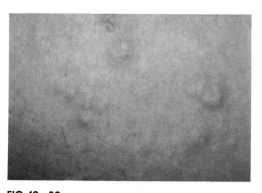

FIG 19–39.
Connective tissue nevus. Raised, skin-colored papules grouped on sacrum.

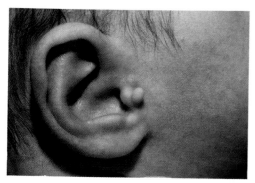

FIG 19–40.
Preauricular skin tag in infant.

lar pits, or auricular sinuses or small ears, or both, are less common. Deafness may accompany congenital malformations of the external ear, or the malformations may be associated with hemifacial microsomia (Goldenhar's syndrome).

Digital Abnormalities

A single crease on one or both upper palms called a *simian crease,* occurs in 2 per 100 live births. It is one feature of Down's syndrome, but also may be observed in a variety of other syndromes, including trisomy 13, the Cornelia de Lange syndrome, Seckel's syndrome, and the cri du chat syndrome. Clinodactyly with inward curvature of a digit is often observed in the fifth finger, and overlapping of the second and third toes is also a frequently observed malformation. Partial or complete fusion (syndactyly) of the second or third toes and clubfoot also occur with relative frequency.

Genital Abnormalities

Hydrocele of one testis and hypospadias are the most common genital anomalies and malformations observed. Malformations of the external genitalia may be clues to urinary tract anomalies, and investigation of the urinary tract may be indicated. They may also be clues to chromosomal abnormalities and may be associated with undescended testes.

Epicanthal Folds

Epicanthal folds of skin on the inner aspect of each eye are frequently observed. They are present in chromosomal abnormalities such as Down's, Turner's, and Klinefelter's syndromes.

Neural Tube Defects

Primary defects in neural tube closures, such as meningomyelocele, encephalocele, and anencephaly, are relatively frequent congenital malformations. In some instances, a tuft of hair that is longer and more pigmented than the adjacent scalp hair overlies the affected area of skull and is a cutaneous clue to an underlying neural tube defect.

Abnormalities of the Lip and Mouth

Pits in the lips have been described in 2 per 100 live births. Cleft lip and cleft palate, or cleft lip alone, are less common. The finding of lip pits and cleft lips or cleft palate, or both, may be a clue to the so-called first arch syndrome, which includes a small jaw and ocular hypertelorism. A number of syndromes are associated with the first arch syndrome, including the Pierre Robin syndrome, the orodigitofacial syndromes, and the Treacher Collins syndrome.

Skin Dimpling

Infants may develop small dimplelike, depressed scars resulting from injury during amniocentesis procedures. The skin covering the lesion appears to be pulled in by absent dermis. The lesion may not be noticed until the infant is several months old and has developed additional subcutaneous fat.

Major Chromosomal Abnormalities

Chromosomal abnormalities occur in 1 of 200 of all live births, in a higher percentage of births resulting in perinatal death, and in up to 50% of spontaneous abortions.

Trisomy 21 (Down's Syndrome)

Trisomy 21 is seen in 1 in 800 live births. Mothers more than 40 years of age have an increased chance of giving birth to a child with Down's syndrome. Cutaneous features are most useful in the recognition of this syndrome. These include prominent epicanthal folds, eyes slanting upward, small ears, simian palmar crease, excessive skin on the back of the neck, and clinodactyly of the fifth fingers. These cutaneous features, plus muscular hypotonia and evidence of congenital heart disease, are the major clinical characteristic. Chromosomal analysis will confirm the diagnosis. Mental retardation may be severe, and growth failure associated with congenital heart disease makes the prognosis poor.

Trisomy 18 and Trisomy 13–15

Trisomy 18 is observed in 1 per 3,000 live births, and trisomy 13–15 occurs in 1 per 5,000 live births. In both of these chromosomal abnormalities, increased parental age has been an associated feature. Babies with trisomy 18 or trisomy 13–15 are small for gestational age, have low-set ears, simian creases, congenital heart disease, and severe mental retardation. The presence of cleft lip and cleft palate associated with these features makes trisomy 13–15 more likely to be diagnosed, while rocker-bottom feet and flexion contractures of the fingers make trisomy 18 more likely. Chromosomal analysis is required for precise diagnosis.

Turner's Syndrome

The most common sex chromosome anomaly is Turner's syndrome, in which only one X chromosome is present (XO). Newborns with Turner's syndrome exhibit webbing of the neck and marked edema of the hands and feet. The neck is often quite short. Coarctation of the aorta may be associated. Chromosomal analysis is necessary to confirm the diagnosis.

Klinefelter's Syndrome

Extra sex chromosomes are characteristic of Klinefelter's syndrome (XXY, XXXY, XXXXY). A low birth weight, undescended testes, and a small penis lead to suspicion of this syndrome. Hypotonia and a variety of other anomalies may also be observed. Mental deficiency is usually severe in this syndrome, and chromosomal analysis is required to confirm the diagnosis.

Ichthyosis

Ichthyosis is a term used to describe excessive scaling of the skin, which may be "fish scale–like." Although normal infants born after 40 to 42 weeks of gestation will display some scaling, as will the dysmature infant, the scaling in the form of ichthyosis is usually generalized and characterized by thick scales. Four major types of ichthyosis have been described. Lamellar ichthyosis and bullous ichthyosis usually are seen at birth with severe scaling. Ichthyosis vulgaris and X-linked ichthyosis may be present in the neonate or may appear later in childhood.

Clinical Features

Ichthyosis Vulgaris.—Ichthyosis vulgaris is inherited as an autosomal dominant disease that may be as frequent as 1 in 250 children. Fine scales usually become prominent by 6 months to 2 years of age. The scales are most prominent on the lower legs (Fig 19–41) and buttocks. Dry, follicular, horny plugs (keratosis pilaris) may be extensive. Palms and soles show an increased number of skin creases. The entire skin surface is dry. Occasionally children may have associated atopic dermatitis, which may be more difficult to treat. The skin in ichthyosis vulgaris usually remains normal throughout the newborn period.

X-Linked Ichthyosis.—X-linked ichthyosis may appear at birth but usually is first seen in infancy with scales on the posterior aspect of the neck, upper part of the trunk, and extensor surfaces of the extremities (Fig 19–42). As the child ages, the scales often become thicker and a dirty-

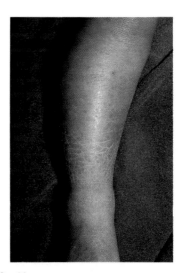

FIG 19–41.
Ichthyosis vulgaris. Prominent scales on lower legs.

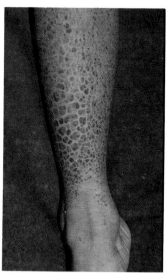

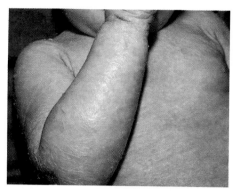

FIG 19–43.
Lamellar ichthyosis. Thickened, shiny skin without erythema in child.

FIG 19–42.
X-linked ichthyosis. Large, dark, platelike scales on lower leg.

yellow or brown color. Scaling is usually mild during the first 30 days of life, and the skin is a normal color. Corneal opacities may be seen on slit lamp examination of the eyes of adults, both in patients and the carrier mothers. Palms and soles are spared, in contrast to the other forms of ichthyosis. An associated steroid sulfatase deficiency has been described with X-linked ichthyosis.

Lamellar Ichthyosis and Congenital Nonbullous Ichthyosiform Erythroderma.— These two names are often used for the same condition. Although both conditions appear to be an autosomal recessive trait, two separate disease entities may exist. The nonbullous congenital ichthyosiform erythroderma patients have generalized fine scales on erythematous skin. The lamellar ichthyosis patients have larger, darker, platelike scales with or without erythematosus skin. Infants with either condition can be born with a collodion membrane. The erythroderma may fade during childhood in some of the infants (Fig 19–43). Ectropion and eclabium may be present and appear shortly after birth in patients with lamellar ichthyosis. The palms and soles in these patients may be greatly thickened. Skin biopsy after the collodion membrane is shed will demonstrate hyperkeratosis but is otherwise not diagnostic.

Bullous Ichthyosis (Congenital Bullous Ichthyosiform Erythroderma, Epidermolytic Hyperkeratosis).—Epidermolytic hyperkeratosis, an autosomal dominant disorder, is characterized by extensive scaling at birth, erythroderma, and recurrent episodes of bullae formation (Figs 19–44 to 19–46). The blisters represent lysis of the epidermal granular layer, and secondary infection with *S. aureus* becomes a major difficulty in the neonatal period and during infancy. As the child ages the involvement becomes more limited in extent. By school age, thick, warty, dirty-yellow scales with malodorous excessive bacterial colonization of the skin will have developed on the palms, soles, elbows, and knees (Fig 19–47). Skin biopsy will reveal enlargement of the granular cell layer with bizarre vacuolization of the epidermal granular cells.

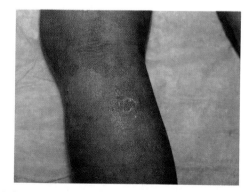

FIG 19–44.
Epidermolytic hyperkeratosis. Thickened skin with infected ruptured bullae.

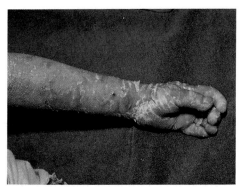

FIG 19–45.
Epidermolytic hyperkeratosis. Thickened skin with large areas of erosion.

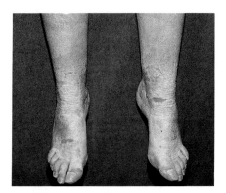

FIG 19–47.
Epidermolytic hyperkeratosis. Thick, malodorous skin on ankles.

Differential Diagnosis

At birth, lamellar ichthyosis and bullous ichthyosis may be difficult to distinguish from one another. The hereditary pattern and skin biopsy may help. As the infants age, the corneal opacities and sparing of the palms and soles will distinguish X-linked ichthyosis, the ectropion and eclabium will distinguish lamellar ichthyosis, and the recurrent bullous episodes will distinguish epidermolytic hyperkeratosis. Measurement of steroid sulfatase activity in red blood cells may be useful in the diagnosis of X-linked ichthyosis.

Ichthyosis vulgaris in its mild form may be difficult to distinguish from dry skin, but the extensive distribution of scales, particularly scaling on the buttocks, increased palmar creases, and skin biopsy, will differentiate ichthyosis vulgaris from dry skin. Scaling disorders similar to lamellar ichthyosis are present in many ichthyosis syndromes associated with neurologic disease.

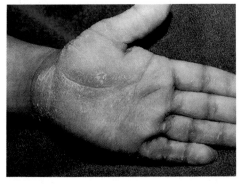

FIG 19–46.
Epidermolytic hyperkeratosis. Hyperkeratosis of palms and fissures at flexural creases.

Pathogenesis

Skin biopsy in the ichthyosis syndromes will often be of diagnostic value. In ichthyosis vulgaris there is a thin or absent granular cell layer in addition to the hyperkeratosis. X-linked ichthyosis demonstrates hyperkeratosis with an otherwise normal-appearing epidermis. Vacuolization and separation of the granular cell layer and blister cavity formation are associated with the hyperkeratosis in bullous ichthyosis. Lamellar ichthyosis may demonstrate hyperkeratosis, acanthosis, and a mild chronic inflammatory infiltrate.

Increased epidermal turnover has been demonstrated in lamellar ichthyosis and bullous ichthyosis, such that excessive numbers of stratum corneum cells are produced. In contrast, X-linked ichthyosis and ichthyosis vulgaris demonstrate normal epidermal turnover, and the accumulated scale is believed to be due to faulty shedding of the stratum corneum. The role of the associated steroid sulfatase deficiency in X-linked ichthyosis is not known.

Treatment

There is no satisfactory treatment for the ichthyosis. In ichthyosis vulgaris and X-linked ichthyosis, hydration of the skin twice daily and the generous use of lubricants will control the dryness and scaling. The use of α-hydroxy acids, such as lactic acid 5% ointment, citric acid 5% ointment, or 12% ammonium lactate lotion (Lac-Hydrin), applied once or more daily, may be helpful in the more severe ichthyoses, although many such patients do as well with bland lubricants alone. In bullous ichthyoses systemic antistaphylococcal antibiotics are required to treat the bullous impetigo in the ichthyosis episodes.

Great caution must be used in applying any therapy to the skin of an infant or child. Because of the larger surface area per body weight, systemic toxicity and side effects can be seen in infants and children, and acidosis can occur as a result of topical therapy. Recognize that both the active medication and the vehicle for the medication could cause significant toxicity in the infant with significant dermatitis or even in the infant with normal skin.

The synthetic retinoids given orally have shown promise in management of ichthyosis, but their use is still experimental.

Patient Education

The genetic nature of the ichthyoses should be emphasized, as well as the methods of controlling these disorders. Good supportive relationships should be established with these patients.

Follow-up Visits

A visit 1 week after discharge from the newborn nursery is useful in evaluating therapy. Thereafter, routine visits for pediatric care and additional visits may be necessary depending on the severity of the ichthyosis.

CHRONIC SKIN CONDITIONS THAT BEGIN IN THE NEWBORN PERIOD

Red, Scaly Newborn

Physiologic Scaling and Redness.—A scaling and often red newborn may be an enigma to the inexperienced observer. A postmature baby may exhibit desquamation that is marked on the hands, feet, and lower part of the trunk, and, if observed during the first day of life when the newborn skin is quite red, may result in an erroneous diagnosis of one of the ichthyoses. Similarly, preterm infants born at 32 weeks of gestational age or earlier will have red or glistening skin that similarly may be confused with ichthyosis. Such changes are transient and are often resolved within the newborn period.

Collodion Baby.—Newborns with an encasement of shiny, tight, inelastic scale are designated as having a collodion membrane (Fig 19–48). The membrane is composed of greatly

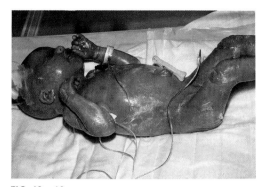

FIG 19–48.
Collodion baby. Erythematous, tight, shiny skin that has been treated with a thick covering of white petrolatum.

thickened stratum corneum that has been saturated with water. As the water content evaporates in extrauterine life, large fissures appear in the membrane and the membrane is shed, revealing red skin underneath. The presence of a collodion membrane does not allow one to predict that the affected baby will necessarily develop ichthyosis, and spontaneous healing may occur. Skin biopsy of the collodion membrane is usually not diagnostic. Most collodion babies do have a form of ichthyosis, and the majority of them develop features of lamellar ichthyosis. Initial presentation as collodion babies has also been reported in bullous ichthyosis, X-linked ichthyosis, and Gaucher's disease.

Harlequin Fetus.—Although harlequin fetus has been considered a more severe form of lamellar ichthyosis, most authorities now believe that it represents a distinct, rare autosomal recessive disease. Harlequin fetus is usually incompatible with extrauterine life. At presentation the infant has massive, dense, platelike scales that produce severe deformities of skeletal and soft tissues, restricting respiration. This has been associated with defects in both lipid and protein metabolism. Recently infants treated with heroic methods have survived with residual severe ichthyosis.

Atopic Dermatitis and Seborrheic Dermatitis

Atopic dermatitis is said to have its onset after the newborn period, with the most frequently observed age of onset being 2 to 3 months. If a dermatitis begins within the newborn period, many authorities designate it *seborrheic dermatitis*. It has now become clear, however, that infants who later develop typical atopic dermatitis may have the onset of their skin eruption within the newborn period. There is significant overlap in infants who have seborrheic and atopic dermatitis, both in distributions of the lesions, which involve the scalp, diaper area, and extensor area, and in the history of pruritus, feeding patterns, food intolerance, and family members with atopic disease. Physiologic overproduction of sebum occurs in the newborn period, giving any dermatitis a greasy feel to the skin surface. It is advisable to designate dermatitis seen in newborns as simply *dermatitis* (see also Chapter 4).

Diaper Dermatitis

Diaper dermatitis occurring in the newborn period is primarily perianal in location and is related to the irritant substances found in stool. Superinfection with *Candida albicans* is frequent in any diaper dermatitis present for more than 72 hours.

Scabies

Infants with scabies may have a generalized dermatitis at initial presentation. They may have only a few or as many as thousands of lesions. Infants usually have involvement of the head and neck. Individual burrows may be obscured and difficult to detect because of the confluence of dermatitis. The scabies mite can be recovered from papules or burrows, with the hands and feet the best sites of recovery.

Histiocytosis X

A generalized dermatitis, particularly that with purpuric papules or petechiae within the dermatitis and involvement of the head and neck, is characteristic of histiocytosis X. The skin eruption may be present at birth, and the presence of chronic draining ears and enlargement of the liver and spleen are useful additional clues in the diagnosis. Skin biopsy will demonstrate the characteristic infiltration with histiocytic cells containing Langerhans-like granules (see also Chapter 12).

Congenital Candidiasis

The presenting symptom of congenital candidiasis may be generalized eczematous skin. Maternal infection of the birth canal with *Candida* is always present. Direct microscopic examination of scales scraped from the skin's surface will demonstrate yeast forms.

Epidermolysis Bullosa

Diagnosis of epidermolysis bullosa in the immediate newborn period may be quite difficult. Many different types of epidermolysis bullosa exist that result in mild to lethal disease (see Chapter 11). The final diagnosis of the disease is dependent on characterization of the site of blister formation within the epidermis, basement membrane, or dermis and the clinical response of the patient. Presence of few or many blisters in the neonate does not define the severity of the disease. Diagnosis should be made with a combination of both light and electron microscopic examination of biopsy specimens and possibly immunofluorescent mapping of antigenic sites within the basement membrane zone. Extreme care must be taken in obtaining and interpreting skin biopsy specimens from newborns to distinguish among these mechanobullous diseases. A shave or ellipse biopsy at the edge of a blister that is less than 12 hours old is preferred. Diagnosis and therapy assistance can be obtained through the National Epidermolysis Bullosa Registry Headquarters (Rockefeller University, 1230 York Ave., New York, NY 10021).

Incontinentia Pigmenti

Clinical Features

Linear rows of blisters on the extremities are seen in incontinentia pigmenti (Fig 19–49). These blistering episodes recur during the first 3 months of life and are replaced by warty linear areas that may last until 1 year of age (Fig 19–50). Rows of brown pigmentation are then left. In addition, swirls of brown pigmentation are found on the trunk and in areas where the blisters and warty lesions did not occur. The pigmentation fades as the child ages and is usually not seen after adolescence.

Incontinentia pigmenti is felt to be an X-linked trait, lethal to the male, which explains the female predominance in this disorder. Mental re-

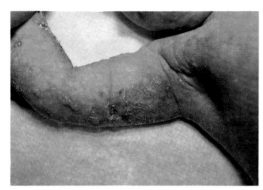

FIG 19–49.
Incontinentia pigmenti. Linear vesicles and crust in a neonate.

tardation, seizures, microcephaly, and other central nervous system disorders occur in 30% of the patients. Ocular and skeletal anomalies may also be noted.

Differential Diagnosis

In the blistering stage, herpes simplex or bullous impetigo may be confused with incontinentia pigmenti, but the linear arrangement of its blisters and appropriate cultures will distinguish it from these two disorders. The warty phase may mimic linear epidermal birthmarks or warts. The hyperpigmentation is uniquely arranged in whorls and is unlikely to be confused with other causes of hyperpigmentation.

Pathogenesis

Skin biopsy demonstrates an inflammatory dermatitis with subcorneal vesicles filled with nu-

merous eosinophils. The warty stage merely demonstrates hyperkeratosis and chronic inflammation in the dermis. In the pigmentary stage, melanin is found free in the dermis or engulfed by dermal macrophages, which accounts for the term *incontinentia pigmenti.* The etiology of this acute dermatitis and its peculiar linear arrangement is not known.

Treatment

There is no satisfactory treatment.

Patient Education

It should be emphasized that the disorder is inherited, and the expected future cutaneous stages should be described.

Follow-up Visits

Routine infant care visits should be scheduled. Additional visits may be necessary dependent on the complications that arise.

Acrodermatitis Enteropathica

Clinical Features

Acrodermatitis enteropathica is an autosomal recessive disorder of zinc metabolism. It is not apparent at birth but begins at 1 to 2 months of age, with acral skin erosions, diarrhea, and failure to thrive. The erosions appear as red, moist areas on the distal extremities, including the hands and feet, and in the perioral and perineal areas (Fig 19–51). Often the cutaneous features precede the diarrhea by several weeks to several months. As the disorder continues, weight loss occurs, as well

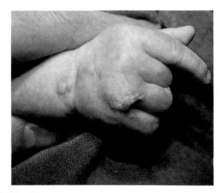

FIG 19–50.
Incontinentia pigmenti. Wartlike lesion on hand of 3-month-old infant.

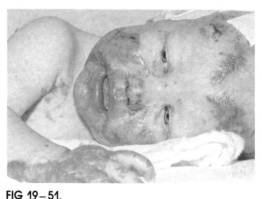

FIG 19–51.
Acrodermatitis enteropathica. Perioral erosions in infant who also had erosions of hands, feet, elbows, and knees.

as photophobia, apathy, alopecia, thrush, and paronychia resulting from *C. albicans* infection. If the child survives the infectious complications of malnutrition, the skin lesions become erythematous plaques with silvery scales that mimic psoriasis.

The diagnosis is made by measuring serum or plasma zinc levels. There are many sources of zinc contamination in rubber stoppers, glass tubes, and other blood-collecting devices that produce falsely high zinc levels. Thus the diagnosis may be obscured. Therefore, blood samples should be collected in acid-washed sterile plastic tubes with use of acid-washed plastic syringes.

Zinc deficiency can also be seen in premature and term infants who are fed a diet deficient in zinc. Occasionally human breast milk can be low in zinc, allowing zinc deficiency in the totally breast-fed infant.

Differential Diagnosis

The lesions are often mistaken for mucocutaneous candidiasis associated with immune deficiency. Plasma or serum zinc levels will distinguish between the two. Often protein-calorie malnutrition states are considered. Lesions usually develop in such patients after 6 months of age, and the nutritional history may distinguish between the two. Intertriginous erosions are the presenting symptoms of histiocytosis X in infancy. Acquired zinc deficiency states, such as seen with prolonged parenteral hyperalimentation, will mimic acrodermatitis enteropathica.

Pathogenesis

Depletion of body zinc stores due to faulty absorption of zinc is responsible for the symptoms and signs of acrodermatitis enteropathica. It is not known whether this depletion results from the lack of a zinc carrier protein or from some defect of zinc absorption in the intestine. Zinc is stored in the same tissues as iron and serves as an important cofactor for a variety of enzymes, such as alkaline phosphatase and carbonic anhydrase. It is believed that zinc deficiency results in impairment of metalloenzyme activity, which produces the clinical features.

Treatment

Oral zinc sulfate, 5 mg/kg/day given twice daily, produces rapid clinical improvement. Apathy disappears within 24 hours, and the skin lesions and diarrhea resolve within 7 to 14 days.

Photophobia, alopecia, and growth failure are reversed in the ensuing months.

Patient Education

The hereditary inability to absorb zinc should be explained. It is not known whether lifetime maintenance with supplemental zinc is required.

Follow-up Visits

A visit 2 weeks after diagnosis is useful to repeat zinc level determinations and to evaluate the response. The measurement of plasma or serum zinc levels at monthly intervals is useful for monitoring supplemental zinc requirements.

BIBLIOGRAPHY

Alper JC, Holmes LB: The incidence and significance of birthmarks in a cohort of 4,641 newborns. *Pediatr Dermatol* 1983; 1:58.

Amir J, Metzker A, Krikler R, Reisner SH: Strawberry hemangioma in preterm infants. *Pediatr Dermatol* 1986; 3:331.

Arlette JP: Zinc and the skin. *Pediatr Clin North Am* 1983; 30:583.

Barsky SH, Rosen S, Geer DE, et al: The nature and evolution of port-wine stains: A computer-assisted study. *J Invest Dermatol* 1980; 74:154.

Brice JEH: Congenital varicella resulting from infection during the second trimester of pregnancy. *Arch Dis Child* 1976; 51:474.

Bruce S, Duffy JO, Wolf JE: Skin dimpling associated with midtrimester amniocentesis. *Pediatr Dermatol* 1984; 2:140.

Burri B, Sweetman L, Nyhan WL: Mutant holocarboxylase synthetase: Evidence for the enzyme defect in early infantile biotin-responsive multiple carboxylase deficiency. *J Clin Invest* 1981; 68:1491.

Cantu JM, Gomez-Bustamente MO, Gonzales-Mendoza A: Familial comedones. *Arch Dermatol* 1978; 114:1807.

Carney RG, Jr: Incontinentia pigmenti. *Arch Dermatol* 1976; 112:535.

Castilla EE, et al: Epidemiology of congenital pigmented naevi: II. Risk factors. *Br J Dermatol* 1981; 104:307.

Curran FP, Al-Salihi FL: Neonatal staphylococcal scalded skin syndrome: Massive outbreak due to an unusual phage type. *Pediatrics* 1980; 66:285.

Dancer SJ, Simmons NA, Poston SM, et al: Outbreak of staphylococcal scalded skin syndrome among neonates. *J Infect* 1988; 16:87.

Dudgeon JA: Congenital rubella. *J Pediatr* 1975; 87:1078.

Duke EMC: Infantile acne associated with transient increases in plasma concentrations of leutinising hormone, follicle-stimulating hormone and testosterone. *Br Med J* 1981; 282:1275.

Eady RAJ, Tidman MJ: Diagnosing epidermolysis bullosa. *Br J Dermatol* 1983; 108:621.

Enjolras O, Riche MC, Merland JJ: Facial port-wine stains and Sturge-Weber syndrome. *Pediatrics* 1985; 76:48.

Esterly NB: Kasabach-Merritt syndrome in infants. *J Am Acad Dermatol* 1983; 8:504.

Esterly NB, Margileth AM, Kahn G, et al: Special symposia: The management of disseminated eruptive hemangiomata in infants. *Pediatr Dermatol* 1984; 1:313.

Fairley JA, Rasmussen JE: Comparison of stratum corneum thickness in children and adults. *J Am Acad Dermatol* 1983; 8:652.

Farber EM, Jacobs AH: Infantile psoriasis. *Am J Dis Child* 1977; 131:1266.

Fiumara NJ: Syphilis in newborn children. *Clin Obstet Gynecol* 1975; 18:183.

Flanagan BP, Helwig EB: Cutaneous lymphangioma. *Arch Dermatol* 1977; 113:24.

Fretzin DF, Arias AM: Sclerema neonatorum and subcutaneous fat necrosis of the newborn. *Pediatr Dermatol* 1987; 4:112.

Frieden IJ: Aplasia cutis congenita: A clinical review and proposal for classification. *J Am Acad Dermatol* 1986; 26:646.

Garden JM, Polla LL, Tan OT: The treatment of port-wine stains by the pulsed dye laser. *Arch Dermatol* 1988; 124:889.

Golitz LE, Rudikoff J, O'Meara OP: Diffuse neonatal hemangiomatosis. *Pediatr Dermatol* 1986; 3:145.

Hanshaw JB, Dudgeon JA: *Viral Diseases of the Fetus and Newborn*. Philadelphia, WB Saunders, 1978.

Harpin VA, Rutter N: Sweating in preterm babies. *J Pediatr* 1982; 100:614.

Hazell M, Marks R: Clinical, histologic, and cell kinetic discriminants between lamellar ichthyosis and nonbullous congenital ichthyosiform erythroderma. *Arch Dermatol* 1985; 121:489.

Heilbron B, et al: Sclerodema in an infant. *Arch Dermatol* 1986; 122:1417.

Heyl T, Raubenheimer EJ: Sucking pads (sucking calluses) of the lips in neonates: A manifestation of transient leukoedema. *Pediatr Dermatol* 1987; 4:123.

Hidano A, Purwoko R, Jitsukawa K: Statistical survey of skin changes in Japanese neonates. *Pediatr Dermatol* 1986; 3:140.

Holbrook KA, Smith LT: Ultrastructural aspects of human skin during the embryonic, fetal, premature, neonatal and adult periods of life. *Birth Defects* 1981; 17:9.

Holmes LB: Congenital malformations. *N Engl J Med* 1976; 295:204.

Honig PJ: Bites and parasites. *Pediatr Clin North Am* 1983; 30:563.

Jacobs AH, Walton RG: The incidence of birthmarks in the neonate. *Pediatrics* 1976; 58:218.

Jarratt M, Ramsdell W: Infantile acropustulosis. *Arch Dermatol* 1979; 115:834.

Jorgenson RJ, Shapiro SD, Salinas CF, et al: Intraoral findings and anomalies in neonates. *Pediatrics* 1982; 69:577.

Kamm LA, Giacola GP: Congenital cutaneous candidiasis. *Am J Dis Child* 1975; 129:1215.

Kibrick S: Herpes simplex infection at term: What to do with mother, newborn, and nursery personnel. *JAMA* 1980; 243:147.

Knauth A, Gordin M, McNelis W, et al: Semipermeable polyurethane membrane as an artificial skin for the premature neonate. *Pediatrics* 1989; 83:945.

Knight PJ, Reiner CB: Superficial lumps in children. What, when, and why? *Pediatrics* 1983; 72:147.

Lane AT: Human fetal skin development. *Pediatr Dermatol* 1986; 3:487.

Lane AT: Development and care of the premature infant's skin. *Pediatr Dermatol* 1987; 4:1.

Lane AT, Rehder PA, Helm K: Evaluations of diapers containing absorbent gelling material with conventional disposable diapers in newborn infants. *Am J Dis Child* 1990; 144:315.

Lau JTK, Ching RML: Mongolian spots in Chinese children. *Am J Dis Child* 1982; 136:863.

Leung AKC, Telmesani AMA: Salmon patches in Caucasian children. *Pediatr Dermatol* 1989; 6:185.

Levy HL, Cothram F: Erythema toxicum neonatorum present at birth. *Am J Dis Child* 1962; 103:617.

Lewis-Jones MS, Evans S, Graham-Brown RAC: Cutis marmorata telangiectatica congenita—a report of two cases occurring in male children. *Clin Exp Dermatol* 1988; 13:97.

Lin AN, Carter M: Epidermolysis bullosa: When the skin falls apart. *J Pediatr* 1989; 114:349.

Lindenauer SM: The Klippel-Trenaunay syndrome. *Ann Surg* 1965; 162:303.

Lipton SV, Brunell PA: Management of varicella exposure in a neonatal intensive care unit. *J Am Acad Dermatol* 1989; 261:1782.

McCray MK, Roenigk HH: Scalp reduction for correction of cutis aplasia congenita. *J Dermatol Surg Oncol* 1981; 7:655.

McWilliams RC, Stephenson JBP: Depigmented

hair. The earliest sign of tuberous sclerosis. *Arch Dis Child* 1978; 53:961.

Mulliken JB, Glowacki J: Hemangiomas and vascular malformations in infants and children: A classification based on endothelial characteristics. *Plast Reconstr Surg* 1982; 69:412.

Murphy WF, Langley AL: Common bullous lesions—presumably self-inflicted—occurring in utero in the newborn infant. *Pediatrics* 1963; 32:1099.

Nanda A, Kaur S, Bhakoo ON, et al: Survey of cutaneous lesions in Indian newborns. *Pediatr Dermatol* 1989; 6:39.

Nordlund JJ, et al: Hypomelanosis of Ito. *Acta Derm Venereol (Stockh)* 1977; 57:261.

Norwood-Galloway A, Lebwohl M, Phelps RG, et al: Subcutaneous fat necrosis of the newborn with hypercalcemia. *J Am Acad Dermatol* 1987; 16:435.

Oranje AP: Blue rubber bleb nevus syndrome. *Pediatr Dermatol* 1986; 3:304.

Paller AS: The Sturge-Weber syndrome. *Pediatr Dermatol* 1987; 4:300.

Philip AG, Hewitt JR: Early diagnosis of neonatal sepsis. *Pediatrics* 1980; 65:1036.

Pollard ZF, Robison HD, Calhoun J: Dermoid cysts in children. *Pediatrics* 1976; 57:379.

Prober CG, Hensleigh PA, Boucher FD, et al: Use of routine viral cultures at delivery to identify neonates exposed to herpes simplex virus. *N Engl J Med* 1988; 318:887.

Ramamurthy R5, Esterly NB: Transient neonatal pustular melanosis. *J Pediatr* 1976; 88:831.

Rand RE, Baden HP: The ichthyoses—a review. *J Am Acad Dermatol* 1983; 8:285.

Rhodes AR: Pigmented birthmarks and precursor melanocytic lesions of cutaneous melanoma identifiable in childhood. *Pediatr Clin North Am* 1983; 30:435.

Rogers M, McCrossin I, Commens C: Epidermal nevi and the epidermal nevus syndrome. *J Am Acad Dermatol* 1989; 20:476.

Rubin L, Leggiadro R, Elie MT, et al: Disseminated varicella in a neonate: Implications for immunoprophylaxis of neonates postnatally exposed to varicella. *Pediatr Infect Dis* 1986; 5:100.

Rudoy RC, Nelson JD: Breast abscess during the neonatal period. A review. *Am J Dis Child* 1975; 129:1031.

Sasaki GH, Pang CY, Wittliff JL: Pathogenesis and treatment of infant skin strawberry hemangiomas: Clinical and in vitro studies of hormonal effects. *Plast Reconstr Surg* 1984; 73:359.

Simpson JR, Lond MB: Natural history of cavernous hemangiomata. *Lancet* 1959; 2:1057.

Smales ORC, Kime R: Thermoregulation in babies immediately after birth. *Arch Dis Child* 1978; 53:58.

South DA, Jacobs AH: Cutis marmorata telangiectatica congenita. *J Pediatr* 1978; 93:944.

Tan OT, Gilchrest BA: Laser therapy for selected cutaneous vascular lesions in the pediatric population: A review. *Pediatrics* 1988; 82:652.

Thomsen RJ: Subcutaneous fat necrosis of the newborn and idiopathic hypercalcemia. *Arch Dermatol* 1980; 116:1155.

Uitto J, Santa Cruz DJ, Eisen AZ: Connective tissue nevi of the skin. *J Am Acad Dermatol* 1980; 3:441.

Vernon HJ, Lane AT, Wischerath LJ, et al: The effect of a semipermeable dressing on transepidermal water loss in premature infants. *Pediatrics,* in press.

Webster SB, Reister HC, Harmon LE: Juvenile xanthogranuloma with extracutaneous lesions. *Arch Dermatol* 1966; 93:71.

West DP, Worobec S, Solomon LM: Pharmacology and toxicology of infant skin. *J Invest Dermatol* 1981; 76:147.

Weston WL, Lane AT, Weston JA: Diaper dermatitis: Current concepts. *Pediatrics* 1980; 66:532.

Whitley RJ, Nahmias AJ, Visintine AM, et al: The natural history of herpes simplex virus infection of mother and newborn. *Pediatrics* 1980; 66:489.

Whitley RJ, Corey L, Arvin A, et al: Changing presentation of herpes simplex virus infection in neonates. *J Infect Dis* 1988; 158:109.

Williams ML, Elias PM: Heterogeneity in autosomal recessive ichthyosis. *Arch Dermatol* 1985; 121:477.

Yates VM, Kerr RE1, MacKie RM: Early diagnosis of infantile seborrheic dermatitis and atopic dermatitis. Clinical features. *Br J Dermatol* 1983; 108:633.

20 Dermato-pharmacology

A great variety of topical and systemic preparations are available for treatment of the skin of pediatric patients. However, the majority of these preparations have not been rigorously investigated as to their efficacy and risk-benefit ratio. This chapter contains an abbreviated formulary of the most useful topical and systemic preparations and the principles of, and rationale for, their use. Specific treatment programs are discussed in the other chapters on each skin disease.

Treatment should be simple and aimed at preserving or restoring the normal physiologic state of the skin. Topical therapy is often preferred because topical medication can be delivered in optimal concentrations at the exact site where it is needed, and effects on internal organs can be minimized. Compounding of preparations or adding medications to commercially available topical preparations is not advised because the ingredients lose their bioavailability.

PERCUTANEOUS ABSORPTION

Absorption of topical medications through the epidermal barrier into the dermis is a complex process. For clinical purposes, however, percutaneous absorption may be simplified and related to skin hydration. In the normal state of hydration of the stratum corneum, the epidermal barrier may be penetrated only by medications passing through a tight lipid barrier between cells.

Hydration of the skin allows binding of water molecules to hydrophilic lipids between stratum corneum cells, so that water-soluble medications may pass between cells. Thus, any of the factors that enhance hydration of the skin enhance percutaneous absorption; for example, plastic wrap, air-tight occlusion, the use of oils or ointments, urea compounds, and propylene glycol all enhance percutaneous absorption. The mechanism of action of occlusive substances is prevention of evaporation of the 200 to 300 mL of body water that normally moves through the stratum corneum daily and that would ordinarily evaporate had it not been for those occlusive coverings. Urea compounds and propylene glycol interact with the lipids between stratum corneum cells. The factors that enhance percutaneous absorption are listed in Table 20–1.

When choosing a topical medication for a child, one selects a preparation that contains two major components, the active medication and the vehicle. Each is important in determining the success or failure of the therapeutic regimen. Often the practitioner selects the correct active medication, but the incorrect vehicle, and thus the treatment program fails.

WATER AND THE SKIN

The outermost layer of the epidermis, the stratum corneum (horny layer), forms a barrier (the epidermal barrier) (see Chapter 1) to the penetration of active medication into the skin. Both excessive environmental humidity (above 90%) and low environmental humidity result in loss of the integrity of the epidermal barrier.

EXCESSIVE ENVIRONMENTAL HUMIDITY

Immersing the skin in water results in uptake of water by the stratum corneum cells and saturation of its intercellular spaces. This water uptake is so great that the stratum corneum triples in

TABLE 20–1.

Factors Enhancing Percutaneous Absorption

Increased water content of stratum corneum
Heat
Inflammation

thickness from 15 μ at 60% humidity to 48 μ at 90% humidity. Further water exposure results in replacement of lipid covalent bonds between the stratum corneum cells by weak hydrogen (water) bonds, and the stratum corneum cells separate. We see this clinically as maceration. Maceration occurs in naturally occluded areas where evaporation of water is usually retarded, such as in the axillae, under the breasts, and in the perineum, scalp, and interdigital webs. Preventing evaporation of water from the skin surface with plastic occlusive wraps, ointments, or oils will also result in maceration.

DEFICIENT ENVIRONMENTAL HUMIDITY

At less than 10% environmental humidity, excessive shrinking of the stratum corneum occurs, resulting in microscopic and macroscopic cracks in the stratum corneum. This is manifested by a dry feel to the skin surface, thin scales with erythema around the borders (eczema craquelé), and dry, inspissated plugs of scale in follicular openings (keratosis pilaris).

SUBSTANCES DESIGNED TO RETAIN WATER ON THE SKIN SURFACE (LUBRICANTS)

On dry, exposed areas of skin, such as the dorsa of the hands and arms, it is desirable to retain water in the stratum corneum. Such lubrication therapy is often all that is necessary to treat chronic dryness and inflammation of the skin successfully (Table 20–2).

TABLE 20–2.

Function of Lubricants

Impede water loss
Retain heat
Increase percutaneous absorption
Reduce scaling

Lubricants are complex mixtures designed to moisturize the skin surface. These preparations are complex in order to make them more efficient at hydrating the skin and to enable them to give a more pleasing cosmetic appearance when applied. The vehicles that are used to provide skin lubrication are usually petrolatum based or are mixtures of lanolin and petrolatum. The vehicles that contain solids and little or no water are called ointments; those with 20% to 50% water are called creams. A list of useful lubricants is found in Table 20–3. All lubricants are best applied to wet skin.

COMPONENTS OF LUBRICANTS AND VEHICLES AND THEIR FUNCTION

Petrolatum, the base for most lubricants, is prepared from the residue remaining in stills after the distillation of petroleum. It usually is a colored solid and must be decolorized to make white petrolatum (petroleum jelly, white soft paraffin). Petrolatum contains a mixture of hydrocarbons, including triglycerides, and is insoluble in water. It retains heat, impedes water loss from the skin surface, and increases percutaneous absorption. It has minor vasoconstrictive activity when applied to the skin, and may enhance reepithelialization of wounds. Petrolatum alone is cosmetically disagreeable, with a greasy film left on the skin surface that frequently results in overheating of the skin and sweat obstruction. The mixing of substances to allow the addition of water to petrolatum will result in a more efficient moisturizing capacity of the skin, with a less greasy feel and more cosmetic acceptance. Substances added to

TABLE 20–3.

Useful Lubricants

Petrolatum based
Moisturel
White petrolatum (Petrolatum White, Vaseline Pure Petroleum Jelly)
Shepard's skin cream
Vaseline Dermatology Formula Lotion
Mixtures of lanolin and petrolatum
Aquaphor ointment base
Eucerin creme
Eucerin lotion
Lubriderm cream
Keri creme

lubricants to increase water-binding capacity include cetyl alcohol, stearyl alcohol, and other stearates.

Addition of cetyl alcohol to petrolatum will increase its water-binding capability from 10% to 50%. Other additives include polyethylene glycol (PEG; Carbowax) of low molecular weight (300–400 daltons) or of high molecular weight (1,540–4,000 daltons) as an agent to disperse the mixture uniformly or for its solvent properties. Addition of cholesterol or polysaccharide macromolecules, such as polysorbate (Tween 20 or 80), as emulsifiers and the addition of yellow wax or white wax (beeswax) for stiffness of the product are common practices. Glycerin, a fatty alcohol derived from triglycerides as a by-product of the manufacture of soap, is a clear, colorless, sticky liquid that takes up water from the skin surface. Its role as an additive to certain creams is unclear.

Bacteriostatic and fungistatic agents are added to preparations that contain water to prolong the life of the product. Popular preservatives include parabens, formaldehyde, or formaldehyde-releasing agents (imidazolinyl ureas); oxyquinoline sulfate; organic quaternary ammonium compounds; chlorobutanol; and hexachlorophene. Fragrances are added to cover any unpleasant smell from the basic product. The added preservatives and fragrances are frequently responsible for irritant or allergic reactions to these lubricants in children. Fragrance- and preservative-free preparations are listed in Table 20–4.

Liquid petrolatum (mineral oil, liquid paraffin) is a fluid phase of petrolatum obtained by distilling the residual petroleum liquid at 330° F and decolorizing it. It is composed of 15 to 20 carbon hydrocarbons, and, because it is in a fluid form at room temperature, it is added to skin preparations in which easy spread on the skin surface is desirable.

Lanolin is a purified fatlike substance obtained from the wool of sheep. It consists of cholesterol esters and oxycholesterol esters and is the external coating of wool, called wool fat or wool wax alcohol. Ordinary lanolin contains 25% to 30% water and is a yellowish-white solid. It must be mixed with other agents such as mineral oil or cetyl alcohol so that it can be spread smoothly on the skin. Lanolin is found in a number of skin lubricants. The function of frequently used ingredients of lubricants and of medicated creams and lotions is listed in Table 20–5. One should not recommend a skin preparation unless he or she is familiar with its ingredients and its therapeutic indications.

OINTMENTS

Ointments spread easily on the skin and are more cosmetically pleasing if they contain some water. White petrolatum, mineral oil, and liquid paraffin are completely water insoluble and have maximal water-retaining (occlusive) properties. However, they often leave a greasy film on the skin and cause excessive heat retention, which make them unacceptable to many patients.

Mixing ointments or oils with a little water makes them spread on the skin more easily and less greasily. The bulk of the lubricants in clinical

TABLE 20–4.

Skin Lubricants That Are Fragrance, Lanolin, and Preservative Free

Fragrance free
  Moisturel
  Aquaphor ointment base
  Eucerin creme
  Eucerin lotion
  White petrolatum (Vaseline Pure Petroleum Jelly, petrolatum white)
Fragrance free, lanolin free
  Moisturel
  White petrolatum
Preservative free, lanolin free
  White petrolatum (Vaseline Pure Petroleum Jelly, Petrolatum White)

TABLE 20–5.

Components of Lubricants and Vehicles and Their Function

Component	Function
Cetyl alcohol, stearates, cholesterol	Additional water binding
Polyethylene glycol (Carbowax)	Dispersants
Yellow wax, white wax	Stiffness
Parabens, formaldehyde releasers	Preservatives
Propylene glycol, alcohol	Solvent
Essential oils	Fragrance
Cholesterol, polysaccharide polymers (Tween, Span)	Emulsifiers

use are emulsifiable with water and contain mostly ointment, with a small amount of water. The water stays in droplet form in the ointment phase, making such lubricants water-in-oil emulsions.

These preparations should be applied to wet skin twice or three times a day for maximal lubrication. (Eucerin, which is composed of lanolin and water, is an inexpensive preparation.) Also useful is mixing equal parts of xipamide (Aquaphor) and water. Patients are instructed to wet the skin with a 5- or 10-minute bath and then apply the lubricants to the wet skin before drying it. These preparations are used successfully on most areas of the skin except the scalp and the axillae.

CREAMS (OIL-IN-WATER EMULSIONS)

When environmental humidity is high and in naturally occluded areas, the use of lubricants that contain more water than oil is desirable. These are the lubricating creams, which contain oil in droplet form in water (oil-in-water emulsions). Such preparations are easily washed from skin surfaces and are cosmetically pleasing. Lubricant creams must be applied every 2 to 3 hours to achieve the same lubricant effect obtained with every 12-hour application of ointment.

SKIN-HYDRATING AGENTS

Certain chemicals act as skin-hydrating agents by adding extra water-binding sites to the skin rather than by simple occlusion. The most effective of these are the urea creams, which dissolve hydrogen bonds and add water-binding sites. The 10% urea creams are the most effective (e.g., Aquacare/HP dry skin cream and Carmol cream). To make a cream, the urea must first be dissolved in water before mixing with oil. High concentrations of urea (20% or more) or improper mixing may result in urea crystals in the preparation, causing severe irritation when applied to the skin.

GELS

Gels are colorless semicolloids that liquefy on contact with the skin. Because of their alcoholic base, they may burn and sting. They permit good penetration of steroids and other medica-

tions and are useful in medications applied to the scalp and in acne preparations. They are the most effective delivery system for benzoyl peroxides for use in acne (Benzagel, Desquam-X, Persa-Gel; see chapter 3) and for the clear, colorless, odorless tar preparations used for psoriasis (Estar gel).

AMOUNT TO DISPENSE AND PATIENT EDUCATION

Therapy often fails because patients apply the topical medication incorrectly. In a comparison of medication application by trained technicians and by patients, it was found that trained technicians applied 1.8 g/m^2 of body surface area, but the self-application group averaged 16.3 g/m^2, with a range of 0.4 to 44.3 g/m^2. Overmedication is common and expensive for the patient.

In Table 20–6 guidelines are presented for the amount to dispense. In Table 20–7 are listed important rules for prescribing topical medication that will result in therapeutic success when followed by the patient.

ANTI-INFLAMMATORY AGENTS

Wet Dressings

Water is an important therapeutic tool, but it is often forgotten that it is also an anti-inflammatory agent. The evaporation of water from the skin surface results in vasoconstriction, relief of pruritus, and debridement of crusts from the skin surface. Water is also the active ingredient in the drying lotions; the anti-infective medications added to these preparations are of little benefit. Infected dermatitis should be treated with systemic antibiotics and wet dressings with use of tap water. Wet dressings can be used in acute dermatitis from any cause. Pruritus is relieved by placing the skin in an environment where the humidity is 90% and allowing it to evaporate to 60% humidity. This slow evaporation of water from the skin surface occurring during a 4- to 6-hour period is the basis of the wet dressing technique.

Either cotton pajamas, leotards, long-sleeved shirts, or cotton gauze can serve as satisfactory wet dressings. In the "two long johns" technique, cotton pajamas and a cotton turtleneck shirt are placed in room temperature water and then wrung out until damp, placed on the skin, and covered with dry pajamas. For inpatient therapy,

TABLE 20–6.

Amount to Dispense

Area	One application (g)	Twice-daily application for 2 wk (g)
Hands, face, head, anogenital area	2	60
One arm, anterior or posterior aspect of trunk	3	80
One leg	4	120
Entire body	30–60	840–1680

cotton gauze, such as 18-inch 20/12 mesh gauze (Parke-Davis No. 30-478, Curity No. 1473), is used on the trunk, folded into 10 to 12 layers, then dampened in the same manner as cotton pajamas. On the extremities, 4-inch 20/12 mesh gauze is used (5 yards is usually sufficient). The gauze is then covered with dry pajamas or dry cotton flannel. One should not apply occlusive dressings such as plastic wrap over the damp dressing because this prevents evaporation. The dressings are completely removed every 4 to 5 hours, redampened, and replaced.

Relief of pruritus is dramatic, as is reduction of erythema. After 24 hours the patient is greatly improved, with maximal benefit occurring at 48 to 72 hours. Treatment beyond this period is of little benefit. Topical steroid creams or ointments, such as mometasone furoate (Elocon) or fluocinolone acetonide 0.01% (Fluonid, Synalar), applied to the skin before the application of wet dressings enhance the wet dressing technique considerably.

Anthralin

Anthralin is a tricyclic hydrocarbon that is useful for the treatment of skin conditions with epidermal hyperplasia, such as psoriasis. It is obtained by the reduction of anthraquinone and is yellowish brown in color. Because it stains and irritates the skin, its use should be restricted to brief periods of time, the "short-contact" anthralin therapy. It is applied to skin lesions of psoriasis for 10 minutes at a time once daily and then washed off with a pH neutral soap such as Dove. Therapy is begun with a 0.1% cream preparation, which is increased to 0.25%, 0.5%, or 1.0% as tolerated. An alternative strategy is to initiate therapy with 1% anthralin use for 5 minutes and increase the contact time each week.

TABLE 20–7.

Rules for Prescribing Topical Medication

1. Prescribe enough medication.
2. Demonstrate to the patient how to apply the medication.
3. Apply lubricants liberally to wet skin.
4. Substitute lubricant therapy for topical steroids whenever possible; do not allow the patient to use the steroid for the lubricant properties of the vehicle when the vehicle alone would suffice.
5. Apply ointments to exposed dry areas, creams to naturally occluded moist areas.
6. Use medications twice daily.
7. Avoid superpotent steroids in prepubertal children.
8. Use only hydrocortisone in diaper area.
9. Do not treat with steroids longer than 2 weeks; prescribe a rest period, using topical lubricants.
10. Monitor growth parameters and cortisol levels in children who have used steroids for long periods.

COAL TAR PREPARATIONS

Coal tars are by-products of the destructive distillation of coal. They contain 48% hydrocarbons and benzene, toluene, naphthalene, anthracene, xylene, phenol, cresols, pyridine ammonia, peroxides, and other aromatic compounds. They are black, stain the skin and clothing, and stink. Their mechanism of action is unknown, but they restore normal keratinization in eczematous and hyperplastic epidermis.

Most tar compounds are derived from coal tars, but oil shale tars (ichthammol), juniper tars (cade oil), or pine tars are sometimes used.

Crude coal tar 1% in petrolatum is the most

commonly used, although concentrations up to 5% have been prescribed. Commercial preparations such as Zetar (3% crude coal tar in Qualatum) are available.

Tars are applied twice daily, always with a downward motion rather than a circular or up-and-down motion, to avoid tar folliculitis. Coal tar concentrates in follicular openings, resulting in a superficial chemical folliculitis. Such chemical folliculitis is rapidly responsive to benzoyl peroxide gels applied twice daily. New colorless and relatively odorless tar preparations have increased the acceptability of tar therapy and have made it a viable alternative to topical steroids. Estar gel and Psorigel are clear and colorless tars in gel vehicles that allow penetration of the skin. They are applied twice daily and are immediately covered with a lubricant, since gels are drying. They are equivalent to crude coal tar 5%.

Coal tar shampoos are useful on the scalp for treatment of scalp psoriasis. Scalp preparations include DHS, Ionil T, Sebutone, Alma-Tar, Pentrax, Vanseb, and Zetar. Coal tar solution, liquor carbonis detergens (LCD), is an alcoholic extract of coal tar. LCD 5% equals crude coal tar 1% in potency. It is used as a shampoo in tincture of green soap or as a bath additive.

TOPICAL GLUCOCORTICOSTEROIDS

Topical glucocorticosteroids are the mainstay of therapy for many inflammatory and hyperproliferative skin diseases. Glucocorticosteroids applied to the skin reduce inflammation by causing vasoconstriction and preventing the egress of inflammatory cells (neutrophils, lymphocytes, monocytes/macrophages, eosinophils) from the bloodstream to tissue sites. Maximal glucocorticosteroid penetration is achieved from ointment vehicles, followed by gels and creams. Penetration is poor with lotions or sprays. A cutaneous anti-inflammatory effect can be achieved with topical glucocorticosteroids without adrenal suppression, which is not the case with systemic steroids.

Potency

The potency of a topical steroid is evaluated by vasoconstriction (blanching) of the skin, which roughly correlates with its anti-inflammatory effects. Although glucocorticosteroid potency can be subdivided further, it is convenient to divide it into four categories (Table 20–8). Numerous moderate-potency glucocorticosteroids are available, with little difference in their effectiveness. Select one low-potency and one moderate-po-

---

TABLE 20–8.

Potency of Topical Glucocorticosteroids

Low potency (anti-inflammatory activity 1)
   Hydrocortisone 1% cream (Nutracort, Penecort,
   Hytone, OTC), 1% ointment
   Desonide 0.05% cream, ointment (Desowen, Tridesilon)
Moderate potency (anti-inflammatory activity 10–99)
   Mometasone furoate 0.1% ointment, 0.1% cream (Elocon)
   Fluocinolone acetonide 0.025% ointment (Synalar, Fluonid)
   Hydrocortisone valerate 0.2% cream, ointment (Westcort)
   Triamcinolone acetonide 0.01% cream, 0.25% lotion, 0.1% ointment
     (Kenalog, Aristocort), 0.5% cream (Aristocort HF)
   Betamethasone valerate 0.1% cream, 0.1% ointment, 0.1% lotion (Valisone)
   Aclometasone dipropionate 0.05% ointment, 0.05% cream (Aclovate)
   Amcinonide 0.1% cream (Cyclocort)
High-potency (anti-inflammatory activity >100)
   Fluocinonide 0.05% cream, gel, ointment (Lidex, Topsyn, Lidex-E)
   Halcinonide 0.1% cream (Halog); amcinonide 0.1% ointment (Cyclocort);
     desoximetasone 0.25% cream (Topicort); betamethasone dipropionate
     0.05% ointment, 0.05% cream (Diprosone, Diprolene)
Highest potency (anti-inflammatory activity >500)
   Betamethasone dipropionate (in optimized vehicle) 0.05% ointment, 0.05%
     cream (Diprolene)
   Clobetasol propionate 0.05% ointment, 0.05% cream (Temovate)
   Diflorasone diacetate 0.05% ointment (Psorcon)

---

tency preparation from the list in Table 20–8 to use for children with inflammatory skin diseases.

Guidelines for Use of Topical Steroids

For most acute, subacute, and chronic dermatitides, select a preparation from the moderate-potency list and treat twice daily for 3 to 10 days until symptoms have subsided. Then begin to apply bland lubricants twice daily, using topical glucocorticosteroids once daily. Eliminate the topical glucocorticosteroid as soon as possible. There are no indications for high-potency topical glucocorticosteroids in children, except for pulse-dose therapy under the direction of an experienced dermatologist.

On the face and scrotum, only low-potency glucocorticosteroids (hydrocortisone 1%) should be used, because the epidermis is thin in these areas and the side effects may be severe (Table 20–9).

High-potency glucocorticosteroids and some moderate-potency glucocorticosteroids, when applied to the skin, may result in tachyphylaxis; that is, after 1 to 3 days of application, maximal vasoconstriction has been achieved and further application results in a rebound vasodilation, manifested by diffuse erythema on the child's face. This is particularly true with the superpotent topical steroids. Simply substitute bland lubricants for such patients, and their skin will return to normal in 1 to 2 weeks.

Systemic side effects have been noted with

TABLE 20–9.
Side Effects of Topical Steroids

Local
  Striae (especially in genital area and axillae)
  Persistent erythema and telangiectasia (face)
  Pustular acneiform eruption (face) (steroid rosacea)
  Atrophic, shiny, erythematous skin
  Telangiectasia, purpura
  Granuloma gluteale infantum
  Folliculitis, miliaria
  Hypertrichosis
  Steroid addiction syndrome
  Allergic contact dermatitis
Systemic
  Suppression of hypothalamic-pituitary-adrenal axis
  Stunted growth in children
  Cataracts and glaucoma
  Glycosuria
  Cushing's syndrome

the short-term use of potent topical glucocorticosteroids, particularly with clobetasol, betamethasone dipropionate, diflorasone, halcinonide or fluocinonide, as well as with the long-term use of moderately potent glucocorticosteroids on 50% of body surface.

Topical Steroid Addiction

Since potent and superpotent topical glucocorticosteroids have become available, a syndrome of topical steroid addiction has been recognized. The syndrome is the result of chronic daily application for longer than 1 month of a potent or moderately potent glucocorticosteroid preparation to the facial skin. As treatment continues, the patient experiences a rebound vasodilation of the facial skin 2 to 6 hours after the application. The face becomes red, and the patient applies the steroid more frequently. Soon burning of the skin is experienced and is relieved only by further steroid applications. Permanent redness of the facial skin eventuates, with thinning and fine wrinkling observed. It is difficult to withdraw the steroid because the patient cannot tolerate the burning sensation, which is relieved only by topical steroids. Substitution of a bland ointment for the topical steroid, plus administration of oral antihistamines, will result in progressive improvement within a 4-week period.

In susceptible infants and children, application of potent or moderately potent glucocorticosteroid preparations to the facial skin may also result in redness and acneiform papules and pustules located on the nose, chin, cheeks, and lower eyelids. This is known as acne rosacea. Abruptly stopping the topical steroid preparation will result in increased numbers of papules and pustules in the following 7 days. Treatment is that recommended for acne, with severe forms requiring systemic antibiotics. Those children who are likely to develop acne are most susceptible.

FORMULARY FOR COMMON PEDIATRIC DERMATOLOGY CONDITIONS

General Skin Care

This formulary is designed to provide information regarding a number of useful skin preparations; it is not intended to be encyclopedic. Formulas for compounding skin mixtures are omitted because low-cost and high-quality preparations from pharmaceutical manufacturers are readily available and are often superior to compounded mixtures.

I. Skin lubricants and moisturizers.

NOTE: Creams and lotions contain water, requiring the addition of preservatives, which are potential allergens. They must be applied more frequently than ointments but are aesthetically more pleasing to apply.

A. Petrolatum based.

NOTE: Petrolatum-based preparations retain heat, feel greasy, and remain on the skin surface for 6 to 12 hours.

1. Moisturel Lotion (petrolatum, water, glycerin, cetyl alcohol, steareth-2, dimethicone, benzyl alcohol, laureth 23, Mg Al silicate, carbomer 934, sodium hydroxide, quaternium-15.
   a. Available in: 8, 12 oz bottles.
   b. Use: Apply to wet skin b.i.d.

2. White petrolatum USP (Vaseline Petrolatum White, Vaseline Pure Petroleum Jelly).
   a. Available in: 30, 75 g tubes.
                    50, 105, 240 g jars.
   b. Use: Apply to wet skin b.i.d.

3. Hydrophilic ointment USP (white petrolatum 86%, cholesterol, stearyl alcohol, white wax).
   a. Available in: 454 g jars.
   b. Use: Apply to wet skin b.i.d.

4. Vaseline Dermatology Formula Lotion (white petrolatum, mineral oil, dimethicone, glycerin water, cetyl alcohol, triethanolamine fragrance, methylparaben, propylparaben, DMDM hydantoin).
   a. Available in: 150, 480 mL bottles.
   b. Use: Apply to wet skin b.i.d.

B. Lanolin-based mixtures with petrolatum.

NOTE: Lanolin products applied to inflamed skin with skin breaks may act as an irritant. Substitute petrolatum-based preparations.

1. Aquaphor Ointment Base (wool wax alcohol, petrolatum, mineral oil, mineral wax).
   a. Available in: 454 g, 2.1 kg jars.
   b. Use: Apply to wet skin b.i.d.

2. Eucerin Creme (wool wax alcohol, petrolatum, mineral oil, mineral wax,

water, 2-bromo-2-nitropropane-1,3-diol).
   a. Available in: 120, 454 g jars.
   b. Use: Apply to wet skin q.i.d.

3. Eucerin Lotion (lanolin alcohol, lanolin acid, glycerin ester, sorbitol, propylene glycol, beeswax, magnesium sulfate, PEG-40, isopropyl myristate, mineral oil, water, preservatives, [thiazolinones]).
   a. Available in: 240, 480 mL plastic bottles.
   b. Use: Apply to wet skin q.i.d.

4. Keri Creme (lanolin alcohol, mineral oil, talc, water, sorbitol, ceresin magnesium, stearate, glyceryl oleate, propylene glycol, isopropyl myristate, fragrance, preservatives).
   a. Available in: 75 g tubes.
   b. Use: Apply to wet skin b.i.d.

5. Lubriderm Creme (water, mineral oil, lanolin, lanolin alcohol, cetyl alcohol, sorbitan laurate, lanolin oil, squalene, PEG-100, glycerin, petrolatum, parabens, quaternium-15, preservatives; scented or unscented).
   a. Available in: 120 g tubes.
   b. Use: Apply to wet skin b.i.d.

C. Urea creams and lotions.

1. Aquacare/HP (urea cream 10%).
   a. Available in: 75 g tubes.
   b. Use: Apply to skin b.i.d.

2. Carmol 10 Lotion (urea lotion 10%) (water, stearic acid, isopropyl palmitate, propylene glycol, cetyl alcohol, PEG-8, xanthan gum, carbromal-940, trolamine, fragrance).
   a. Available in: 180 mL bottles.
   b. Use: Apply to skin b.i.d.

D. Soaps and soap substitutes.

NOTE: For children with sensitive skin, soap substitutes are preferred. If soap is to be used, it should be neutral pH.

1. Cetaphil lotion cleanser—cetyl alcohol.
   a. Available as: Solution in 4 and 16 oz bottles.
   b. Use: Massage into dry skin, until it foams, then massage foam into skin.

2. Moisturel Sensitive Skin Cleanser (so-

dium laureth sulfate, laureth 6 carboxylic acid).
  a. Available as: 8.75 oz plastic pump bottle.
  b. Use: Lather into wet skin, rinse off.
  3. Dove.
    a. Available as: Neutral pH unscented 4.75 oz bar.
    b. Use: Lather into wet skin, rinse off.

II. Hair and scalp preparations.
  A. Antimicrobial shampoos.
    1. Selenium sulfide suspension (Exsel, Selsun; selenium sulfide 2.5% in water, bentonite, ethylene glycol, titanium dioxide, preservatives [captan], fragrance).
      a. Available in: 120 mL bottles.
      b. Use: Massage 5 to 10 mL into wet scalp for 2 to 3 minutes; rinse out. Preferred for prophylaxis in household contacts of epidemic scalp ringworm.
    2. Zinc pyrithione (Denorex, Head & Shoulders, Sebulon) (zinc 1%–2% in water plus anionic detergent and fragrance).
      a. Available in: 120, 210, 330, 450 mL bottles.
      b. Use: Massage 5 to 10 mL into wet scalp for 2 to 3 minutes; rinse out.
  B. Tar shampoos (Sebutone, T-Gel, DHS-T) (tar 0.5% to 1% in detergent shampoos).
    a. Available in: 120, 240-mL bottles.
    b. Use: Massage into wet scalp for 2 to 3 minutes; rinse out.
  C. Keratolytic shampoos (salicylic acid–sulfur) (Sebulex, Ionil, Vanseb) (salicylic acid 2%, sulfur 2% in detergent shampoo).
    a. Available in: 4, 8 oz bottles.
    b. Use: Massage into wet scalp for 2 to 3 minutes; rinse out.
  D. Keratolytic scalp preparations.
    NOTE: All keratolytic agents are irritating to the skin and mucous membranes, and contact with eyes, nose, and mouth should be avoided. Sunburn may occur more readily after use of these agents, and areas greater than 10% of the skin surface should not be treated because of possible percutaneous absorption.

Skin lubricants are useful adjuncts when keratolytics are used.
    1. Phenol and saline solution (phenol, glycerin, sodium chloride, water, mineral oil, fragrance).
      a. Available in: 120, 240 mL bottles.
      b. Use: Massage into scalp at bedtime; shampoo out, with thorough rinsing, in the morning.
    NOTE: All of these hair preparations are valuable in the management of scaling of the scalp; severe scaling conditions such as psoriasis may require phenol and saline solution treatments.
  E. Detergent shampoos.
    A large variety of commercial over-the-counter shampoos are available. Their main ingredients are water, sodium lauryl sulfate as an emulsifier and dispersing agent, and fragrance. The sodium lauryl sulfate may act as an irritant. For dry scalp or cradle cap, such preparations may be used daily. Massage the shampoo in for 20 minutes, then rinse out.

III. Keratolytic agents.
  These preparations are used for excessive thickening of the palms and soles, the ichthyoses and follicular plugging states. The mechanism of action is unknown, but faulty cell-to-cell adherence is the major effect.
  A. Retinoic acid, tretinoin (Retin-A).
    a. Available in:
      0.01% gel: 15, 45 g tubes.
      0.025% gel: 15, 45 g tubes.
      0.025% cream: 20, 45 g tubes.
    b. Use: Apply b.i.d.
  B. Lactic acid.
    a. Available in:
      5% lotion (Lac V; LactiCare Lotion): 120 mL bottles. 12% ammonium lactate lotion (Lac-hydrin lotion): 150, 360 mL bottles.
    b. Use: Apply b.i.d.
  C. Salicylic acid: 3%–6% ointment.
    1. Whitfield's Ointment USP (salicylic acid 3%, benzoic acid 6% in polyethylene glycol ointment).
      a. Available in: 30 g tubes.
    2. Keralyt Gel (salicylic acid 6%, propylene glycol 60% in alcohol).

a. Available in: 28.4 g tubes.

b. Use: Apply once daily.

IV. Agents that reduce sweating.

A. Aluminum chloride solutions.

1. Aluminum chloride hexahydrate 20% in alcohol (Drysol).

a. Available in: 37.5 mL bottles.

b. Use: Apply to dry skin at bedtime for 2 to 7 consecutive nights.

NOTE: Very irritating to the axillae.

2. Aluminum chlorohydrate spray (Arid Extra Dry, Unscented).

a. Available in: 120 mL spray cans.

b. Use: Spray b.i.d.

B. Glutaraldehyde 10% solution (must be compounded).

NOTE: Restricted for use on feet only. Stains skin brown. Allergic contact dermatitis may occasionally result.

V. Sunscreens.

The potency of sunscreens is determined by a sun protection factor (SPF), which represents the multiples of time to sunburn. At least, SPF 15 should be recommended. A large number of sunscreens are available; only a few are listed. Sunscreens that are fragrance free and nonstinging to children's skin are preferred.

NOTE: PABA, cinnamates, and salicylates protect in the sunburn range of 280 to 320 nm ultraviolet light, but not in the longer wavelengths, such as those responsible for porphyrias, drug phototoxicity, or some forms of polymorphous light eruption (325–400 nm). Benzophenones will protect in wavelengths of 200 to 365 nm, but sunblocks and sun avoidance are the best strategies for ultraviolet A sensitivity.

A. Fragrance free.

1. PreSun For Kids. (Octyl methoxycinnamate, oxybenzone, octyl salicylate).

a. Available as: SPF 29 in 4 oz bottles.

b. Use: Apply to dry skin ½ hour before sun exposure.

2. Presun lip protector sunscreen (octyl dimethyl PABA; oxybenzone).

a. Available as: SPF 15 lipstick.

b. Use: Apply to lips several times during sun exposure.

B. With fragrance.

1. Johnson's Baby Sunblock (octyl methoxycinnamate, octyl salicylate, oxybenzone, titanium dioxide).

a. Available as: SPF 15 cream or lotion in 4 oz bottles.

b. Use: Apply to dry skin ½ hour before sun exposure.

2. Coppertone sunblock lotion SPF 44 (Ethylhexyl *p*-methoxycinnamate, 2-ethylhexyl salicylate, padimate O, oxybenzone).

a. Available as: SPF 44 lotion in 4 oz bottles.

b. Use: Apply ½ hour before sun exposure.

3. PreSun 39 creamy sunscreen (octyl dimethyl PABA, oxybenzone).

a. Available as: SPF 39 cream in 4 oz bottles.

b. Use: Apply ½ hour before sun exposure.

VI. Sunblocks.

1. Zinc oxide ointment.

a. Available in: 15 g tubes.

2. Zinc oxide 20%, red veterinary petrolatum 3%, cinoxate 1.4% (RV Paque).

a. Available in: 120 mL bottles.

b. Use: Apply before sun exposure.

3. Beta carotene (Solatene).

a. Available in: 30 mg capsules (do not prescribe generic).

NOTE: In subjects with erythropoietic protoporphyria, oral beta carotene therapy results in dramatic relief of sun intolerance. Small amounts may be converted to vitamin A in the liver, and additional vitamin A should not be administered.

b. Use: In children, 30–120 mg/day is the recommended dose, with response of sun sensitivity and yellow skin color as a useful end point of therapy.

VII. Anti-inflammatory and antipruritic agents.

A. Water and evaporative lotions.

Evaporation of fluid from the skin surface results in vasoconstriction and relief of erythema as well as a cooling sensation and the relief of itch. Water in the form of wet dressings, compresses, or baths is as efficacious as alcoholic lotions, such as calamine lotion.

B. Topical glucocorticosteroids: A complete list can be found in Table 20–8. A low-potency and a moderate-potency preparation are listed here.
  1. Low potency: Hydrocortisone 1% cream, ointment.
     a. Available in: 30, 120 g tubes.
     b. Use: Apply b.i.d. to q.i.d.
  2. Moderate potency: Mometasone furoate 0.1% cream, ointment.
     a. Available in: 15, 45 g tubes.
     b. Use: Apply once daily.

VIII. Coal tars.
  A. Coal tar 1% ointment USP.
     a. Available in: 454 g jars.
     b. Use: Apply b.i.d.; wash off with mineral oil.
  B. Tar gels.
     1. Estar 5%.
        a. Available in: 90-g tubes.
        b. Use: Apply b.i.d.
           NOTE: Instruct patient on proper application (see Chapter 9) to avoid folliculitis.

IX. Anthralin (Dritho-Creme, Anthra-Derm) 0.1%, 0.25%, 0.5%, 1.0%.
     a. Available in: 50, 42.5 g tubes.
     b. Use: Begin with lowest concentration. Apply for 10 minutes once daily; then wash off. Increase duration or concentration weekly.

X. Antihistamines.
  1. Diphenhydramine hydrochloride (Benadryl). An ethanolamine derivative, Benadryl is associated with a high likelihood of sedation. Effective in urticaria or other pruritic conditions.
     a. Available in:
        Elixir (12.5 mg/5 ml): 120, 240 ml bottles. Capsules: 25, 50 mg.
     b. Use: 4–6 mg/kg/day, not to exceed 300 mg; give t.i.d. or q.i.d.
  2. Hydroxyzine hydrochloride (Atarax): Drug of choice for dermographism and heat- and exercise-induced urticaria. Effective in other pruritic states. Has mild tranquilizing effects.
     a. Available in:
        Syrup (10 mg/5 ml): 240 mL bottles.
        Tablets: 10, 25, 50 mg.
     b. Use: 2–4 mg/kg/day; give b.i.d. or t.i.d.
  3. Chlorpheniramine maleate (Chlor-Trimeton). An alkylamine derivative, it is sold over the counter and is inexpensive.
     a. Available in:
        Syrup (2 mg/5 mL): 120 mL bottles.
        Tablets: 4, 8 mg.
     b. Use: 0.2–0.4 mg/kg/day; give b.i.d. to t.i.d.
  4. Terfenadine (Seldane): Nonsedating H_1 receptor antagonist.
     a. Available in: 60 mg capsules.
     b. Use: 60 mg (if weight >30 kg); give every 12 hours.
  5. Astemizole (Hismanal): Long-acting nonsedating H_1 receptor antagonist.
     a. Available in: 10 mg tablets.
     b. Use: 10 mg once daily in children older than 12 years.

XI. Oral glucocorticosteroids (prednisone). Used in acute dermatoses, certain collagen vascular diseases, autoimmune bullous diseases. Not recommended in chronic dermatitis.
     a. Available in:
        Syrup (5 mg/5 mL; Liquid Pred): 120, 240 mL bottles.
        Tablets: 2.5, 5, 20 mg.
     b. Use: 0.5–2.0 kg/day; give as single AM dose. If necessary to treat longer than 3 weeks, attempt alternate-day therapy.
        NOTE: Absolute contraindications to oral glucocorticosteroid use are ocular herpes simplex and untreated tuberculosis. Alternative agents should also be used in a child with acute or chronic active infection, diabetes mellitus, hypertension, peptic ulcer, psychosis, renal insufficiency, or congestive heart failure. Known side effects, including Cushing's syndrome, may be minimized by limiting therapy to less than 3 weeks' duration.

XII. Nonsteroidal anti-inflammatory agents.
Used in erythema nodosum and for prevention of pain and redness of sunburn. All

agents are well absorbed and highly protein bound. All are associated with toxic epidermal necrolysis.

1. Ibuprofen (Advil, Medipren, Nuprin, PediaProfen).
   a. Available as: Tablets: 200 mg. Suspension (PediaProfen): 100 mg/5 mL.
   b. Use: 200 mg tablets t.i.d. in patients older than age 12 years. 5–10 mg/kg t.i.d. for children 6 months to 12 years.
2. Indomethacin (Indocin).
   a. Available as: Capsules: 25 mg, bottles of 100.
   Oral suspension (25 mg/5 mL): 237 mL bottles.
   b. Use: 25 mg b.i.d. in patients older than 14 years.

XIII. Antibacterial agents.

A. Topical antiseptics.
For skin cleansing and surgical scrub, these agents are effective in reducing numbers of skin bacteria. They may provide a cumulative antibacterial effect.
1. Chlorhexidine (Hibiclens Antimicrobial Skin Cleanser): Useful for daily handwashing in a child with skin infections.
   a. Available as: Chlorhexidine gluconate 4%, 120 mL bottles.
   b. Use: Surgical scrub or cleansing once daily.
2. Povidine-iodine (Betadine).
   a. Available in: Skin cleanser, 120 mL bottles.
   b. Use: Surgical scrub or cleansing once daily.

B. Topical antibiotics.
Topical antibiotics are best used as prophylaxis. For established skin infections, oral antibiotics should be given (see also Antiacne Agents).
1. Bacitracin: Polypeptide antibiotic that interferes with bacterial cell wall growth. Effective against a wide variety of gram-positive and gram-negative bacteria.
   a. Available in: Ointment (500 U/g): 15, 30 g tubes.
   b. Use: Apply to cleansed area of skin q.i.d.
2. Neomycin Aminoglycoside antibiotic effective against gram-negative bacteria. Group A streptococci are often resistant. Allergic contact dermatitis is a major problem with this topical antibiotic, in contrast to bacitracin.
   a. Available in: Neosporin Ointment, Myciguent (3.5 mg/g): 15, 30, 120 gm tubes.
   b. Use: Apply to cleansed area of skin q.i.d.
3. Mupirocin (Bactroban): Effective antistaphylococcal agent, but should be reserved for children with burns, epidermolysis bullosa, or immunosuppression. Because of bacterial resistance to this agent, routine use for impetigo may result in mupirocin-resistant staphylococcal infection in the community.
   a. Available in: 2% ointment, 15 g tubes.
   b. Use: Apply three times daily.

C. Oral antibiotics: For common bacterial skin infections, group A streptococci.
1. Phenoxymethyl penicillin V: Penicillin inhibits bacterial cell wall mucopeptides. Penicillin V has the advantage of being resistant to inactivation by gastric acid and is better absorbed. It can be given with meals. Should not be prescribed for patients with a history of penicillin allergy.
   a. Available in:
   Tablets: 125, 250, 500 mg.
   Oral solution (125 or 250 mg/5 mL): 100, 200 mL bottles.
   b. Use: 25 mg/kg/day, divided in three or four doses, for 10 days.
2. Erythromycin (see also Chapter 3): Erythromycin is the drug of second choice in streptococcal infections and should be used in penicillin-allergic children.
   a. Available in:
   Tablets: 125, 250 mg.
   Suspension: (200 or 400 mg/5 mL): 200 mL bottles.
   b. Use: 30–50 mg/kg/day, in divided in three or four doses, for 10 days.
3. Dicloxacillin. Isoxazolyl penicillin that resists destruction by the en-

zyme penicillinase (β-lactamase) with a mechanism of action similar to that of penicillin. It should not be used in penicillin-allergic children.
  a. Available in:
    Capsules: 250, 500 mg.
    Suspension (62.5 mg/5 mL): 100 mL bottles.
  b. Use: 12.5 mg/kg/day, in three or four divided doses, for 10 days.
4. Cephalosporins. In penicillin-allergic children, a cephalosporin may be considered despite the possibility that 5% of children who are penicillin allergic may also be allergic to cephalosporins. Cephalosporins inhibit bacterial cell wall synthesis. They are expensive.
  Cefaclor.
  a. Available in:
    Capsules: 250, 500 mg.
    Oral suspension (125 mg/5 mL): 100, 200 mL bottles.
  b. Use: 20 mg/kg/day, divided in three or four doses.
  Cephradine.
  a. Available in: Capsules: 250, 500 mg.
    Oral suspension (125 or 250 mg/5 mL).
  b. Use: 25–50 mg/kg/day, divided in three or four doses.
    NOTE: Adverse reactions, such as urticaria, angioedema, severe diarrhea, nausea, and vomiting, should prompt discontinuation of the drug and reexamination of the child.
5. Tetracycline (see also Chapter 3). A useful agent in acne vulgaris but not in common skin infections. Causes staining of teeth in preadolescents. Gastrointestinal tract upset is common. Must be taken on an empty stomach. Chelates heavy metals and should not be given with iron or calcium.
  a. Available as: Capsules: 250, 500 mg, bottles of 100.
  b. Use in acne: 500 mg–1.0 g, divided in two doses.

XIV. Antifungal agents.
  A. Topical antifungal agents. Each of the following agents is effective against all dermatophytes, *Candida albicans,* and *Pityrosporum orbiculare.*
    1. Clotrimazole (Lotrimin).
      a. Available in:
        1% cream: 15, 30, 45, 90 g tubes.
        1% solution: 10, 30 mL plastic bottles.
      b. Use: Apply to affected areas b.i.d.
    2. Ciclopirox olamine (Loprox).
      a. Available in: 1% cream: 15, 30, 90 g tubes.
      b. Use: Apply to affected areas b.i.d.
    3. Miconazole nitrate (Monistat-Derm).
      a. Available in:
        2% cream: 15, 30, 90 g tubes.
        2% lotion: 30, 60 mL bottles.
      b. Use: Apply to affected areas b.i.d.
    4. Econazole nitrate (Spectazole).
      a. Available in: 1% cream: 15, 30, 85 g tubes.
      b. Use: Apply to affected areas b.i.d.
    5. Ketoconazole (Nizoral).
      a. Available in: 2% cream: 15, 30 g tubes.
      b. Use: Apply to affected areas b.i.d.
    6. Haloprogin (Halotex).
      a. Available in:
        1% cream: 15, 30 g tubes.
        1% solution: 10, 30 mL plastic bottles.
      b. Use: Apply to affected areas b.i.d.
    7. Tolnaftate (Tinactin): Effective only against dermatophytes.
      a. Available in:
        1% cream: 15 g tubes.
        1% solution: 10 mL bottles, OTC.
      b. Use: Apply b.i.d.
    8. Nystatin (Nilstat, Mycostatin): Effective only against *C. albicans* and yeasts.
      a. Available in: Cream or ointment (100,000 U/g): 15, 30 g tubes.
      b. Use: Apply b.i.d.
    9. Selenium sulfide (Selsun): Effective against tinea versicolor, spores of *Trichophyton tonsurans.*
      a. Available in: 2.5% lotion, 120 mL bottles.
      b. Use: Apply for 10 minutes daily for 7 days.
        NOTE: OTC 1.5% selenium is not effective.

B. Oral antifungal agents.
  1. Griseofulvin (Fulvicin, Grifulvin, Grisactin, Gris-PEG). Griseofulvin is effective against all dermatophytes except *C. albicans* and *P. orbiculare.* It is a microtubule poison and arrests rapidly dividing cells. It is the drug of choice for tinea capitis. It is poorly absorbed from the gastrointestinal tract. Giving griseofulvin with ice cream or other fatty meals enhances absorption. It is contraindicated in children with porphyria or hepatocellular failure. A fungal culture should be obtained before initiating therapy.
     a. Available in: 125, 250, 500 mg tablets.
     b. Use: 20 mg/kg/day for 6–8 weeks for tinea capitis.
  2. Ketoconazole (Nizoral). Effective against dermatophytes, *C. albicans, P. orbiculare,* and many deep fungi. Hepatotoxicity restricts its use in children, and this agent should be considered only when no alternative is available. Complete blood cell count and liver and renal function tests should be obtained before and 2 weeks after therapy is started, and again whenever signs and symptoms develop.
     a. Available in: 200 mg tablets.
     b. Use: 3–6 mg/kg/day.
        NOTE: exact protocols in children have not been devised, and long-term therapy (more than 6–8 weeks) is not advised.

XV. **Antiviral agents.**
  A. Topical antiviral agents (acyclovir [Zovirax]).
     Selective inhibitor of herpesvirus–specific DNA polymerase, must be activated by virus-specific thymidine kinases. It is somewhat effective against cutaneous herpes simplex virus (HSV) infections. For severe HSV infections, oral or intravenous acyclovir should be used.
     a. Available in: 5% ointment: 15 g tubes.
     b. Use: Apply to lesions every 3 hours (six times daily) for 7 days.

Apply with finger cot or rubber glove to avoid autoinoculation.
  B. Systemic antiviral agents (acyclovir [Zovirax]).
     Currently available in intravenous and oral (capsule) forms. Indicated for treatment of primary HSV infection, HSV infection in immunocompromised hosts, eczema herpeticum, and varicella-zoster virus (VZV) infections in immunocompromised children. It is best to initiate therapy within 72 hours of cutaneous lesions. Contraindicated in renal disease or drug hypersensitivity.
     a. Available in:
        Sterile vials for intravenous use (500 mg/10 mL).
        200 mg capsules.
     b. Use:
        IV: 10 mg/kg/day for 7 days.
        200 mg capsules: for HSV infection: 10/mg/kg/day, in four doses, for 5 days.
        for VZV infection: 20 mg/kg/day, in four doses, for 5 days.

XVI. **Scabicides and pediculicides.**
  A. Gamma benzene hexachloride (GBH) (Kwell).
     Drug of choice for scabies and pediculosis. Kills adult mites, nits, and ova. Concern about percutaneous absorption in infants and pregnant women and subsequent CNS toxicity has resulted in increased caution with this agent. It is used with caution in pregnancy, and may be used with close supervision in infants.
     a. Available in: 1% cream: 57 g tubes.
        1% lotion: 59 ml bottles.
        1% shampoo: 59 mL bottles.
     b. Use: For scabies: apply from neck down; wash off in 4–6 hours. Persistent itching for up to 2 weeks after successful treatment can be expected. Pruritus is not an indication for retreatment.
        For pediculosis: apply to skin and hair; wash off in 4–6 hours.
        For pediculosis capitis: massage 5–10 mL GBH shampoo into scalp hair and leave on for 10 minutes. Shampoo out with a commercial shampoo. Residual pediculicidal

activity remains for five or six subsequent hair washings. Mechanical removal of remaining nits may be necessary.

B. *N*-Ethyl-*o*-crotonotoluidide (crotamiton; Eurax). Effective alternative scabicide to GBH.

   a. Available in:
     10% cream: 60 g tubes.
     10% lotion: 60 mL bottles.

   b. Use: Apply from neck down daily for 2 days; wash off 48 hours after initial application.

C. Permethrin (Nix).
Synthetic pyrethroid; effective pediculicide and ovicide.

   a. Available in: 1% creme rinse, 2 oz bottles.

   b. Use: After shampoo and towel dry, massage creme rinse into scalp thoroughly for 10 minutes, then rinse out.

D. Pyrethrins (RID, A-200 Pyrinate).
Effective pediculicide as naturally occurring pyrethrins.

   a. Available as: 2% or 3% liquid: 60, 120 mL bottles.
     4% gel: 30 g tubes.

   b. Use: Apply to wet hair and leave on for 10 minutes. Shampoo out with commercial shampoo. Mechanical nit removal may be required.

XVII. Wart therapy.

Specific antihuman papillomavirus (HPV) therapy is unavailable. Instead, agents that destroy viable keratinocytes, including keratinocytes containing HPV, are used. Even under ideal circumstances, the recurrence rate is 15%, as would be expected from nonspecific cytotoxic therapy.

A. Salicylic acid 16.7% and lactic acid 16.7% in flexible collodion (Duofilm, Viranol, Salactic).
Treatment of choice for many types of warts. Preparation should not be used on the face or areas where the epidermis is thin.

   a. Available in: 10, 15 mL bottles.

   b. Use: Apply 4 drops with a toothpick to the wart once daily, allowing each drop to dry. Cover with plastic strip bandage. Every 3–4 days, soak off dead wart tissue; 3–6 weeks required for response.

B. Salicylic acid 40% plaster (Mediplast).
Treatment of choice for plantar warts. Must not be used on areas of thin epidermis, such as the face.

   a. Available as: Individually wrapped rectangular plaster.

   b. Use: Cut plaster to size of wart; remove paper backing and apply gummed side to wart; secure in place with adhesive tape. Leave in place for 5 days; avoid getting wet. Replace every 5 days. Two to 5 weeks required for successful therapy.

C. Salicylic acid 17% solution (Occlusal, Wart-Off).
Not so potent as preparations listed in *A*, above.

   a. Available in: 10 mL bottles.

   b. Use: As in *A*, above.

D. Liquid nitrogen.
Store in metal container (e.g., metal thermos bottle). Apply to wart via spray or with a cotton swab with a loose, pointed tip. Touch center of lesion with the swab, using light pressure, or spray until an ice ball extending 1 to 3 mm beyond the margin of the wart is formed. Warts >8 mm in diameter should not be frozen. Freezing should be maintained for 25 to 30 seconds. In 1 to 3 days a blister, sometimes hemorrhagic, forms on the wart. A second freezing 5 to 7 days later may be required.

   a. Available as:
     Liquid nitrogen in metal tanks from medical or veterinary supply firms.
     Spray delivery device in metal thermos (CryAc).

E. Cantharidin (Cantharone).
Vesicant obtained from Spanish fly that produces a blister under the wart. It has the advantage of being relatively painless. Treatment of choice for periungual warts.

   a. Available as: Cantharidin 0.7% in flexible collodion, 7.5 mL bottles.

   b. Use: Apply with a toothpick to wart; allow to dry; then cover with tape for 24 hours. Remove tape and wash the area. Do not use cantharidin on the face, perineum, or axillae.

F. Podophyllin 25% in alcohol.

Podophyllin is a metaphase inhibitor used to treat warts on moist surfaces. It is a powerful caustic, and if overused can result in areflexic coma and death. Use should be limited to venereal warts, and it should be applied only by a health care provider.

    a. Available only by compounding podophyllin 25% in alcohol. Podophyllin 25% in tincture of benzoin is available commercially, but difficult to wash off.

    b. Use: Apply directly to wart, carefully avoiding normal mucosa. Wash off thoroughly with soap and water in 4 hours to prevent severe tissue necrosis. Must not be used in pregnant adolescents.

G. Trichloroacetic acid.

Strong acid that causes tissue necrosis when applied to skin. Useful for office treatment of molluscum and common warts.

    a. Available in: 50% saturated solution for plantar warts; 35%, 30%, or 25% solutions for common warts or molluscum; must be compounded.

    b. Use: Apply 1–2 drops with toothpick to wart, wiping immediately with an alcohol swab. Trichloroacetic acid is slow acting and painful. Repeat treatment every 5–7 days may be necessary. Instruct patient to soak the wart 3 days after therapy and remove whitish dead skin.

XVIII. Anti-acne agents. For complete listing of anti-acne agents, see Table 3–4.

A. Isotretinoin (13-*cis*-retinoic acid; Accutane).

Indicated for treatment of nodulocystic acne resistant to standard therapeutic regimens. In female patients with childbearing potential, must be used only in exceptional circumstances (see Chapter 3).

    a. Available as: 10, 20, 40 mg tablets, packages of 10.

    b. Use: 0.5–1.0 mg/kg/day for 4 months; then at least 8-week interval before next use. Typical dose in male adolescent, 40 mg b.i.d. for 4 months.

    WARNING: Should not be used in female patients of childbearing potential except under unusual circumstances. Be certain patient follows warnings on package. Warn about excessive mucocutaneous dryness.

BIBLIOGRAPHY

Arndt KA: *Manual of Dermatologic Therapeutics.* Boston, Little, Brown, 1989.

Balfour HH Jr, England JA: Antiviral drugs in pediatrics. *Am J Dis Child* 1989; 143:1307.

Bickers DR: The carcinogenicity and mutagenicity of coal tar—a perspective. *J Invest Dermatol* 1981; 77:173.

Fleischer AB, Resnick SD: The effect of antibiotics on the efficacy of oral contraceptives: A controversy revisited. *Arch Dermatol* 1989; 125:1562.

Fritz KA, Weston WL: Indications for systemic corticosteroid therapy in children. *Pediatr Dermatol* 1984; 1:236.

Lane AT: Development and care of the premature infants' skin. *Pediatr Dermatol* 1987; 4:1.

Lester RS: Topical formulary for the pediatrician. *Pediatr Clin North Am* 1983; 30:749.

Leyden JJ: Retinoids and acne. *J Am Acad Dermatol* 1988; 19:164.

Lucky AW: Principles of the use of glucocorticosteroids in the growing child. *Pediatr Dermatol* 1984; 1:226.

Lynfield YL, Schecter S: Choosing and using a vehicle. *J Am Acad Dermatol* 1984; 10:56.

Krochmal L, Wang JCT, Patel B, et al: Topical corticosteroid compounding: Effects on physicochemical stability and skin penetration rate. *J Am Acad Dermatol* 1989; 21:979.

Lichtenstein J, Flowers F, Sheretz EF: Nonsteroidal anti-inflammatory drugs. Their use in dermatology. *Int J Dermatol* 1987; 26:80.

Morelli JG, Weston WL: Soaps and shampoos in pediatric practice. *Pediatrics* 1987; 80:634.

Rasmussen JE: Advances in nondietary management of children with atopic dermatitis. *Pediatr Dermatol* 1989; 6:210.

Shah VP, Peck CC, Skelly JP: "Vasoconstriction"—

skin blanching–assay for glucocorticoids—a critique. *Arch Dermatol* 1989; 125:1558.

Sheretz EF: Pharmacology. I. Topical therapy in dermatology. *J Am Acad Dermatol* 1989; 21:108.

Sheretz EF: Pharmacology. II. Systemic drugs in dermatology. *J Am Acad Dermatol* 1989; 21:298.

Simons FER, Watson WTA, Simons KJ: The phamacokinetics and pharmacodynamics of terfenadine in children. *J Allergy Clin Immunol* 1987; 80:884.

Stoughton RB, Wullich K: The same glucocorticoid in brand-name products: Does increasing the concentration result in greater biologic activity? *Arch Dermatol* 1989; 125:1509.

Sunscreens. *Med Lett Drugs Ther* 1988; 30:61.

Tree S, Marks R: An explanation for the "placebo" effect of bland ointment bases. *Br J Dermatol* 1975; 92:195.

West DP, Worobeck S, Solomon LM: Pharmacology and toxicity of infant skin. *J Invest Dermatol* 1981; 76:147.

Williams ML, Sagebiel RW: Sunburns, melanoma and the pediatrician. *Pediatrics* 1989; 84:381.

Yohn JJ, Weston WL: Topical glucocorticosteroids. *Curr Probl Dermatol* 1990; 2:31–63.

Index

Appendix

PROBLEM-ORIENTED DIFFERENTIAL DIAGNOSIS INDEX

This index allows the health care provider to diagnose skin conditions based on examination of the skin. The diagnoses are listed in order from the commonest to the rarest, and separate differential diagnosis lists are provided for newborns and for infants and children. Use of the problem-oriented algorithm from Chapter 2 is recommended for this section.

Blistering (Vesiculobullous) Lesions

Newborns

1. Impetigo, 41–43
2. Burns, 48, 129
3. Miliaria, 136–137
4. Herpes simplex, 82–87
5. Dermatitis, acute, 26–40
6. Sucking blisters, 227
7. Friction blisters, 137–138
8. Epidermolysis bullosa, 138–142
9. Lymphangioma, 153, 237–238
10. Incontinentia pigmenti, 250–251
11. Acrodermatitis enteropathica, 251–252
12. Aplasia cutis congenita, 243–244
13. Varicella, 87–90
14. Scalded skin syndrome, 47–48
15. Bullous ichthyosiform erythroderma, 247, 248

Infants and Children

1. Impetigo, 41–43
2. Burns, 48, 129
3. Dermatitis, acute, 26–40
4. Friction blisters, 137–138
5. Viral blisters, 141
   a. Herpes simplex virus, 82–87
   b. Varicella-zoster, 87–90
   c. Hand-foot-and-mouth disease, 90–91
6. Papular urticaria, 71–72
   a. Insect bites
      Spider, 68–69
      Tick, 67–68
7. Miliaria, 136–137
8. Erythema multiforme (Stevens-Johnson syndrome), 126–129
9. Epidermolysis bullosa, 138–142
10. Linear IgA dermatosis, 133–134
11. Polymorphous light eruption, 119–122
12. Scalded skin syndrome, 47–48
13. Toxic epidermal necrolysis, 126–129
14. Acute parapsoriasis, 105–107
15. Lymphangioma, 153, 237–238
16. Bullous tinea pedis, 58–59
17. Fixed drug eruption, 215–219
18. Bullous pemphigoid, 126–143
19. Pemphigus vulgaris, 126–143
20. Dermatitis herpetiformis, 134–136
21. Diabetic bullae, 126–143
22. Kerion, 56
23. Lupus erythematosus, 109–112
24. Lichen planus, 107–109
25. Incontinentia pigmenti, 250–251
26. Bullous ichthyosiform erythroderma, 247, 248
27. Porphyria cutanea tarda
28. Epidermolysis bullosa acquisita, 138–142

NOTE: Molluscum contagiosum appears as shiny white dome-shaped papules, which although solid may be mistaken for blisters.

Mucosal Erosions or Blisters

Newborns

1. Herpes simplex virus, 82–87
2. Aphthous stomatitis, 131–132

B. Raised
   1. Milia, 224
   2. Microcomedones of acne, 17
   3. Molluscum contagiosum, 95–96

Infants and Children
A. Flat
   1. Pityriasis alba, 28–29, 199
   2. Tinea versicolor, 60–61
   3. Vitiligo, 197–199
   4. Postinflammatory hypopigmentation, 199–200
   5. Scleroderma (morphea), 210–212
   6. Lichen sclerosis et atrophicus, 212–213
   7. Ash leaf macules, 195–196
   8. Piebaldism, 195
   9. Waardenburg's syndrome, 196–197
   10. Chédiak-Higashi syndrome, 197
   11. Hypomelanosis of Ito, 196–197
   12. Halo nevus, 204–205
B. Raised
   1. Microcomedones of acne, 17
   2. Milia, 224
   3. Keratosis pilaris, 38–39
   4. Molluscum contagiosum, 95–96

Brown Lesions
Newborns
A. Flat
   1. Mongolian spot, 238
   2. Café au lait spot, 201
   3. Junctional nevus, 200–203
   4. Nevus of Ota, 202–203
   5. Freckles, 200
   6. Lentigo, 200–203
   7. Postinflammatory hyperpigmentation, 200–203
   8. Transient neonatal pustular melanosis, 225–226
   9. Linear and whorled hypermelanosis, 202
B. Raised
   1. Congenital pigmented intradermal nevus, 204
   2. Skin tags, 245

Infants and Children
A. Flat
   1. Freckles, 200
   2. Café au lait spots, 201
   3. Junctional nevus, 200–203
   4. Mongolian spot, 238
   5. Postinflammatory hyperpigmentation, 200–203

   6. Tinea versicolor, 60–61
   7. Melasma, 225–226
   8. Diffuse endocrine hyperpigmentation, 208
   9. Incontinentia pigmenti, 250–251
   10. Becker's nevus, 202
   11. Nevus of Ota, 202–203
   12. Lentigo, 200–203
B. Raised
   1. Intradermal nevus, 204
   2. Dermatofibroma, 148
   3. Spindle and epithelioid cell nevus, 204–205
   4. Urticaria pigmentosa, 160–167
   5. Juvenile xanthogranuloma, 150–151
   6. Blue nevus, 204–205
   7. Skin tags, 245
   8. Melanoma, 205–206
   9. Lentigo, 200–203
   10. Flat warts, 93
   11. Pyogenic granuloma, 153
   12. Hemangioma, 234–236

Yellow Lesions
Newborns
1. Carotenemia, 195–209
2. Sebaceous gland hyperplasia, 224–225
3. Sebaceous nevus, 241–242
4. Juvenile xanthogranuloma, 150–151
5. Mastocytomas, 166
6. Goltz's syndrome, 195–209
7. Nevus lipomatosis, 206–207

NOTE: In a baby with jaundice any skin lesion containing fluid may be yellow.

Infants and Children
1. Jaundice, 195–209
2. Juvenile xanthogranuloma, 150–151
3. Urticaria pigmentosa, 166–167
4. Sebaceous nevus, 241–242
5. Mastocytomas, 166
6. Carotenemia, 195–209
7. Xanthomas, 151–153
8. Necrobiosis lipoidica diabeticorum, 154
9. Goltz's syndrome, 195–209
10. Nevus lipomatosis, 206–207

Red Papules and Nodules
Newborns
1. Erythema toxicum, 225
2. Furuncles, 45–46
3. Insect bites, 67–68
4. Erysipelas, 43–44

5. Ectodermal dysplasia, 184–185
6. Progeria, 176–188
7. Congenital hypothyroidism, 176–188
8. Atrichia congenita, 176–188
9. Marinesco-Sjögren syndrome, 176–188
10. Cartilage-hair hypoplasia, 176–188
11. Follicular atrophoderma, 176–188

Infants and Children

A. Acquired circumscribed hair loss, 176–184
   1. Alopecia areata, 176–178
   2. Tinea capitis, 54–57, 178–180
   3. Traction alopecia, 181–182
   4. Kerion, 56
   5. Pyoderma, 41–53
   6. Varicella, 87–90
   7. Lichen planus, 107–109
   8. Lupus erythematosus, 109–112
   9. Darier's disease, 70, 172–173
   10. Porokeratosis of Mibelli, 115
   11. Physical trauma (abrasions, cuts), 176–188
   12. Chemical or thermal burns, 176–188
   13. Radiation injury, 176–188
   14. Psoriasis, 98–103
   15. Scleroderma, 176–188
   16. Secondary syphilis, 105
B. Acquired diffuse hair loss, 176–184
   1. Hypothyroidism, 176–184
   2. Hypopituitarism, 176–184
   3. Hypoparathyroidism
   4. Diabetes mellitus
   5. Androgenetic alopecia (male-pattern baldness), 176–184
   6. Hypervitaminosis A, 176–184
   7. Acrodermatitis enteropathica, 251–252
   8. Marasmus
   9. Heparin or coumarin therapy
   10. Antithyroid drugs
   11. Antimetabolites, 102
   12. Thallium poisoning
   13. Any congenital hair loss that persists, 176–184

Nail Disease

Newborns

A. Thick nails, 189–191
   1. Unknown cause

B. Thin or atrophic nails, 191–192
   1. Ectodermal dysplasia, 191
   2. Epidermolysis bullosa, 138–142
   3. Incontinentia pigmenti, 250–251
   4. Nail-patella syndrome, 191
   5. Acrodermatitis enteropathica, 251–252
   6. Anonychia with or without ectrodactyly, 191
   7. Focal dermal hypoplasia, 191–192
   8. Ellis–van Creveld syndrome, 191–192
   9. Turner's syndrome, 191–192
   10. Dyskeratosis congenita, 191–192
   11. Trisomy 13, 246
   12. Trisomy 18, 246
   13. Periodic shedding of nails, 191–192
   14. Coffin-Siris syndrome, 191–192
   15. Hallermann-Streiff syndrome, 191–192
   16. Progeria

Infants and Children

A. Thick nails, 189–191
   1. Psoriasis, 98–103
   2. Lichen planus, 107–109
   3. Onychomycosis, 60
   4. Twenty nail dystrophy, 190
   5. Pachyonychia congenita, 190
   6. Ectodermal dysplasia, 191
   7. Norwegian scabies
   8. Dermatitis, 26–40
   9. Palmoplantar keratodermas (hereditary forms)
B. Thin or atrophic nails, 191–192
   1. Trauma
   2. Lichen planus, 107–109
   3. Erythema multiforme major (Stevens-Johnson syndrome), 126–129
   4. Raynaud's phenomenon
   5. Vascular disease
   6. Drug eruptions, 215–222
   7. Twenty nail dystrophy, 190
   8. Any congenital cause